THE WASHINGTON MANUAL OF TRANSPLANT NEPHROLOGY

THE WASHINGTON MANUAL® OF TRANSPLANT NEPHROLOGY

Edited by

Tarek Alhamad, MD, MS-PH, MBA
Associate Professor of Medicine
Medical Director of Transplant Nephrology
Division of Nephrology
Department of Internal Medicine
Washington University School of Medicine
St. Louis, Missouri

Executive Editor

Thomas M. Ciesielski, MD
Associate Professor of Medicine
Division of General Medicine & Geriatrics
Department of Internal Medicine
Washington University School of Medicine
St. Louis, Missouri

Wolters Kluwer

Philadelphia • Baltimore • New York • London
Buenos Aires • Hong Kong • Sydney • Tokyo

Acquisitions Editor: James Sherman
Development Editor: Ariel Winter, Cindy Yoo
Editorial Coordinator: Chester Anthony Gonzalez
Editorial Assistant: Jaida Lively
Marketing Manager: Kirsten Watrud
Production Project Manager: Frances Gunning
Manager, Graphic Arts & Design: Stephen Druding
Manufacturing Coordinator: Bernard Tomboc
Prepress Vendor: TNQ Technologies

9 8 7 6 5 4 3 2 1

Printed in the United States of America

Library of Congress Cataloging-in-Publication Data

ISBN-13: 978-1-975210-82-3

Cataloging in Publication data available on request from publisher.

---

shop.lww.com

MPP0923

In honor of my parents (Abdul Salam Alhamad and Fawzieh Ammar) who are in their eighties and continue to live in Damascus, Syria. You've been my foundation throughout this journey.

To my wife, Basma Elabdullah, for her continuous endless care. Thank you for providing the stability and encouragement I've needed to bring this book to life.

To my brave kids, Hamzah and Taleah, for their dedication to learning. I hope this book inspires you to reach to your dreams.

To all immigrants who had to leave their country to seek a better life, you can overcome any obstacles with determination and courage.

Contributors

Tarek Alhamad, MD, MS-PH, MBA
Associate Professor of Medicine
Medical Director of Transplant Nephrology
Division of Nephrology
Department of Internal Medicine
Washington University School of Medicine
St. Louis, Missouri

Su-Hsin Chang, MD
Associate Professor of Surgery
Division of Public Health
Department of Surgery
Washington University School of Medicine
St. Louis, Missouri

Raja S. Dandamudi, MD
Assistant Professor of Medicine
Division of Pediatric Nephrology
Department of Pediatrics
Washington University School of Medicine
St. Louis, Missouri

Rowena Delos Santos, MD
Associate Professor of Medicine
Division of Nephrology
Department of Internal Medicine
Washington University School of Medicine
St. Louis, Missouri

Vikas R. Dharnidharka, MD, MPH
Professor of Medicine
Division of Pediatric Nephrology
Department of Pediatrics
Washington University School of Medicine
St. Louis, Missouri

Casey A. Dubrawka, PharmD
Pharmacist
Solid Organ Transplantation
Barnes-Jewish Hospital
St. Louis, Missouri

Karen Flores, MD
Assistant Professor of Medicine
Division of Nephrology
Department of Internal Medicine
Washington University School of Medicine
St. Louis, Missouri

Joseph Gaut, MD, PhD
Professor of Pathology and Immunology
Division of Anatomic and Molecular Pathology
Department of Pathology and Immunology
Washington University School of Medicine
St. Louis, Missouri

Ige A. George, MD, MS
Associate Professor of Medicine
Division of Infectious Diseases
Department of Internal Medicine
Washington University School of Medicine
St. Louis, Missouri

Seth Goldberg, MD
Associate Professor of Medicine
Division of Nephrology
Department of Internal Medicine
Washington University School of Medicine
St. Louis, Missouri

Mohamed M. Ibrahim, MD
Transplant Nephrology Fellow
Division of Nephrology
Department of Internal Medicine
Washington University School of Medicine
St. Louis, Missouri

Abdullah Jalal, MD
Nephrology Fellow
Division of Nephrology
Department of Internal Medicine
Washington University School of Medicine
St. Louis, Missouri

Anuja Java, MD
Associate Professor of Medicine
Division of Nephrology
Department of Internal Medicine
Washington University School of Medicine
St. Louis, Missouri

Sri Mahathi Kalipatwapu, MD
Transplant Nephrology Fellow
Division of Transplant Nephrology
Department of Internal Medicine
Washington University School of Medicine
St. Louis, Missouri

Shun Kawashima, MD, PhD
Fellow
Renal Division
Department of Internal Medicine
Brigham and Women's Hospital
Brookline, Massachusetts

Charbel C. Khoury, MD
Assistant Professor of Medicine
Division of Nephrology
Department of Internal Medicine
Washington University School of Medicine
St. Louis, Missouri

Petra Krutilova, MD
Endocrine Fellow
Division of Endocrinology
Department of Internal Medicine
Washington University School of Medicine
St. Louis, Missouri

Hrishikesh S. Kulkarni, MD
Assistant Professor of Medicine
Division of Pulmonary and Critical Care Medicine
Department of Internal Medicine
Washington University School of Medicine
St. Louis, Missouri

Jessica Lindemann, MD
General Surgery Resident
Division of Transplant Surgery
Department of Surgery
Washington University School of Medicine
St. Louis, Missouri

Chang Liu, MD
Associate Professor of Medicine
Division of Laboratory & Genomic Medicine
Department of Pathology and Immunology
Washington University School of Medicine
St. Louis, Missouri

Andrew Malone, MD
Associate Professor of Medicine
Division of Nephrology
Department of Internal Medicine
Washington University School of Medicine
St. Louis, Missouri

Armaghan-e-Rehman Mansoor, MD
Infectious Disease Fellow
Division of Infectious Diseases
Department of Internal Medicine
Washington University School of Medicine
St. Louis, Missouri

Gary Marklin, MD
Chief Medical and Research Officer
Mid-American Transplant
St. Louis, Missouri

Abraham J. Matar, MD
General Surgery Resident
Division of Transplantation
Department of Surgery
Emory University
Atlanta, Georgia

Neha Mehta-Shah, MD, MSCI
Associate Professor of Medicine
Division of Oncology
Department of Internal Medicine
Washington University School of Medicine
St. Louis, Missouri

Massini Merzkani, MD, MSc
Assistant Professor of Medicine
Division of Nephrology
Department of Internal Medicine
Washington University School of Medicine
St. Louis, Missouri

Nidia Messias, MD
Associate Professor of Medicine
Division of Anatomic and Molecular Pathology
Department of Pathology and Immunology
Washington University School of Medicine
St. Louis, Missouri

Haris F. Murad, MD
Assistant Professor of Medicine
Division of Nephrology
Department of Internal Medicine
Washington University School of Medicine
St. Louis, Missouri

Naoka Murakami, MD, PhD
Assistant Professor of Medicine
Renal Division
Department of Internal Medicine
Harvard Medical School
Brookline, Massachusetts

Nicole Nesselhauf, PharmD, BCPS, BCTXP
Pharmacist
Solid Organ Transplantation
Barnes-Jewish Hospital
St. Louis, Missouri

Ronald F. Parsons, MD
Associate Professor of Surgery
Division of Transplantation
Department of Surgery
Washington University School of Medicine
St. Louis, Missouri

April Pottebaum, PharmD, BCOP
Pharmacist
Solid Organ Transplantation
Barnes-Jewish Hospital
St. Louis, Missouri

Kristin Progar, PharmD
Pharmacist
Transplant Nephrology
Barnes Jewish Hospital
St. Louis, Missouri

Gaurav Rajashekar, MD
Transplant Nephrology Fellow
Division of Nephrology
Department of Internal Medicine
Washington University School of Medicine
St. Louis, Missouri

Maamoun Salam, MD
Associate Professor of Medicine
Division of Endocrinology
Department of Internal Medicine
Washington University School of Medicine
St. Louis, Missouri

Manli Shen, MD
HLA Fellow
Division of Laboratory & Genomic Medicine
Department of Pathology and Immunology
Washington University School of Medicine
St. Louis, Missouri

Ojaswi Tomar, MD
Nephrology Fellow
Division of Nephrology
Department of Internal Medicine
Washington University School of Medicine
St. Louis, Missouri

Jason R. Wellen, MD, MBA
Professor of Surgery
Division of General Surgery
Department of Surgery
Washington University School of Medicine
St. Louis, Missouri

Helen Wijeweera, NP
Nurse Practitioner
Division of Nephrology
Department of Internal Medicine
Washington University School of Medicine
St. Louis, Missouri

Parker C. Wilson, MD, PhD
Assistant Professor of Medicine
Division of Anatomic and Molecular Pathology
Department of Pathology and Immunology
Washington University School of Medicine
St. Louis, Missouri

Jennifer Yu, MD
Assistant Professor of Medicine
Division of General Surgery
Department of Surgery
Washington University School of Medicine
St. Louis, Missouri

Preface

The field of transplant nephrology has undergone numerous advancements over the past few decades. The advances in histocompatibility testing, biomarkers, immunosuppressive protocols, surgical techniques, and antiviral therapies have resulted in better outcomes for kidney transplant recipients. The management of these recipients requires a thorough understanding of the interactions of immunosuppressive medications, the recipient's immune system, and the overall balance between the risk of allograft rejection and infections.

The first edition of *The Washington Manual® of Transplant Nephrology* provides a guide to transplant providers and trainees who care for kidney transplant recipients. The manual brings original high-standard medical literature formatted into a "bullet style" layout, transforming pages of text into an easily accessible layout.

Written by experts in immunology, nephrology, surgery, pharmacy, pathology, HLA medicine, and statistics, *The Washington Manual® of Transplant Nephrology* provides complete coverage of the growing field of transplant nephrology with an abundance of algorithms, tables, and illustrations for fast visual guidance. Several chapters were written in collaboration among transplant nephrologists, pharmacists, and pathologists, which adds a more thorough review of these topics.

I hope that *The Washington Manual® of Transplant Nephrology* will be an essential resource for the providers and trainees who participate in the care of kidney transplant recipients. This includes physicians, nurse practitioners, pharmacists, and transplant coordinators. I hope the readers find this publication to be a relevant, informative, and useful tool in their clinical day-to-day practice and a good resource to enhance knowledge and improve practice.

I would like to acknowledge and thank the authors for all the time and effort they vested in this publication. I thank Drs. Benjamin Humphreys and Victoria Fraser for their support and mentorship. I appreciate the continued support from the leaders of the Transplant Center, including Dr. John Lynch, Dr. Katherine Henderson, Martha Stipsits, Gene Ridolfi, and Heather Wertin. Last, but not least, I want to acknowledge the wonderful collaboration with our transplant surgery team under the leadership of Drs. William Chapman and Jason Wellen.

Department Chair's Note

It is a pleasure to present the first edition of *The Washington Manual® of Transplant Nephrology*. This pocket-size book and online resource is an excellent reference for medical students, interns, residents, and other practitioners who need ready access to practical clinical information to care for patients with kidney transplants. The science underlying transplant immunology, clinical care of kidney transplant patients, and the prevention of opportunistic infections has increased dramatically since the first renal transplant was performed decades ago. *The Washington Manual® of Transplant Nephrology* provides current scientific and clinical information to aid physicians and other clinical providers to evaluate, assess, and treat patients with kidney transplants.

I want to personally thank the authors, who include fellows and attendings—most of who are from Washington University School of Medicine and Barnes-Jewish Hospital. Their commitment to patient care and education are unsurpassed, and their efforts and skill in compiling this manual are evident in the quality of the final product. In particular, I would like to acknowledge our editor, Dr. Tarek Alhamad, and the executive editor, Dr. Thomas M. Ciesielski, who have worked tirelessly to produce this manual. I believe this manual will meet its desired goal of providing timely and practical knowledge that can be directly applied at the bedside and in outpatient settings to improve patient care for patients with kidney and pancreas transplants.

Victoria J. Fraser, MD
Adolphus Busch Professor of Medicine
Chair, Department of Medicine
Washington University School of Medicine
St. Louis, Missouri

Contents

1 Cells and Soluble Mediators in the Immune System

Hrishikesh S. Kulkarni

GENERAL PRINCIPLES

- Most end-stage diseases involve a majority of the organ (or both organs) resulting in organ failure. Hence, solid organ transplantation remains dependent on suitable allograft availability to replace organ function.
- Establishing **tolerance** promotes allograft function in the host.
- Multiple triggers, such as infections, result in the breakdown of this tolerance, resulting in **alloimmune responses**, which remain a major impediment to the long-term success of solid organ transplantation. These alloimmune responses occur because proteins expressed in the (donor) allograft trigger immune responses by the host.
- Immune responses vary based on their temporal nature, as well as components that form the basis of this response (**Table 1-1**).[1]
- **Innate immune responses** are more immediate, yet nonspecific. These responses include cellular components such as myeloid cells (neutrophils, monocytes, macrophages, eosinophils, and dendritic cells [DCs]), as well as natural killer (NK) cells, which can be derived from common lymphoid progenitors and are considered separate from myeloid lineage. An important fluid phase component of the innate immune response is the complement system.
- **Adaptive immune responses** are facilitated by T and B lymphocytes, which have unique pathways for development that contribute to their subtypes and functions.
- Many immune cells secrete soluble proteins called **cytokines**, which may disrupt tolerance, and/or directly worsen allograft function.
- In the absence of appropriate **regulation**, these immune responses result in **rejection**, ultimately resulting in **graft failure**.

INNATE IMMUNITY

- Transplantation of an allograft activates innate immunity. This activation occurs within the first few hours of surgery primarily due to **ischemia-reperfusion injury (IRI)**, which is driven by ischemic time (particularly **cold ischemic time**, which is the time between cross-clamping of the donor organ and its reperfusion in the recipient).[2]
- IRI results in the release of **danger-associated molecular patterns (DAMPs)**,[3] which activate **pattern recognition receptors** (PRRs) to release danger signals (**Figure 1-1**).[4]
- DAMPs may be **intracellular**, which are released upon cellular injury, such as ATP, heat shock proteins, HMGB1, and mitochondrial DNA. DAMPs may also be extracellular, such as fragments of heparan sulfate, fibronectin, and hyaluronan.
- Correspondingly, during infection, **pathogen-associated molecular patterns (PAMPs)** can also activate PRRs to activate the innate immune response.
- There are many types of PRRs (>100) that recognize DAMPs and PAMPs. These receptors are germline encoded; as a result, cells of the same lineage have identical

TABLE 1-1 Differences Between the Innate and Adaptive Immune System

	Innate Immune System	Adaptive Immune System
Time to initiation	Minutes to hours	Days
Duration of response	Days	Weeks
Receptor diversity	Conserved germline receptors	Highly specialized due to genetic recombination
Antigen specificity	Not as specific; recognize conserved patterns across damaged cells (DAMPs) and pathogens (PAMPs)	Exquisite specificity of antigen recognition

DAMPs: damage-associated molecular patterns; PAMPs: pathogen-associated molecular patterns.

receptors. One such PRR is the **toll-like receptor** (TLR).[4] There are many TLRs and they have different cellular locations—some are on the surface and some are inside the cell. Different ligands bind to different TLRs; for example, gram-negative bacteria bind to TLR4, whereas mitochondrial DNA binds to TLR9.

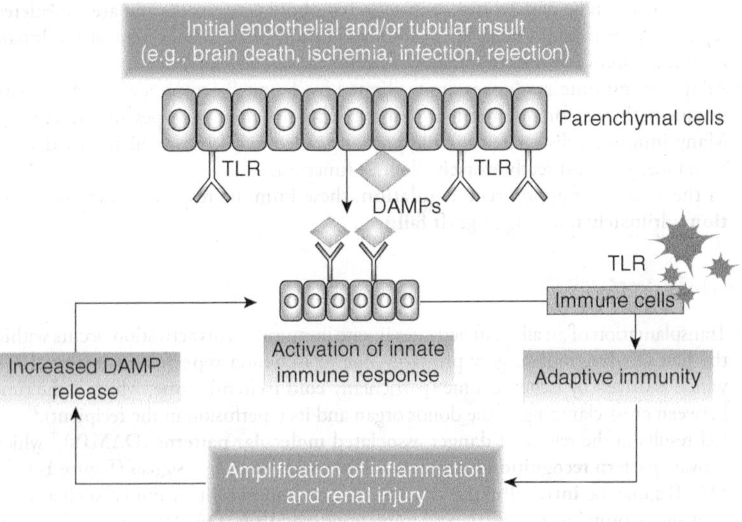

Figure 1-1. Non–antigen-dependent injury amplifies inflammatory responses. DAMPs such as HMGB1 and HSPs are released by injury to the graft epithelium and microvascular endothelium, and activate locally expressed sensing receptors (e.g., TLRs). The activation of innate immunity results in an adaptive immune response amplifying the injury. DAMP, danger-associated molecular pattern; HMGB1, high-mobility group box protein-1; HSP, heat shock protein; TLR, Toll-like receptor. (Reproduced with permission from Leventhal JS, Schröppel B. Toll-like receptors in transplantation: sensing and reacting to injury. *Kidney Int.* 2012;81(9):826-32.)

- DAMPs bind to TLRs on cells of the innate immune system such as neutrophils and monocytes and recruit them to the transplanted organ, as well as result in proinflammatory cytokine secretion from these cells.
- Although one purpose of such an evolutionary conserved response (i.e., attracting immune cells to an inflamed site) is to clear debris, a massive neutrophilic or monocytic influx can also result in allograft injury.
- Long-term, persistent activation of PRRs can result in impaired tolerance, especially due to activating cells of the adaptive immune system.
- Thus, components of the innate immune system are activated within minutes to hours, and last for days, before the adaptive immune system takes over.
- Although there are some clear differences between the innate and adaptive immune system (**Table 1-1**), the boundaries are becoming increasingly blurred. These emerging areas of investigation include aspects of immunological memory and allorecognition.[5,6] For example, innate immunity was thought to have no memory, but innate lymphoid cells (ILCs) recall exposure to prior antigens and cytokines. Similarly, recent work suggests that the innate immune system is able to recognize allogeneic nonself.
- Finally, cells in the innate immune system are dynamic, as their phenotypes and functions vary based on cell maturation, tissue localization, and the cytokine milieu.

Complement System

- There are many cells that comprise the innate immune system. However, the complement system is a key component of innate immunity that is functional in the fluid phase. It is activated within minutes of an insult, even before innate immune cells are mobilized.
- The complement cascade is a family of over 60 proteins present in the circulation, and can be activated via three pathways—the classical pathway, lectin pathway (LP), and alternative pathway—via assembly of different proteins.
- Each of these three pathways is triggered by certain components on the surface of pathogens or damaged cells, which facilitate assembly of molecules that are subsequently cleaved by proteases (**Figure 1-2**).[7]
- In certain cases, a component can activate more than one pathway. For example, pentraxin-3—which is associated with graft failure after solid organ transplantation—can activate both the classical and LPs of complement.
- The three pathways for complement activation converge to form the **C3 convertase**, which cleaves C3 to C3a and C3b. Subsequently, C3b also contributes to the formation of a **C5 convertase**, which cleaves C5 to C5a and C5b.
- **Convertase-independent C5 cleavage** also occurs in a setting of acute inflammation via proteases such as thrombin.
- C5b interacts with C6, C7, C8, and C9 to form the **membrane attack complex (MAC)**, which perturbs cell membranes and promotes cell lysis.
- At each step, there are membrane- and fluid-phase inhibitors (also known as **complement regulatory proteins**) that prevent the uncontrolled activation of the cascade.
- A genetic (e.g., polymorphism) or acquired deficiency of these inhibitors (e.g., via downregulation) predisposes the graft to damage due to MAC formation.
- Sublytic MAC formation can also increase NLRP3-mediated inflammasome activation, which predisposes to cellular injury.
- Complement has been implicated in **hyperacute rejection** during ABO-mismatched organ transplantation or in presensitized recipients. In this scenario, antibodies

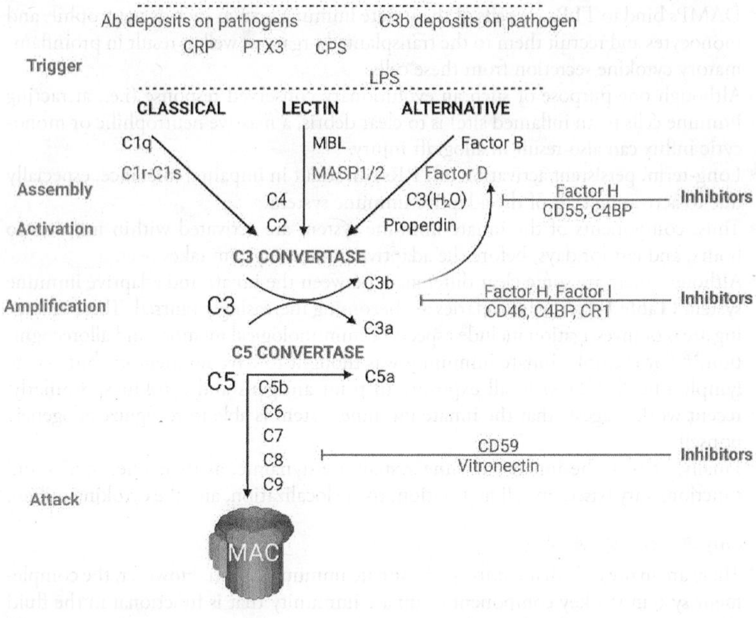

Figure 1-2. The complement cascade. The three pathways for complement cascade activation converge to form the C3 convertase (C4bC2a for CP and LP; C3bBb for AP), which cleaves C3 to C3a and C3b. Both C3b and C4b covalently bind to a target. C3b can also bind to Factor B to subsequently form the AP convertase, thereby amplifying the cascade. Figure created with BioRender.com. Abbreviations: Ab, antibody; C4BP, C4-binding protein; CPS, capsular polysaccharide; CRP, C-reactive protein; MASP, mannose-binding protein-associated serine protease; MBL, mannose-binding lectin; LPS, lipopolysaccharide; PTX3, pentraxin-3. (Reproduced with permission from Sahu SK, Kulkarni DH, Ozanturk AN, Ma L, Kulkarni HS. Emerging roles of the complement system in host-pathogen interactions. *Trends Microbiol.* 2022;30(4):390-402.)

against donor blood group antigens or donor HLA antigens bind to endothelial cells of the allograft, activating the complement cascade, thereby resulting in endothelial injury, activation of the coagulation cascade, occlusion of blood vessels in the graft, and subsequently, graft failure.

- The complement system is also implicated in antibody-mediated rejection (**AMR**), when donor-specific antibodies target the endothelium and result in graft failure. C4d deposition is a hallmark of AMR, although C4d-negative AMR has also been reported.
- Complement activation fragments such as C3a and C5a influence adaptive immune responses, thus also modifying transplant outcomes independent of MAC formation.

Neutrophils

- In addition to the complement system, neutrophils are one of the first responders to infection and injury.[8]
- Neutrophils are produced in the bone marrow and mobilized into the circulation (via factors such as granulocyte colony–stimulating factor), before extravasating into the allograft during the first few hours after transplantation.

- A hierarchal set of signals guide neutrophils into the allograft and orient them toward the site of tissue injury (**Figure 1-3**). Many of these signals are initiated through different forms of **inflammatory cell death**, which occur in the setting of IRI.[2] Many cell types also mediate neutrophil recruitment into the allograft via cytokine secretion, especially monocytes, macrophages, and DCs; in some cases, these involved cell types may be donor derived.
- Once the neutrophils reach the site of injury, DAMPs such as mitochondrial formylated peptides enable them to precisely identify dying cells and remove tissue debris.
- Neutrophils have multiple effector functions that are important for host defense yet augment tissue inflammation and injury:
  - Release of proteolytic enzymes such as matrix metalloproteinases and elastases result in tissue breakdown, but exposes alloantigens.

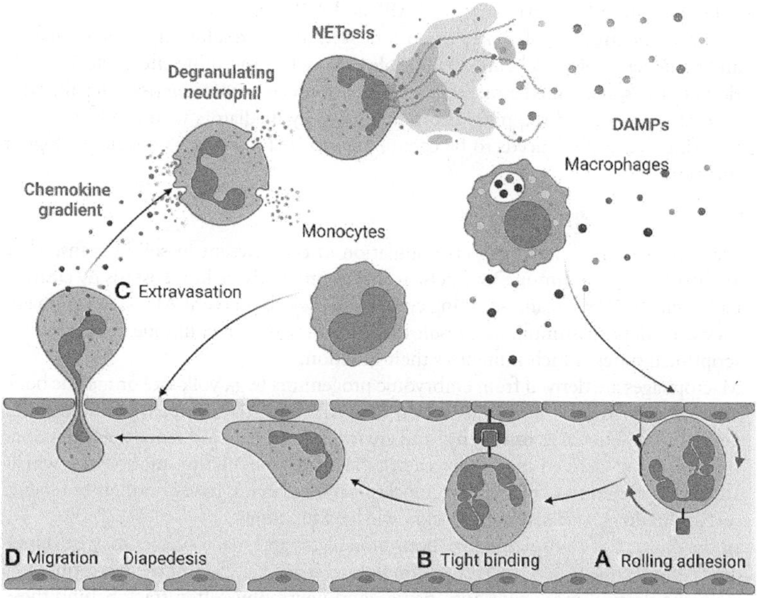

Figure 1-3. **A hierarchal set of signals guide neutrophils into the allograft and orient them in the direction of tissue inflammation.** A, **Rolling adhesion:** The upregulation of integrins and selectins on the endothelial surface, by DAMPs, and cytokines secreted by monocyte and macrophage equivalents allow for neutrophil adhesion to vascular beds near the site of injury. For example, a sialyl-Lewis X moiety on neutrophils binds to E-selectin in the endothelium. B, **Tight binding:** LFA-1 on neutrophils binds to ICAM-1 on the endothelium. C, **Extravasation/diapedesis:** Cytokines, such as IL-1β released by monocytes, facilitate neutrophil extravasation through the endothelium into the interstitial space by loosening tight junctions. D, **Migration:** Gradients of chemokines, such as IL-8, guide neutrophils within the interstitial space through the healthy tissue toward the sites of injury. Upon reaching the sites of injury, neutrophils degranulate to release their contents such as proteolytic enzymes and can also form neutrophil extracellular traps (through a process called NETosis). (Created with www.biorender.com.)

- Chemokine release (e.g., interleukin [IL]-8) brings in more neutrophils to clear the bacteria and debris, but perpetuates inflammation.
- Neutrophil extracellular traps (NETs) are expulsions of chromatin intended to trap bacteria, but damage the tissue and worsen graft function.
- Reactive oxidant species are generated especially after uptake of mitochondrial DAMPs but perpetuate injury.

- Additionally, neutrophils enhance the adaptive immune response by:
  - Facilitating the maturation of antigen-presenting cells (APCs) via a tumor necrosis factor (TNF)–mediated mechanism.
  - Upregulating the expression of costimulatory molecules and major histocompatibility complex (MHC) receptors to promote alloantigen presentation to T cells.
  - Transporting donor antigens from injured tissues to peripheral lymph nodes, given they have antigen-presenting capabilities themselves.
  - Inducing T-cell recruitment to the allograft through the release of cytokines such as CCL1, CCL2, and CCL5.
  - Expressing B-cell–stimulating factors that promote plasma cell proliferation and differentiation (e.g., via release of BAFF and APRIL).
- However, neutrophils also play important roles in the resolution of inflammation and tissue repair after ischemia in multiple organs, by promoting efferocytosis, secretion of proresolving mediators, release of microvesicles promoting tissue repair, cytokine scavenging, and trapping of proinflammatory mediators within NETs.[9] Thus, targeting neutrophils needs to be carefully optimized in order to promote allograft function.

Monocytes and Macrophages

- Macrophages are a heterogenous population of cells present in solid organs. They are best known as immune sentinels, as they promote tissue homeostasis by clearing pathogens and debris, and secreting cytokines. They also serve as APCs. Additionally, they can adapt to stimuli, as a result of which they display a unique range of transcriptional states, which influences their function.[10]
- Macrophages are derived from embryonic progenitors (e.g., yolk sac) or may be bone marrow derived (also known as spleen derived). Both the source from where they develop (also known as **ontogeny**) and environmental cues influence their function.
- Bone marrow–derived macrophages originate from circulating monocytes, which are often referred to as classical or nonclassical monocytes, based on their ontogeny, surface markers, and historically acknowledged functions.
- In the context of transplantation, both monocytes and macrophages may be donor derived or recipient derived.[11] For example, IRI is associated with the recruitment of recipient classical monocytes into tissues, and neutrophils often track behind these classical monocytes. Classical monocytes can then give rise to both tissue-resident macrophages and DCs, which present antigens and influence adaptive immune responses.
- However, recent studies have shown that donor nonclassical monocytes respond to inflammatory cell death signals in tissues (such as the lung) to secrete chemokines, which play an important role in recruiting both classical monocytes and neutrophils into the allograft.[8] Thus, understanding what is the source of the cellular infiltration and their downstream effects is key to modulating their function.
- Additionally, there are inherent differences in the role of monocytes and macrophages among solid organ transplants. Whether certain pathways are conserved across organs versus being tissue specific is only just beginning to be understood. For

example, donor-derived macrophages play an important role in neutrophil extravasation and worsen graft function in thoracic transplantation, but may be protective in the kidney.

- Current immunosuppression such as calcineurin inhibitors and steroids affect monocyte differentiation and cytokine production, in addition to inhibiting T-cell activation.
- An emerging concept in myeloid cells (such as neutrophils, monocytes, and macrophages) relevant to transplantation is **trained immunity (Figure 1-4)**.[6] The injury associated with donor organ procurement, storage, and engraftment triggers DAMP release, which results in temporary epigenetic and metabolic reprogramming of myeloid cells, known as training. For example, trained macrophages have a heightened inflammatory response upon reexposure to donor graft antigens thus resulting in more potent alloimmunity.
- This trained immunity amplifies T-cell activity by enhancing stimulatory factor production, enhancing antigen presentation, and promoting the differentiation of monocytes.
- Our knowledge of how these cells influence allograft function is likely to improve over the next decade due to new technologies such as next generation sequencing. Specifically, our understanding of their spatiotemporal modulation of graft function is just beginning.

Dendritic Cells

- DCs are innate immune cells developing in the bone marrow that are considered the most effective APCs, even more than neutrophils and macrophages.

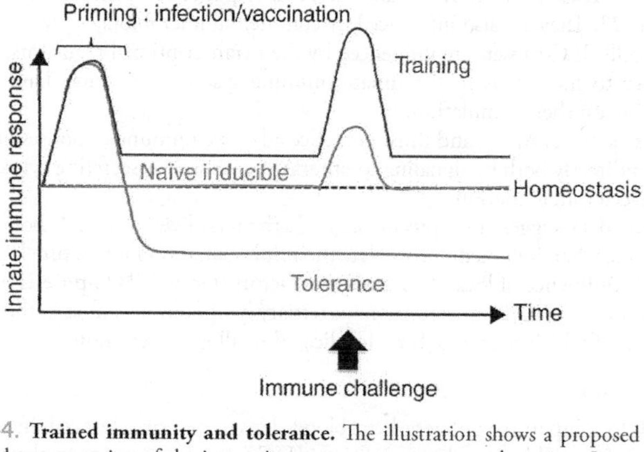

Figure 1-4. **Trained immunity and tolerance.** The illustration shows a proposed model of differential programming of the innate immune system posttransplantation. Innate immune responses during and after donor organ procurement, storage, and engraftment can lead to immunological reprogramming and a decreased/refractory (tolerance/immunoparalysis) or heightened ("trained") immunity, which might accordingly translate into increased or decreased susceptibility to subsequent inflammatory episodes. Trained immunity occurs due to epigenetic and metabolic reprogramming of these cell types, thereby allowing altered responses to subsequent heterologous stimuli. (Reproduced with permission from Quintin J, Cheng SC, van der Meer JWM, Netea MG. Innate immune memory: toward a better understanding of host defense mechanisms. *Curr Opin Immunol.* 2014;29:1-7.)

- There are at least two types of DCs: (a) classical dendritic cells (cDCs), which can be either cDC1 or cDC2, and (b) plasmacytoid dendritic cells (pDCs).[12]
- cDCs are monocyte derived; they are migratory cells, whose differentiation can occur either in the bone marrow, or in the organ where they infiltrate.
- Like many other myeloid cells, their function is dependent on their maturation, tissue location, and environmental cues.
- In the context of transplantation, DCs modulate **allorecognition**.[5] As a result, they serve as a bridge between innate and adaptive immunity. The mechanisms of allorecognition are discussed in **Chapter 2, Transplant Immunobiology**.
- Lesser is known about the role of pDCs in the context of transplantation. pDCs resemble plasma cells, and are less efficient than cDCs in presenting antigens to T cells. However, pDCs can promote T regulatory cell generation, and may have a role in tolerance.

Innate Lymphoid Cells

- ILCs are the innate counterparts of T cells that are tissue resident, do not have T-cell receptors (TCRs), and are devoid of conventional lineage markers.[13]
- A major function is ILCs is to maintain epithelial integrity and secrete cytokines to promote tissue repair.
  - **Group 1 ILCs** produce cytokines such as interferon-gamma (IFN-γ) and TNF-α in response to IL-12, IL-15, and IL-18. They promote immunity to viruses, fungi, and intracellular bacteria and parasites.
  - **Group 2 ILCs** produce type 2 cytokines, such as IL-4, IL-5, and IL-13 and amphiregulin, a member of the epidermal growth factor family that is important in tissue remodeling and repair. Group 2 ILCs preferentially respond to certain type 2 stimuli such as IL-25 and IL-33.
  - **Group 3 ILCs** produce IL-17 and IL-22 in response to cytokines such as IL-1β and IL-23. They are also influenced by commensal microbiota.
- Like T cells, ILC subsets are influenced by their transcriptional regulators.
- Contrary to most cells in the innate immune system, ILCs may have memory depending on their stimulation.
- ILCs also serve as APCs, and thus, influence adaptive immune responses directly, as well as indirectly both by signaling to other APCs, as well as secreting cytokines that direct T-cell differentiation.
- Emerging data suggest ILC precursors from the fetal liver and adult bone marrow enter tissue when inflamed to complete their differentiation into mature ILC subsets under the influence of local environmental factors (termed "**ILC-poiesis**").
- ILCs are involved in the organization for tertiary lymphoid structures in the allograft, as a result of which they have been implicated in allograft rejection.

Natural Killer Cells

- NK cells form up to 10% of peripheral blood-derived mononuclear cells in recipients.
- They are activated by the absence of self-MHC Class I molecules on the target cell surface to produce IFN-γ, TNF-α, perforins, and granzyme B to destroy those cells (called **missing-self hypothesis**). This activity of NK cells complements $CD8^+$ T cells because those cells are activated when exposed to nonself peptides on MHC Class I molecules.
- NK cells contribute to IRI, as receptor ligands for NK cells (i.e., NKG2D) are upregulated on endothelial and epithelial cells following IRI.[14]

- NK cells also participate in antibody-dependent cellular cytotoxicity as they express Fc-gamma receptors (i.e., CD16 or FcγRIIIA); these effects are complement independent.
- Allograft infiltrating NK cells may also potentiate alloimmune T cells and promote rejection. On the other hand, NK cells may promote tolerance via depleting donor APCs.
- NK cells also play key roles in the protection against infection, especially CMV.

ADAPTIVE IMMUNITY

- Adaptive immune responses occur within days to weeks of transplantation, and are comprised of T- and B-cell responses.[15]
- T and B lymphocytes recognize their targets via TCRs and B-cell receptors (BCRs).
- TCRs are highly polymorphic surface receptors, which guarantee maximal functional flexibility. Most of the TCRs are comprised of **alpha/beta chains**, which recognize peptide:MHC complexes, and are key for adaptive immune responses. Some TCRs also have gamma/delta chains, which recognize unconventional (non-MHC) antigens.
- BCRs are comprised of immunoglobulins, which are tetramers made of two heavy and two light chains. BCR can either be on the surface and have an intracellular signaling component, or be soluble, thereby contributing to **humoral immunity**.
- The set of TCR and BCR in a single individual is called a **repertoire**.
  - **Sequence repertoire** is all the possible sequences of TCR alpha or beta chains, or BCR heavy and light chains, and their potential pairings.
  - **Ligand repertoire** is all the possible ligands that can be targeted.
- Their diversity rests in a random combination of germline VDJ gene segments (**combinatorial diversity**) and random addition or deletion at junctional site of segments (**junctional diversity**). These changes occur during T- and B-cell maturation.
- When a surface TCR or BCR recognizes an antigen, it transduces signals to the cytosol thereby inducing transcription factors and influences its target gene expression.
- The type of cellular response to receptor stimulation differs according to the stage of maturation of the T or B lymphocyte.

T Lymphocytes

- T cells arise in the bone marrow but migrate to the thymus for maturation into $CD4^+$ and $CD8^+$ T cells.
- In the context of transplantation, the presence of alloreactive memory T cells endangers graft survival due to both acute and chronic cellular rejection, as they respond to HLA epitope differences between the donor and recipient. For example, $CD8^+$ T cells encountering APCs presenting mismatched HLA Class I antigens kill the target cell that expresses this antigen. At the same time, $CD4^+$ T cells contribute to rejection by recruiting other effector cells such as $CD8^+$ T cells, macrophages, NK cells, and B cells.
- On encountering antigens present on APCs, naïve T cells go through multiple phases, such as priming and expansion, resolution and contraction, and memory (**Figure 1-5**).[16]
  - **Priming and expansion:** Naïve T cells divide and differentiate into effector cells that produce cytokines and proteins to execute their functions. For example,

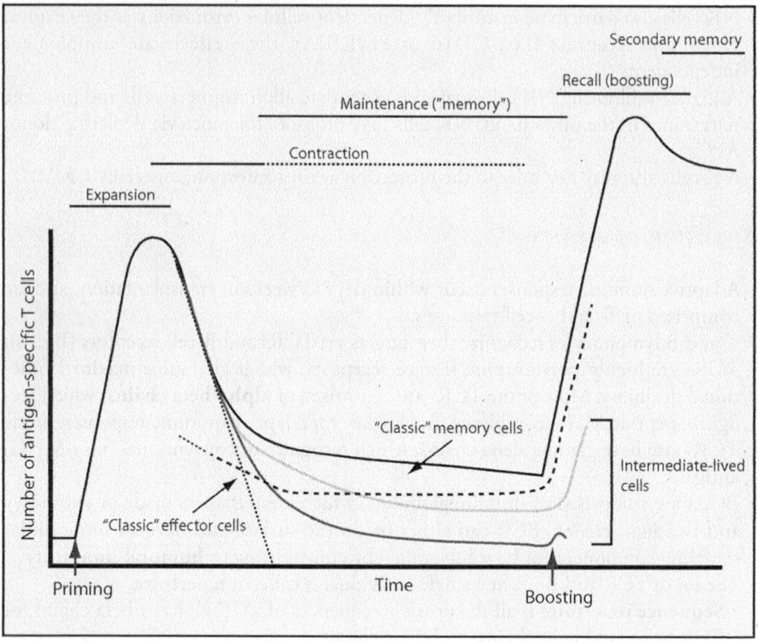

Figure 1-5. **Development of T-cell memory.** The figure shows numbers of antigen-specific T cells (black line) at various stages after priming and boosting of a prototypical acute immune response, similar to what would be occurring postallotransplantation or an infection posttransplant. During the primary response, the fate of typical effector (dotted line) and memory (dashed line) cells is shown. Also shown are populations of intermediate longevity that may also contribute to protection form reinfection (dark gray and light gray lines). (Reproduced with permission from Jameson SC, Masopust D. Diversity in T cell memory: an embarrassment of riches. *Immunity*. 2009;31(6):859-71.)

cytotoxic $CD8^+$ T cells produce granzymes and perforins and induce death of a target cell expressing a cognate foreign antigen on a Class I MHC molecule.

- **Resolution and contraction:** Subsequently, a majority of the effector T cells die.
- **Memory:** T cells are maintained long term as resident, effector and central memory cells. These subtypes are affected by environmental cues and underlying transcriptional factors and are distinguished by their location and functions.
  - **Resident memory T cells** are present in the mucosal surface and do not reenter the circulation. They serve as immune sentinels to offer immediate protection through their own effector functions and their ability to recruit and reactivate other immune cells.
  - **Effector memory T cells** migrate between tissues and secondary lymphoid organs (e.g., lymph nodes) and provide immune surveillance.
  - **Central memory T cells** are present in the secondary lymphoid organs and can rapidly expand and differentiate following a rechallenge.
- $CD4^+$ (helper) T cells, along with $CD8^+$ T cells, make up a majority of the T lymphocytes.

- After their activation and differentiation, $CD4^+$ T cells execute multiple functions such as activating other innate immune cells, B lymphocytes, $CD8^+$ T lymphocytes and nonimmune cells, as well as regulating immune function. There are multiple subsets of $CD4^+$ helper T cells, which are influenced by the environmental cytokine milieu, transcriptional factors, and epigenetic modifications:
  - **Type 1 helper cells (Th1)** produce IL-2 and IFN-γ and have been implicated in the protection against intracellular pathogens, especially due to their ability to activate phagocytes.
  - **Type 2 helper cells (Th2)** produce IL-4, IL-5, and IL-13 and are conventionally acknowledged in their role for host defense against parasites, as they can influence eosinophils, mast cells, basophils, and B lymphocyte function.
  - **Type 17 helper cells (Th17)** produce IL-17 and IL-22 and are known to clear extracellular pathogens including fungi, due to their ability to attract neutrophils.
- **Regulatory T cells (Tregs)** are a distinct subset of $CD4^+$ T cells that promote tolerance via multiple pathways, one being IL-10 production. Both central and peripheral Tregs exist. **Central Tregs** develop in the thymus when high-affinity, tissue-restricted self-antigens presented by medullary thymic epithelial cells or bone marrow-derived APCs drive $CD4^+$ T cells toward Treg precursors. Subsequently, cytokines such as IL-2 or IL-15 drive the precursors toward fully committed central Tregs (also known as thymic Tregs). **Peripheral Tregs** develop when $CD4^+$ T cells in tissues are presented with certain antigens by DCs in presence of cytokines such as TGF-β, retinoic acids, and short-chain fatty acids.
- Further details regarding T-cell immune responses, including recognition, costimulation, differentiation, and memory are covered in Chapter 2, Transplant Immunobiology.

B Lymphocytes

- APCs such as DCs present HLA peptides to T cells, which provide signals to naïve B cells *that have the same antigen on their Ig receptor.*
- The **naïve B cell** then proliferates to form **short-lived plasma cells** secreting IgM, but also undergoes **somatic hypermutation** to identify the optimal antigen-binding BCR-expressing clone. The strongest clones undergo **class switching** of their immunoglobulins to IgG and further differentiate into more short- and middle-lived plasma cells, which produce high-affinity IgG against the epitope.
- These high-affinity IgG-producing clones also differentiate into **memory B cells**, which persist in secondary lymphoid organs and can later redifferentiate into the specific high-affinity plasma cells if a very similar antigen is encountered.[17]
- A small proportion of the highly specific, high-affinity IgG-producing clones differentiate into **long-lasting plasma cells** that persist in the bone marrow, contributing a constant small supply of specific antibodies.
- **T-cell–independent B-cell activation** can also occur, for example, in response to acute bacterial infections, when B cells encounter lipopolysaccharide on the bacteria.
- In the context of transplantation, naïve B cells are activated by $CD4^+$ T cells that have previously encountered APCs with donor-derived antigens. These naïve B cells now form plasma cells producing donor-specific antibodies.
- B cells have both antibody-mediated and direct effects on the allograft:
  - **Antibody-mediated effects on the allograft** include inactivation, opsonization, complement activation, and chemotaxis.
  - **Direct effects on the allograft** include antigen presentation via MHC Class II (as B cells also serve as APCs), immune activation, and immunomodulation.

TABLE 1-2 Effects of Immunosuppressants on Different Immune Cell Types

Drug	T Cells	B Cells	Plasma Cells	APCs	Complement	Antibodies
Steroids	++	+	–	++	–	±
ATG	+++	+	+	+	–	±
IL-2 antagonists Basiliximab	+++	++	–	+	–	–
Alemtuzumab	+++	++	+	±	–	±
Calcineurin inhibitors TAC/CYA	+++	+	–	±	–	–
Antiproliferatives MMF/AZA	++	++	(+)	+	–	(+)
mToR inhibitors SIR/EVE	++	++	(+)	++	–	(+)

APC, antigen-presenting cell; ATG, antithymocyte globulin; AZA, azathioprine; CYA, cyclosporine; EVE, everolimus; MMF, mycophenolate mofetil; SIR, sirolimus; TAC, tacrolimus. The symbols refer to an effect on inhibiting a specific component of the immune system (+) or the lack thereof (–), and the number of symbols refers to the degree of effect.
Adapted with permission from Dr. Simon Urschel, University of Alberta, Stollery Children's Hospital.

- Donor-specific antibodies are now known risk factors for chronic rejection, although they can result in **acute AMR**, due to their ability to:
  - Induce complement activation
  - Promote antibody-mediated cytotoxicity via Fc receptor on macrophages/NK cells
  - Modulate endothelial cell signaling and proliferation via mTOR signaling
- It is important to know the surface markers on these different cell types to understand how they respond to therapy. For example, plasma cells lack CD20 as a result of which they are not depleted with rituximab, an anti-CD20 monoclonal antibody. On the other hand, proteosomal inhibitors affect memory B cells in addition to naïve B cells and plasma cells and reduce antibody levels more quickly.
- Further details regarding B-cell immune responses, including recognition, differentiation, and memory, are covered in Chapter 2. Understanding how our immunosuppression practices affect cell types in both the innate and adaptive immune systems will be key to optimally modulating their effects (**Table 1-2**).

REFERENCES

1. Murphy K, Weaver C, Berg L. *Innate immunity: the first lines of defense.* In *Janeway's Immunobiology*. 10th ed. W. W. Norton & Company; 2022:37-78.
2. Frye CC, Bery AI, Kreisel D, Kulkarni HS. Sterile inflammation in thoracic transplantation. *Cell Mol Life Sci.* 2021;78(2):581-601.
3. Kulkarni HS, Scozzi D, Gelman AE. Recent advances into the role of pattern recognition receptors in transplantation. *Cell Immunol.* 2020;351:104088.

4. Leventhal JS, Schröppel B. Toll-like receptors in transplantation: sensing and reacting to injury. *Kidney Int.* 2012;81(9):826-32.
5. Quintin J, Cheng SC, van der Meer JWM, Netea MG. Innate immune memory: towards a better understanding of host defense mechanisms. *Curr Opin Immunol.* 2014;29:1-7.
6. Ochando J, Ordikhani F, Boros P, Jordan S. The innate immune response to allotransplants: mechanisms and therapeutic potentials. *Cell Mol Immunol.* 2019;16(4):350-6.
7. Sahu SK, Kulkarni DH, Ozanturk AN, Ma L, Kulkarni HS. Emerging roles of the complement system in host-pathogen interactions. *Trends Microbiol.* 2022;30(4):390-402.
8. Shepherd HM, Gauthier JM, Terada Y, et al. Updated views on neutrophil responses in ischemia-reperfusion injury. *Transplantation.* 2022;106(12):2314-24.
9. Peiseler M, Kubes P. More friend than foe: the emerging role of neutrophils in tissue repair. *J Clin Invest.* 2019;129(7):2629-39.
10. Chen S, Lakkis FG, Li XC. The many shades of macrophages in regulating transplant outcome. *Cell Immunol.* 2020;349:104064.
11. Kopecky BJ, Frye C, Terada Y, Balsara KR, Kreisel D, Lavine KJ. Role of donor macrophages after heart and lung transplantation. *Am J Transplant.* 2020;20(5):1225-35.
12. Macri C, Pang ES, Patton T, O'Keeffe M. Dendritic cell subsets. *Semin Cell Dev Biol.* 2018;84:11-21.
13. Withers DR, Mackley EC, Jones ND. Innate lymphoid cells: the new kids on the block. *Curr Opin Organ Transplant.* 2015;20(4):385-91.
14. Calabrese DR, Lanier LL, Greenland JR. Natural killer cells in lung transplantation. *Thorax.* 2019;74(4):397-404.
15. Duneton C, Winterberg PD, Ford ML. Activation and regulation of alloreactive T cell immunity in solid organ transplantation. *Nat Rev Nephrol.* 2022;18(10):663-76.
16. Jameson SC, Masopust D. Diversity in T cell memory: an embarrassment of riches. *Immunity.* 2009;31(6):859-71.
17. Ionescu L, Urschel S. Memory B cells and long-lived plasma cells. *Transplantation.* 2019;103(5):890-8.

2 Transplant Immunobiology

Shun Kawashima and Naoka Murakami

GENERAL PRINCIPLES

- The immune system has evolved to recognize self from nonself and plays a critical role to maintain tolerance and eliminate foreign pathogens (e.g., bacteria, virus, and fungus).
- Innate and adaptive immune systems consist of various cell types, soluble mediators, and complement systems. Innate and adaptive immune systems react to environmental signals (e.g., ischemia and tissue damage) and non–self-antigens (e.g., allograft and pathogens), and both contribute to alloimmune response in transplantation (discussed in Chapter 1).
- Immune response against allo-antigens follows three steps: (1) recognition and presentation of allo-antigens, (2) activation, differentiation and proliferation of allo-reactive immune cells (T cells, natural killer [NK] cells, and myeloid cells), and (3) effector phase in the allograft that causes rejection.

ALLO-ANTIGEN RECOGNITION BY ADAPTIVE IMMUNE SYSTEM

Major Histocompatibility Complex/Human Leukocyte Antigen

- Major histocompatibility complex (MHC) is a key signaling molecule in antigen recognition in adaptive immune system. Human MHC is specifically called human leukocyte antigen (HLA). HLA molecules are encoded on chromosome 6 in human genome.
- MHC molecules are highly polymorphic, as an evolutionary consequence to increase the variety of peptides that can be presented to T cells, and due to this polymorphism, donor's HLA molecules are recognized by transplant recipient's T cells as non–self-antigens (allo-antigen) and play a critical role in transplant rejection.
- Individuals inherit one set, or haplotype, of HLA class I and class II molecules from each parent. The MHC genes (genotype) then encode for the MHC molecules located on the surface of cells.
- MHC molecules all have a peptide-binding groove, immunoglobulin like region, transmembrane, and intracytoplasmic region. The peptide binding region is where molecules of self or foreign antigens are presented to T cells.
- To generate MHC-restricted T-cell epitopes, protein antigens are processed into linear stretches of approximately 15 to 25 amino acids via proteolytic degradation in the late endosomes or lysosomes.
- **HLA class I molecules** encode for HLA A, B, and C and are expressed in all nucleated cells, consisting of one alpha chain (polymorphic) and one beta chain (shared) (**Figure 2-1**). They primarily interact with $CD8^+$ T cells.
- **HLA class II molecules** encode for HLA DR, DQ, and DP and are expressed on antigen-presenting cells (such as dendritic cells [DCs], monocytes/macrophages, and B cells), consisting of two polymorphic alpha chains (**Figure 2-1**). They primarily interact with $CD4^+$ T cells.
- In kidney transplantation, the importance of HLA A, B, and DR loci are well described.[1] The larger number of HLA mismatches is associated with worse allograft survival in

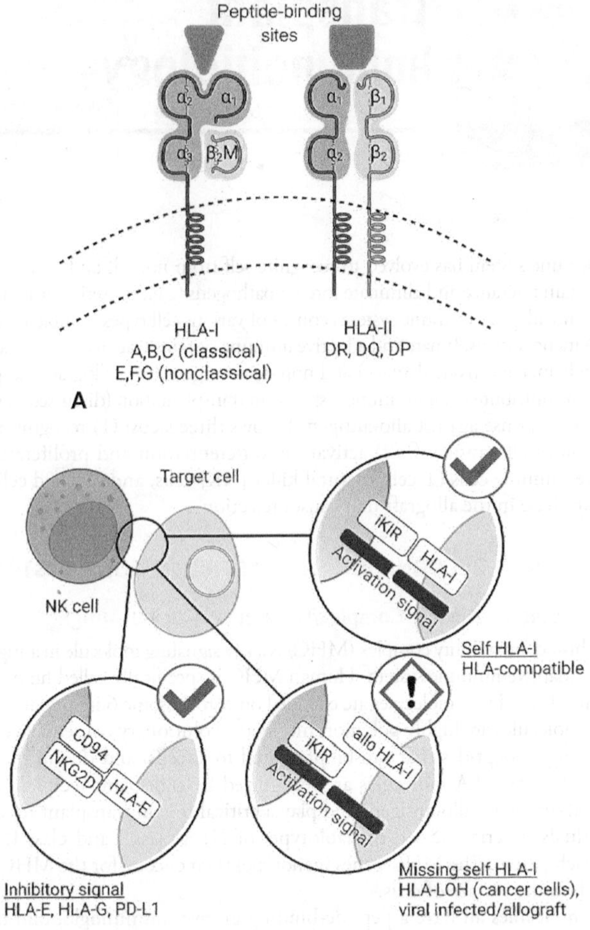

Figure 2-1. **Alloantigen presentation by MHC molecules and mode of recognition by NK cells.** Panel A: Schematic figure of the human MHC molecules. The MHC class I molecule consists of polymorphic a chain, which is noncovalently bound to a nonpolymorphic beta2 microglobulin chain (b2m). The MHC class II molecule consists of alpha and beta chain, both of which are polymorphic. Panel B: Schematic figure of the antigen recognition of NK cells. NK cells interact with cells through KIR receptor. Missing-self signal (middle panel) activates NK cells and to contribute to rejection. HLA, human leukocyte antigen; KIR, killer cell immunoglobulin-like receptors; MHC, major histocompatibility complex; NK, natural killer. (Created with www.biorender.com.)

multiple organs. Additionally, a genetic mismatch of non-HLA haplotypes is also associated with an increased risk of allograft dysfunction independent of HLA incompatibility.

- MHC class I chain-related gene A, encoding a polymorphic nonconventional MHC class I molecule, is also found to be an immunogenic polymorphic antigen that contributes kidney transplant rejection.

- Mismatches in non-MHC antigens are also known to provoke alloimmune response: such angiotensin II type 1 receptor and LIM zinc finger domain containing 1 (LIMS1) loci.
- Interaction between MHC molecules and T-cell receptor (TCR) is essential for T-cell activation (signal 1). T cells encounter allo-antigens via recognition of non–self-peptides presented on self MHC, or self- or non–self-peptides presented on allogenic MHC. MHC molecules are required to present these HLA peptides to T lymphocytes and are highly polymorphic (i.e., there are many different alleles in the different individuals inside a population).
- Once T cells recognize donor HLA, they are activated to differentiate to different subtypes of T cells (such as memory, effector, and helper T cells) and can also activate B cells to provoke alloimmune response (see details in Chapter 1, Cells and Soluble Mediators in the Immune System).
- See Chapter 3, The Science of Histocompatibility Testing and Cross-matching, for clinical application of MHC molecules.

Alloantigen Recognition Pathway

- There are three proposed mechanisms by which T-cell allorecognition occurs (**Figure 2-2**).[2]

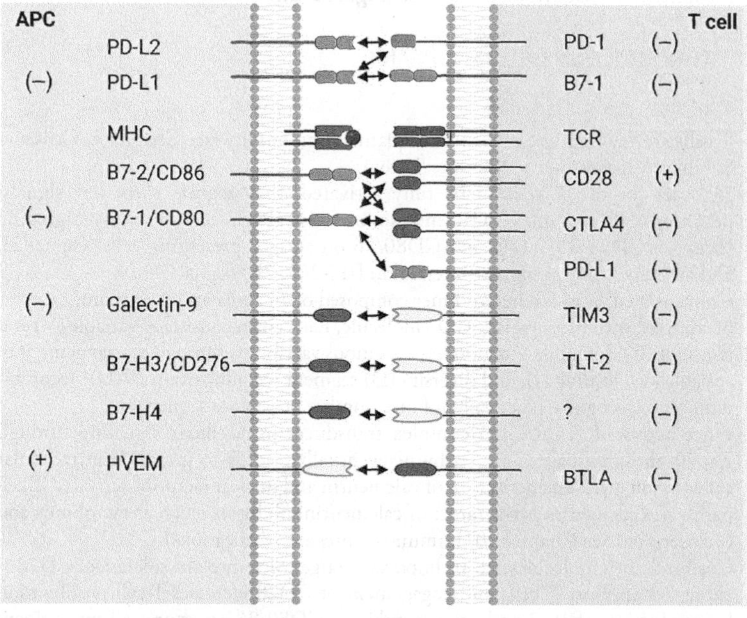

Figure 2-2. **Costimulatory molecules in the interface of APCs and T cells.** Schematic of costimulatory molecules of CD28 and TNF superfamily. Signals transduced to cells can either be stimulatory (+) or inhibitory (–). APC, antigen-presenting cell; BTLA, B- and T-lymphocyte attenuator; CTLA4, cytotoxic T-lymphocyte associated protein 4; HVEM, herpes virus entry mediator; MHC, major histocompatibility complex; PD-1, programmed cell death receptor-1; TCR, T cell receptor; TIM3, T-cell immunoglobulin and mucin-domain containing-3; TLT-2, triggering receptor expressed on myeloid cell-like transcript 2; TNF, tumor necrosis factor. (Created with www.biorender.com)

- **Direct allorecognition:** Donor DCs activated by damage-associated molecular patterns migrate to the recipient draining lymph nodes or their spleen, and present peptide:MHC complexes in the context of donor MHC molecules to recipient T cells. These recipient T cells traffic back to the allograft as cytotoxic effector T cells and contribute to graft rejection (in hours to days).
- **Semidirect allorecognition (cross-dressing):** Recipient DCs (rather than donor DCs) acquire intact donor MHC molecules by capturing donor-derived extracellular vesicles, thereby activating recipient T-cell responses shortly after transplantation (~days to weeks).
- **Indirect allorecognition:** Recipient DCs internalize donor antigens such as HLA and process them via their antigen-presenting pathway, subsequently representing them on MHC molecules to recipient T cells (~weeks to years).

- DCs demonstrate a process known as **trogocytosis**, whereby they extract surface molecules from other antigen-presenting cells and express them on their own cell surface. This process results in recipient DCs carrying intact donor HLA molecules on the surface.
- NK cells are activated by "missing-self" signals. If NK cells interact with cells that lack self MHC class I molecules (such as cells in allograft, xenotransplant organs, or cancer cells that downregulate expression of MHC class I molecules), NK cells are activated and elicit cytotoxic response (**Figure 2-2**).[3]

IMMUNOBIOLOGY OF TRANSPLANT

T-Cell Activation Signaling

- T cells are key immune cells for transplant allo-immunity (see Chapter 1, Cells and Soluble Mediators in the Immune System).
- In order for the T cells to be fully activated, they require three key signals: peptide:MHC complex/TCR interaction (signal 1), costimulatory signaling (between CD28 on T cells and CD80/86 on antigen-presenting cells) (signal 2), and cytokine survival signals (interleukin [IL]-2/IL-2R) (signal 3).
- Conventional TCR is a heterodimer composed of an alpha and beta chain, as a part of complex with the invariant CD3 molecule. Each chain consists of variable (V) and constant (C) domains. V region has enormous variability, through rearrangement of variable (V), joining (J), and diversity (D) segment recombination (V(D)J recombination), to recognize practically infinite number of peptide sequences.
- Once activated, TCR/CD3 complex transduces intracellular signaling through Zap70-phospholipase C-IP_3 pathway, eventually leading to increased intracellular calcium ion level, and activation of calcineurin and nuclear factor of activated T-cell pathway. Calcineurin is the target of calcineurin inhibitors (such as tacrolimus and cyclosporine. See Chapter 10, Immunosuppressive Medications).
- Costimulatory molecules are an important target of transplant tolerance. CD28 is expressed on most T cells and engagement of CD28 increases T-cell proliferation by production of IL-2 and other cytokines. CD80/86 are expressed on antigen-presenting cells, and their expression levels are upregulated by inflammatory stimuli, such as infection or ischemia.
- Belatacept (cytotoxic T-lymphocyte–associated protein 4 [CTLA4]-Ig) is a clinically used costimulatory blockade. It inhibits T cell's interaction by competing CD28 engagement with CD80/86. Other monoclonal antibody therapies to directly block CD28 signaling are also under development (see Chapter 10, Immunosuppressive Medications, for details).

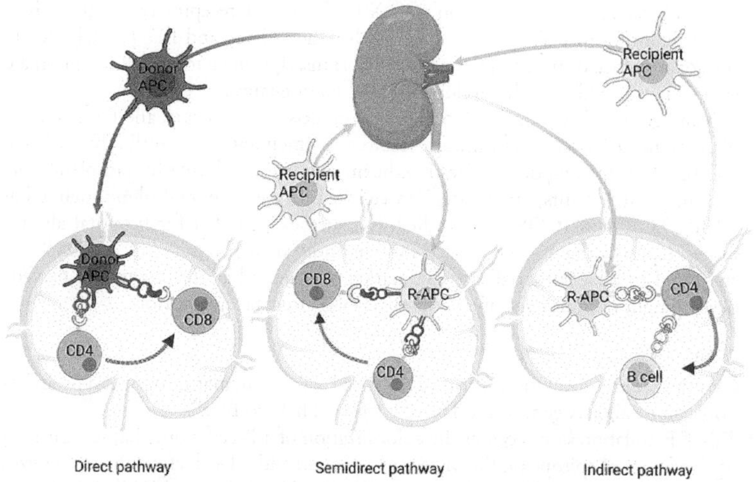

Figure 2-3. **Alloantigen recognition pathways.** In direct pathway (left), recipient T cells recognize intact allogeneic MHC molecules on donor APCs. In semidirect pathway (middle), recipient APCs obtain intact recipient MHC molecules and present to recipient T cells. In indirect pathway (right), recipient T cells recognize allo-peptides presented in the context of self (recipient) MHC molecules. The allo-peptides are derived from donor MHC molecules that have been digested and presented to the cell surface by recipient APCs. APC, antigen presenting cell; R-APC, recipient APC; MHC, major histocompatibility complex. (Created with www.biorender.com)

- Numerous coinhibitory molecules have been reported that transduce negative signals once engaged with their receptors (**Figure 2-3**). These coinhibitory receptors play key roles to maintain immune tolerance (such as feto-maternal tolerance, autoimmune disease, and transplantation) and cancer immunity.
- Targeted therapy against coinhibitory molecules has been used as cancer immunotherapy, also known as immune checkpoint blockade, such as antiprogrammed cell death protein-1 (PD-1) and anti-CTLA4.[4] Transplant recipients receiving immune checkpoint blockade are at higher risk of acute rejection. This observation suggests the critical roles of coinhibitory molecules in maintaining tolerance against allograft.

T-B COLLABORATION IN ALLOGRAFT REJECTION

Follicular Helper T Cells

- Naïve CD4$^+$ T cells are precursors of phenotypically and functionally distinct subsets of T cells, such as effector T cells (type 1 helper [Th1], type 2 helper [Th2], and type 17 helper [Th17] cells) and regulatory T cells (Treg) (Chapter 1, Cells and Soluble Mediators in the Immune System). T follicular helper cells (Tfh) promote humoral response in secondary lymphoid tissues, while T follicular regulatory cells inhibit them.[5]
- Tfh differentiation begins after initial activation by DCs in secondary lymphoid tissues. Modest TCR stimulation and CD28 ligation favors effector T-cell differentiation, while potent TCR activation and signaling through both CD28 and inducible costimulatory (ICOS), as well as IL-2, are required for Tfh differentiation.

- Tfh is characterized by expression of C-X-C chemokine receptor type 5 (CXCR5), which helps localize Tfh cells to the lymph node follicle, and PD-1, likely due to the consequence of potent TCR activation. Transcription factor B cell lymphoma 6 (Bcl-6) is required for Tfh development and maintenance.
- Tfh and germinal centers develop in mouse models of skin, heart, and kidney transplantation. Deletion of Tfh lineage resulted in amelioration of antibody-mediated rejection in animal models, suggesting the importance of Tfh cells in transplantation.
- In transplant patients, circulating Tfh cells (cTfh) in peripheral blood, defined as $CD4^+CXCR5^+$ or $ICOS^+$, are studied as a surrogate marker for humoral alloimmune response, due to lack of access to lymphoid tissues in patients. cTfh cells are suggested to be a potential early biomarker of humoral alloreactivity and precede development of donor-specific antibody (DSA) after transplantation.

Germinal Center Reaction

- Germinal center formation is critical for B-cell activation, maturation, and proliferation against alloantigen, where Tfh cells provide help to B cells.
- This T-B collaboration requires the colocalization of a B-cell clone that recognizes a conformational epitope on the surface of a protein and a T-cell clone that recognizes a linier peptide derived from the same antigen and bound to an MHC class II molecule on the B-cell clone.
- Antigen-activated B cells move to T/B border, where B cells meet with cognate Tfh cells. Some B cells differentiate to short-lived plasma blasts, while other cells further moved into follicles to form germinal center, where B cell proliferates and undergoes somatic hypermutation and class switching.
- Memory B cells arise both outside the germinal center (extrafollicular) as well as in the early stages of germinal center response. The roles of extrafollicular memory B cells in transplantation are not fully understood.
- The initiation and maintenance of germinal center reactions required the reciprocal induction of the transcription factor Bcl-6 and B-lymphocyte–induced maturation protein-1 in both germinal center B cells and cognate Tfh cells (**Figure 2-4**).

Immunologic Monitoring

- Clinical diagnosis of allograft rejection relies on monitoring kidney function (creatinine) and histopathological analysis of allograft biopsy, an invasive and costly procedure.
- Historically, multiple attempts have been made to monitor alloreactivity ex vivo.
- DSA: monitoring humoral alloimmune response by measuring DSA using single antigen bead assay is now widely used. See Chapters 3 and 13 for details.
- A classic, experimental way to monitor cellular alloimmune response is mixed lymphocyte reaction, where recipient peripheral T cells are cocultured with irradiated donor cells, and T-cell proliferation are monitored by thymidine incorporation or carboxyfluorescein succinimidyl ester dilution assay. This technique is also applied for enzyme-linked immunosorbent spot assay, where the frequency of alloreactive T cells producing interferon gamma can be quantified.[6]
- ImmuKnow assay is a commercially available test to estimate $CD4^+$ T-cell activation status by measuring adenosine triphosphate production after various immunological (non-donor-specific) stimuli. However, its use in predicting allograft rejection is limited.
- Donor-derived cell-free DNA is also a commercially available test to monitor allograft rejection. See Chapter 12, Cellular Rejection, for details.

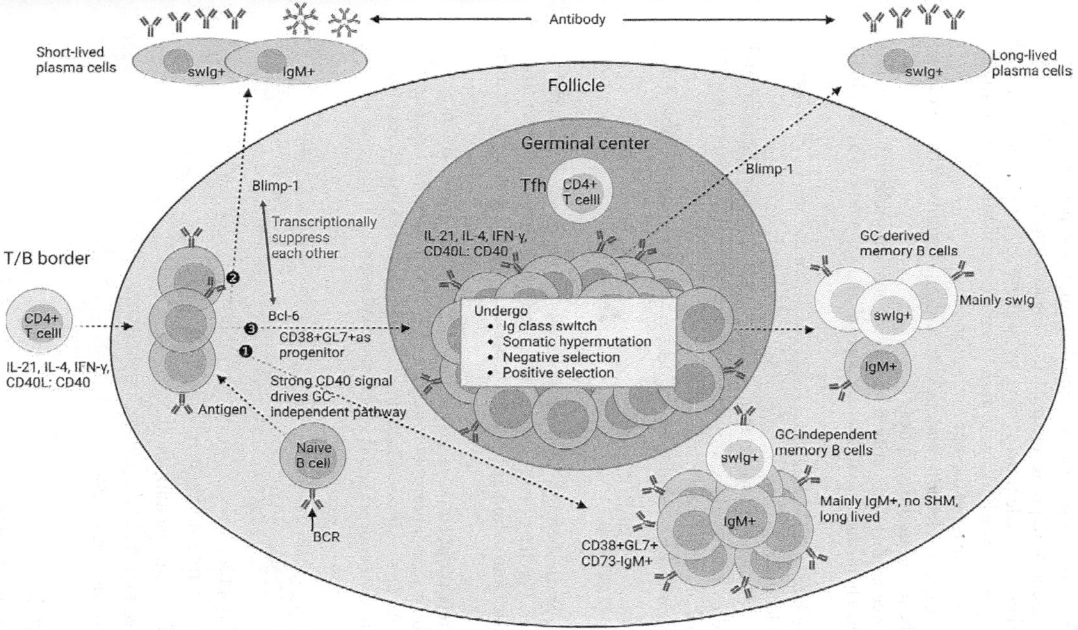

Figure 2-4. **Germinal center response and B-cell development after alloantigen encounter.** B-cell differentiation in response to alloantigen. After B-cell activation via antigen, naïve B cells migrate to T/B border of the follicle and T cell area. The activated B cells receive signals through CD40-CD40L interaction and cytokine signaling through corresponding receptors through interacting with cognate $CD4^+$ T cells. B cells then proliferate and differentiate to memory B cells, migrating to the follicle, or upregulate Blimp-1, migrate out of the follicle to short-lived plasma cells, or upregulate Bcl-6 and migrate deep into the follicles to establish germinal centers (GCs). In the GC, B cells proliferate robustly and undergo $CD4^+$ T-cell–dependent affinity maturation. Failure to receive signals from $CD4^+$ T cells results in death, whereas cells that receive signals can exit the GC as long-liver plasma cells or memory B cells. Most GC-derived memory B cells express isotype switched Ig (swIg), whereas most GC-independent memory B cells express IgM. Bcl-6: B-cell lymphoma 6; BCR, B cell receptor; Ig, immunoglobulin; Tfh, follicular helper T cells. (Created with www.biorender.com.)

Tolerance

- Tolerance is the mechanism that immune system does not respond against particular antigens (e.g., self-antigens, fetus antigens, and microbiome).
- During T-cell development, two crucial tolerance mechanisms prevent immune responses against self-antigens: central tolerance and peripheral tolerance.
- **Central tolerance** occurs in the thymus, through negative and positive selection. T cells that have undesirable response against self-antigens expressed on thymic epithelial cells are deleted or made unresponsive by negative selection. Then, those T cells that can recognize non–self-antigens in the context of self MHC are positively selected and allowed to leave the thymus to circulation.
- The process of the negative selection is not perfect, and small number of autoreactive T-cell clones can be found in the periphery.
- **Peripheral tolerance** is, therefore, critical to prevent autoimmunity. This is maintained by several mechanisms: clonal deletion, anergy, and suppression by coinhibitory signaling.
- Treg cells, characterized as $CD4^+CD25^+CD127^-Foxp3^+$, are the key T-cell subset to drive peripheral tolerance.
- Transplant tolerance has been sought as an ultimate goal of transplantation, and practically defined as a state that transplant recipients do not reject transplanted organ without need of immunosuppression.
- Multiple preclinical and clinical studies are ongoing to achieve tolerance (**Table 2-1**).[7]

XENOTRANSPLANTATION

- Due to the serious organ shortage, xenotransplantation has been sought as a potential source of organs. Pigs have been used for preclinical study of xenotransplantation due to the organ size close to humans', relatively large litter size and short maturation period.
- Major barriers of xenotransplantation are (1) hyperacute rejection due to xenorecognition (e.g., unique glycosylation molecules, alpha(1-3)-Gal, expressed on pig cells and pig MHC molecules), (2) acute humoral rejection due to cross-species incompatibilities, (3) infection concerns, and (4) ethical challenges.

TABLE 2-1 Approaches to Transplant Tolerance (Preclinical and Clinical)

Mixed chimerism approach
Combined bone marrow and kidney transplant
Mobilized $CD34^+$ stem cell infusion
Autologous, ex vivo expanded polyclonal Treg infusion
Mesenchymal stromal cells infusion
DCreg infusion
CAR Treg infusion
Low-dose IL-2/engineered IL-2
Nanoparticle-based donor antigen delivery

CAR, chimeric antigen-receptor; DCreg, regulatory dendritic cells; IL, interleukin; Treg, regulatory T cells.

TABLE 2-2 Targets of Gene Modification in Xenotransplantation

Gene	Function/Mechanism
Porcine Genes	
1,3-galactosyltransferase (GGTA1)	aGal epitope
CMP-N-acetylneuraminic acid hydroxylase	Neu5Gc epitope
b-1, 4N-acetygalactosaminyl transferase	SDa epitope
Porcine endogenous retrovirus (PERV)	PERV xenozoonosis
Human Genes	
Membrane cofactor protein (CD46)	Inactivation of complement factors C3b abd C4b
Decay accelerating factor (DAF)	Complement decay
Thrombomodulin (TBM)	Anticoagulation
Endothelial cell protein C receptor (EPCR)	Anticoagulation
Integrin-associated protein (CD47)	Macrophage activation and phagocytosis
Hemeoxygenase-1 (HO-1)	Anti-inflammatory
Membrane attack complex (C5b-9) inhibitory protein	Inhibition of C5b-9
Tissue factor pathway inhibitor	Antagonize the function of tissue factor

- Gene editing technology, clustered regularly interspaced short palindromic repeats-Cas9 system, enabled removal and modification of antigenic and immunomodulatory molecules on pig-derived organs (**Table 2-2**).
- In early 2022, several cases of heart and kidney xenotransplantations were performed for either living or brain-dead recipients. In kidney transplant case, transplanted pig kidneys produced urine for a few hours, but histological analysis revealed endothelial injury. More mechanistic analysis is needed before clinical application of xenotransplantation.[8]
- In addition, these initial cases of xenotransplantation brought us ethical concerns. Strict informed consent process and pre-delineated plan to share the results of clinical trials to the public are critical in the future trials of xenotransplantation.[9]

REFERENCES

1. Yeung MY. Histocompatibility assessment in precision medicine for transplantation: towards a better match. *Semin Nephrol.* 2022;42(1):44-62.
2. Duneton C, Winterberg PD, Ford ML. Activation and regulation of alloreactive T cell immunity in solid organ transplantation. *Nat Rev Nephrol.* 2022;18(10):663-76.
3. Callemeyn J, Lamarthée B, Koenig A, Koshy P, Thaunat O, Naesens M. Allorecognition and the spectrum of kidney transplant rejection. *Kidney Int.* 2022;101(4):692-710.
4. Waldman AD, Fritz JM, Lenardo MJ. A guide to cancer immunotherapy: from T cell basic science to clinical practice. *Nat Rev Immunol.* 2020;20(11):651-68.

5. Zhang H, Sage PT. Role of T follicular helper and T follicular regulatory cells in antibody-mediated rejection: new therapeutic targets? *Curr Opin Organ Transplant.* 2022;27:371-5.
6. Hricik DE, Augustine J, Nickerson P, et al. Interferon gamma ELISPOT testing as a risk-stratifying biomarker for kidney transplant Injury: results from the CTOT-01 multicenter study. *Am J Transplant.* 2015;15(12):3166-73.
7. Leventhal JR, Mathew JM. Outstanding questions in transplantation: tolerance. *Am J Transplant.* 2020;20(2):348-54.
8. Carrier AN, Verma A, Mohiuddin M, et al. Xenotransplantation: a new era. *Front Immunol.* 2022;13:900594.
9. Reese PP, Parent B. Promoting safety, transparency, and quality in xenotransplantation. *Ann Intern Med.* 2022;175(7):1032-4.

3 The Science of Histocompatibility Testing

Manli Shen and Chang Liu

GENERAL PRINCIPLES

- HLAs are the **main immunologic barriers** to kidney transplantations due to their extreme diversity in human populations, the broad tissue expression of these antigens, and their strong immunogenicity.
- During T cell- and antibody-mediated graft rejections, mismatched donor HLA antigens are the molecular targets of alloreactive T cells and anti-HLA antibodies, respectively; therefore, contemporary histocompatibility testing focuses on assessing HLA mismatch in donor-recipient pairs and recipients' humoral response to donor HLA.
- The physiological function of HLA antigens is to present non-self-peptides to T cells to launch adaptive immunity against pathogens or neoantigens on autologous cells; while the diversity of HLA antigens at individual and population levels maximizes the capacity of peptide presentation, the chance is high for any random donor-recipient pair to be HLA mismatched.
- HLA antigens are divided into class I (HLA-A, B, C) and class II (HLA-DR, DQ, DP) molecules (**Figure 3-1**, left panel); their structural and functional differences are:
  - Class I HLA antigens comprise heavy chains (α chain) heterodimerized with β-2-microglobulin and present cytosolic peptides to $CD8^+$ T cells; they are expressed in all nucleated cells.
  - Class II HLA antigens comprise heterodimerized α and β chains and present peptides derived from phagocytosed antigens to $CD4^+$ T cells; they are primarily

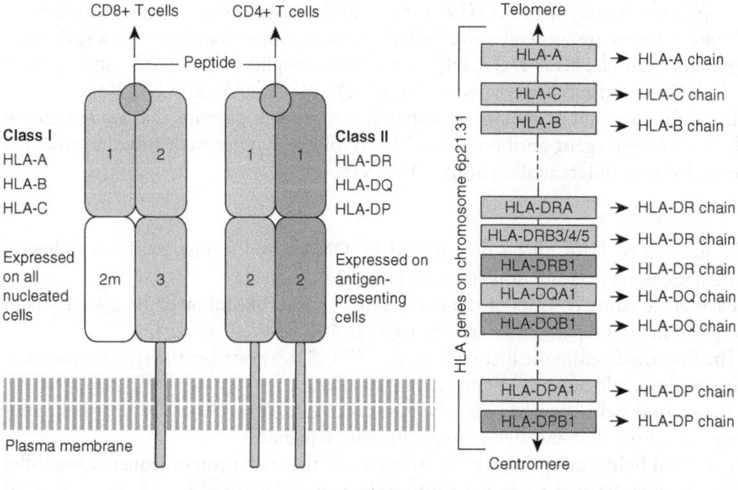

Figure 3-1. **Class I and II HLA molecules and genes.**

expressed in antigen-presentation cells, including dendritic cells, macrophages, and B cells, but may also be induced in endothelial cells and T cells under inflammatory conditions.

HLA POLYMORPHISM AND NOMENCLATURE

Coding for HLA

The diverse HLA antigens in human populations are encoded by the most polymorphic group of genes in the human genome.[1]

- These genes are clustered in the human Major Histocompatibility Complex (MHC) region on the short arm of chromosome 6 (**Figure 3-1, right panel**).
- Class I HLA genes, *HLA-A*, *B*, and *C*, encode the α chains of class I HLA antigens, while the nonpolymorphic *B2M* gene on chromosome 15 encodes the β-2-microglobulin.
- Class II HLA genes encode the α and β chains of class II HLA antigens:
  - *HLA-DRA* and *DRB1* genes encode the α and β chains of the HLA-DR antigen, respectively; one additional copy of *HLA-DRB3*, *DRB4*, or *DRB5* gene is present on some HLA haplotypes and encodes the β chains of HLA-DR52, DR53, and DR51 antigens.
  - *HLA-DQA1* and *DQB1* genes encode the α and β chains of the HLA-DQ antigen, respectively.
  - *HLA-DPA1* and *DPB1* genes encode the α and β chains of the HLA-DP antigen, respectively.

Serological Definition

HLA antigens used to be defined serologically using antisera or monoclonal antibodies of known antigen specificities.

- The World Health Organization Nomenclature committee recognizes a list of HLA antigens, including 28 HLA-A, 62 HLA-B, 10 HLA-C, 24 HLA-DR, and 9 HLA-DQ antigens.
- Examples of HLA antigens: HLA-A2, HLA-Cw7, HLA-DQ2. "w" stands for "workshop" and was only kept for HLA-C to be distinguished from complement factors.
- Some antigens are subsequently divided into subgroups of antigens, or **a split antigen**; for example, HLA-DQ7, DQ8, and DQ9 are splits of the broader specificity of HLA-DQ3 and can be reported as HLA-DQ7(3), DQ8(3), and DQ9(3).
- Each HLA antigen represents a group of heterogeneous proteins that are recognized by the same reagent antibodies used for serologic typing; each unique protein is encoded by a different allele at the DNA level.

Naming of HLA

The naming of HLA alleles determined by DNA-based typing methods follows a systematic nomenclature implemented in 2010.[2]

- Each allele name consists of the gene name, an asterisk, followed by 2 to 4 sets of digits ("fields") separated by colons, e.g., *HLA-A*02:01:01:01*.
- **The first field** before the first colon (e.g., *HLA-A*02*) describes the type corresponding to the serologic antigen encoded by an allele.
- **The second field**, together with the first field (e.g., *HLA-A*02:01*), describes a subtype, or allele, that encodes a unique protein sequence.
- **The third field** distinguishes alleles that encode the same protein sequence but differ by synonymous nucleotide substitutions in exons.

- **The fourth field** distinguishes alleles that only differ by sequence variants in introns or the 5′ or 3′ untranslated regions.
- **Suffixes** may be added to an allele to indicate its expression status; for example, "L" for antigens expressed at low levels, "N" for nonexpressed antigens, "S" for soluble or secreted antigens, and "Q" for antigens with questionable expressions.

HLA Catalog

A large and growing number of HLA alleles are cataloged in the IPD-IMGT/HLA database (Immuno Polymorphism Database-ImMunoGeneTics/Human Leukocyte Antigens).[1]

- As of June 2022, a total of 7,562, 9,000, 7,513, 3,298, 2,278, and 2,067 unique alleles have been named at *HLA-A, B, C, DRB1, DQB1*, and *DPB1* genes, respectively; the class II genes encoding the α chains and HLA-DRB3/4/5 β chains are less polymorphic.
- Of all the alleles at the two-field resolution in the IPD-IMGT/HLA database (version 3.31.0), 74% are rare, observed less than five times in over 8 million individuals; the rest are categorized as common (≥1 in 10,000; 4.7% of total), intermediate (≥1 in 100,000; 4.4%), or well documented (≥5 occurrences; 16.9%) in the common, intermediate, and well-documented alleles 3.0 catalog.

HLA Equivalences in Kidney Transplantation

Although DNA-based HLA typing has largely replaced serologic typing, serologic antigen names equivalent to molecular typing results are widely used for kidney transplantation.

- Tables of HLA antigen equivalences are provided in Organ Procurement and Transplantation Network (OPTN) Policies to allow the comparison of serologic and molecular terms.
- The serologic equivalents of specific HLA alleles can also be looked up online at the IPD-IMGT/HLA database.[1]
- HLA-DQA1, DPA1, DPB1 antigens, and those encoded by most newer alleles have not been characterized serologically and, therefore, do not have corresponding serologic equivalents.

OVERVIEW OF HISTOCOMPATIBILITY TESTING FOR KIDNEY TRANSPLANTATION

- Histocompatibility testing is essential in evaluating the immunologic barrier to kidney transplantation, the risk of hyperacute or acute rejection, and the presence of antibody-mediated rejection (AMR).
- Histocompatibility testing addresses several practical questions to facilitate clinical decision-making (**Table 3-1**):
  - Is the donor-recipient pair mismatched for important HLA antigens?
  - Does the recipient have preformed anti-HLA antibodies due to previous sensitization events?
  - Does the recipient have preformed donor-specific anti-HLA antibodies (DSA) that may increase the risk of rejection?
  - Is the donor-recipient pair serologically compatible?
  - Does the recipient have DSA at the time of suspected AMR?

TABLE 3-1 Clinical Questions Addressed by Histocompatibility Testing

Clinical Questions	Laboratory Test
Pre- and peri-transplantation assessment	
• Is the donor-recipient pair HLA-mismatched?	• Intermediate- or high-resolution HLA typing of the donor and recipient DNA
• Is the recipient sensitized to HLA and to what extent?	• Anti-HLA antibody screen and identification by SPI
• Is the donor-recipient pair at risk for anti-HLA AMR?	• Virtual crossmatch to determine the presence of DSA
• Is the donor-recipient pair serologically compatible?	• Physical crossmatch, including CDC crossmatch and FCXM
Posttransplantation Assessment	
• Does the patient have circulating DSA to support the diagnosis of AMR? • Does the patient have circulating DSA as a risk factor for poor prognosis?	• Anti-HLA antibody screen by SPI and DSA interpretation

AMR, antibody-mediated rejection; CDC, complement-dependent cytotoxicity; DSA, donor-specific anti-HLA antibody; FCXM, flow cytometric crossmatch; HLA, human leukocyte antigen; SPI, solid-phase immunoassays.

- Several histocompatibility tests and data analyses are performed at **different times spanning the pre- and posttransplant periods** as detailed in the following sections:
  - HLA typing by DNA-based methods (pretransplant)
  - HLA antibody screen (pretransplant)
  - Virtual crossmatch (pretransplant)
  - Physical crossmatch: complement-dependent cytotoxicity (CDC) crossmatch and flow cytometric crossmatch (FCXM; pretransplant or retrospective)
  - HLA antibody screen for the detection of DSA (posttransplant)

HLA TYPING

Rationales

- HLA typing of donor-recipient pairs **establishes the extent of HLA mismatch** as a risk factor for rejection and allo-sensitization; donor HLA typing also enables the virtual crossmatch for organ allocation and identification of DSAs.
- HLA typing methods have evolved since the discovery of HLA, from serologic techniques to DNA-based methods.
  - HLA phenotyping by reagent antibodies of known specificity, i.e., serologic typing, is laborious and cannot reliably differentiate the diverse HLA antigens in the population.
  - DNA-based HLA typing, including polymerase chain reaction (PCR) and sequencing-based methods, has replaced serologic typing as the current standard of care.

- Genotype-phenotype relationship: DNA-based HLA typing can predict the phenotype (i.e., HLA antigens expressed) but does not directly assess the expression and posttranslational modification of HLA antigens.
- Donors and recipients must be typed for HLA-A, B (including Bw4 and Bw6), C, DR, DR51, DR52, DR53, DQA1, DQB1, DPA1, and DPB1 per current policies of the OPTN.[3]
- **Many alleles at adjacent HLA genes are in linkage disequilibrium**, especially among HLA-DRB1, DRB3/4/5, and DQB1, and between HLA-B and C.
  - Some alleles are more likely to be found on one parental chromosome and be inherited together as a haplotype; for example, the most common haplotype in European whites is *HLA-A*01:01~C*07:01~B*08:01~DRB1*03:01~DQB1*02:01.*
  - One direct implication of the linkage association is that donor-patient pairs that are matched for HLA-B and DRB1 are likely to be matched for HLA-C and DQB1 as well.
  - Common linkage associations among certain HLA alleles also allow histocompatibility laboratories to detect erroneous typing results with unexpected haplotypes.
- Specimens for HLA typing: DNA-based HLA typing is performed using genomic DNA extracted from buccal swabs or EDTA--anticoagulated peripheral blood.
- Several DNA-based HLA typing methods generate results of different resolutions at the antigen or allele levels as described below.

Low-to-Intermediate Resolution HLA Typing

- Histocompatibility laboratories must perform low- to-intermediate resolution **(LR) HLA typing of at least serologic split-level resolution** per current OPTN policies.[3] For example, HLA-DQ7, DQ8, and DQ9 are known splits of HLA-DQ3, and LR HLA typing must be able to differentiate HLA-DQ7, DQ8, and DQ9; a typing of HLA-DQ3 is unacceptable.
- **Table 3-2 provides an example of LR HLA typing result in molecular** and serologic equivalent nomenclatures.
  - The numbering of serologic equivalents is consistent with the first field of the LR DNA-based HLA typing for most antigens, e.g., HLA-A2 (serologic equivalent) and *HLA-A*02* (molecular).
  - When split antigens exist, the numbering of serologic equivalents may differ from the first field of the LR molecular HLA typing, e.g., HLA-B64 and B65 are splits of B14 (B*14), B60 and B61 are splits of B40 (B*40), and Cw9 and Cw10 are splits of Cw3 (C*03); in these cases, serologic equivalent adds information to the molecular typing result.
- LR HLA typing detects informative **sequence variants at selected positions of HLA genes** rather than sequencing these genes at single-base resolution.
  - Each type may include many possible alleles of various frequencies, which is called **ambiguity**.
  - For example, *HLA-A*02* (or HLA-A2) may include tens or hundreds of alleles such as *HLA-A*02:01, A*02:03, A*02:06*, etc., depending on the typing method.
  - While all LR HLA typing methods must achieve the serologic split-level resolution, they may differ in the number of ambiguous alleles for each type.
  - In general, the more sequence variants examined in a typing assay, the less ambiguous alleles will be included in the typing results.
- LR HLA typing is commonly achieved by **real-time PCR (RT-PCR)** and **reverse sequence-specific oligonucleotide (rSSO)**.

- **RT-PCR** uses multiple sequence-specific primer pairs to determine the presence or absence of informative sequence variants in HLA genes by PCR, typically on a 384-well tray; the fluorescent signals from PCR reactions are detected and analyzed in real time to generate LR HLA genotypes.
  - RT-PCR can be completed in 2 hours to enable rapid allocation of deceased-donor kidneys and is used in most organ procurement organization (OPO) laboratories.
  - The throughput of RT-PCR is low (i.e., one tray for each donor) and may be unsuitable for typing a batch of many patients and donors.
  - The resolution of RT-PCR used for deceased-donor typing is relatively low and may not be able to distinguish certain common alleles.
- **rSSO** hybridizes biotinylated amplicons from HLA genes with an array of microsphere particles (Luminex beads) coated with sequence-specific oligonucleotide probes; phycoerythrin (PE)-conjugated streptavidin binds to biotin and allows detection of hybridization-positive beads on the Luminex platform; the positive hybridization pattern is analyzed by software to generate LR HLA genotypes.
  - rSSO can be completed in 4 to 5 hours and is suitable for typing deceased donors or a batch of donor and recipient samples.
  - We routinely type kidney transplant candidates and living donors with this method during pretransplant evaluation at our medical center.
  - Some rSSO assays (e.g., LABType CWD) evaluate a sufficient number of sequence variants per HLA gene to be able to distinguish most common alleles at *HLA-A*, *B*, *C*, and *DRB1* genes.

High-Resolution HLA Typing

- High-resolution (HR) HLA typing is increasingly performed to support kidney and other solid-organ transplantations.
- HR typing adds value to the following aspects of donor-recipient compatibility assessment:
  - HR typing allows in-depth evaluation of their HLA molecular mismatch at the level of amino acid residues or structural epitopes.
  - HR typing of donors enables the identification of DSA against a subset of proteins in an antigen group encoded by specific alleles ("allelic DSA").
  - HR typing of recipients allows differentiating allelic antibodies and autologous reactivities detected in their serum samples.
- HR typing is best achieved by sequencing the entire HLA genes, or at least the most polymorphic exons of HLA genes, at single-base resolution.
- HR typing results are typically reported as 2-field alleles that encode unique protein sequences (**Table 3-2**).
- Sanger sequencing was the gold standard but is limited by low throughput and typing ambiguity.
- Next-generation sequencing (NGS) is the current standard of care for HR HLA typing and can efficiently type many samples in a multiplexed sequencing run at **2-field or 3-field resolution** with few ambiguous alleles.
  - The process of NGS-based HR HLA typing:
    - Enrich HLA genes by PCR amplification or hybridization-based capture.
    - Prepare pooled sequencing library that includes DNA fragments ligated with sample-specific barcode and sequencing adapters.
    - Sequence the library on NGS platforms.
    - Analyze the sequencing reads by validated bioinformatic pipelines to determine health metrics for quality assurance and HR HLA typing.

TABLE 3-2 An Example of Low- to Intermediate-Resolution (LR) and High-Resolution (HR) HLA Typing Results and Their Serological Equivalents

HLA Genes	LR Typing Result	HR Typing Result	Serologic Equivalent
HLA-A	*HLA-A*02*	*HLA-A*02:01*	HLA-A2
	*HLA-A*31*	*HLA-A*31:01*	HLA-A31
HLA-B	*HLA-B*15*	*HLA-B*15:01*	HLA-B62, Bw6
	*HLA-B*40*	*HLA-B*40:01*	HLA-B60, Bw6
HLA-C	*HLA-C*02*	*HLA-C*02:02*	HLA-Cw2
	*HLA-C*03*	*HLA-C*03:04*	HLA-Cw10
HLA-DRB1	*HLA-DRB1*01:03*	*HLA-DRB1*01:03*	HLA-DR103
	*HLA-DRB1*14*	*HLA-DRB1*14:01*	HLA-DR14
HLA-DRB3/4/5	*HLA-DRB3*02*	*HLA-DRB3*02:01*	HLA-DR52
HLA-DQB1	*HLA-DQB1*05*	*HLA-DQB1*05:03*	HLA-DQ5
	*HLA-DQB1*03*	*HLA-DQB1*03:01*	HLA-DQ7
HLA-DQA1	*HLA-DQA1*01*	*HLA-DQA1*01:01*	–
	*HLA-DQA1*05*	*HLA-DQA1*05:01*	
HLA-DQB1	–	*HLA-DPB1*02:01*	–
		*HLA-DPB1*04:01*	

- HR typing by NGS can typically be completed **within 3 to 4 days and requires batching to be cost effective**, which hinders its application in deceased donor typing for organ allocation; newer technologies such as rapid nanopore sequencing may enable this application soon.[4]
- All living and deceased kidney donors are typed at high resolution by NGS at our center to facilitate the identification of DSA in the posttransplant setting (see below).

- HR typing may be inferred based on LR typing and known HLA haplotypes in the population, which has been used in research to study the impact of HLA disparity on graft outcomes; however, inferred HLA typing may lack the accuracy required for clinical application.

HLA Mismatch and Transplant Outcome

- HLA mismatch is an important prognostic factor, not a contraindication, for kidney transplantation; on the other hand, the benefit of HLA matching has been evidenced by the superior long-term graft outcomes after kidney transplantations from identical twins, HLA-matched siblings, or HLA-matched unrelated donors.
- Multiple registry-based and single-center cohort studies demonstrated an association between worsened long-term transplant outcomes and HLA-A, B, and DR antigen mismatches.[5]
  - Each incremental HLA antigen mismatch, out of HLA-A, B, and DR, was significantly associated with 6% higher risk of overall graft failure (HR: 1.06; 95% CI: 1.05-1.07), based on multivariate analyses from 11 studies (289,987 adult recipients).

- For the impact of different antigens, each incremental HLA-DR antigen mismatch was significantly associated with 12% higher risk of overall graft failure (HR: 1.06; 95% CI: 1.05-1.07), based on multivariate analyses from seven studies; the effect of HLA-A and B mismatch on overall graft failure was studied in fewer studies and was not as pronounced.
- Each incremental HLA antigen mismatch was also associated with **increased death-censored graft failure** (HR: 1.09; 95% CI: 1.06-1.12) and **all-cause mortality** (HR: 1.04; 95% CI: 1.02-1.07), based on over 100,000 recipients from four cohorts.
- A metaanalysis of 18 studies in 26,018 pediatric recipients also showed that HLA-DR mismatch and combined HLA-A and B mismatch significantly increase the risk of graft failure, rejection, and all-cause mortality.[6]

- Beyond HLA-A, B, and DR mismatch, limited data suggest that mismatches in other HLA antigens such as HLA-C and DQ may independently increase the risk of rejection; HLA-DP mismatch may be tolerated without increased risk of rejection or graft loss.[7]
- Unlike unrelated hematopoietic stem cell transplantations, where we can search among millions of HLA-typed registry donors to identify well-matched donors, routine HLA matching is impractical for kidney transplantation; however, **two approaches can increase the number of transplantations between better-matched donor-recipient pairs:**
  - Additional allocation points are assigned to candidates with 0 HLA-A, B, and DR mismatch or 0 to 1 HLA-DR mismatch with a donor, which helps prioritize HLA-matched candidates during organ allocation; up to four points can be assigned for 0 HLA-A, B, DR mismatches in pediatric candidates under 10 years of age.
  - Paired kidney donation in a pool of donor-recipient pairs may implement an algorithm to improve the HLA matching in multiple pairs while simultaneously resolving other constraints such as preformed anti-HLA antibodies and ABO incompatibility.
- To customize the care for individual candidates, **the benefit of a better HLA match should be balanced with other factors** in waitlist management.
  - The haplotype frequency of the candidate may dictate the likelihood of a well-matched donor in the population.
  - Prolonged wait time is not justified for the sole purpose of an HLA-matched kidney.
  - A better HLA-matched organ may be far away, and the long-distance transportation may increase the cold ischemia time.
  - Broadly sensitized candidates are likely to require a well-matched kidney to avoid preformed antibodies against diverse, non-self-HLA antigens.

ANTI-HLA ANTIBODY TESTING

Rationales

- Approximately 30% of kidney transplant candidates are sensitized to HLA due to prior sensitization events such as blood transfusions, pregnancies, and previous transplantations.
- Exposure to foreign HLA antigens during sensitization events triggers the production of anti-HLA antibodies to immunogenic epitopes shared among groups of **cross-reactive antigens**.[8]

- The immunogenicity and antibody recognition of HLA antigens are likely to be driven by patches of functional epitopes (or "**eplets**") consisting of one or more polymorphic residues within a 3 to 3.5 Angstrom radius on the surface of an antigen.
- **HLAMatchmaker** (www.epitopes.net) is the most widely used computer program that predicts and analyzes HLA eplets in relation to histocompatibility testing results[9]; note that we use the more general term, epitope, interchangeably with eplet in this chapter.
- HLA Epitope Registry (www.epregistry.com.br) is an online database that compiles serologic data supporting antibody-verified HLA epitopes; users can also perform epitope analysis at the website using HLA typing and antibody testing results.[10]
- HLA antigens display multiple immunogenic epitopes on their surfaces; different antigens may share epitopes and form overlapping cross-reactive groups.
- Serum reactivity to a shared epitope creates a distinct pattern encompassing all or most antigens within a cross-reactive group.
- An epitope shared broadly among a large group of cross-reactive HLA antigens is considered a **public epitope**; for example, the HLA-Bw4 epitope is shared among approximately half of the HLA-B antigens and several HLA-A antigens.

- Anti-HLA antibodies are the leading cause of hyperacute, acute, or chronic AMR:
  - The detection, identification, and monitoring of preformed anti-HLA antibodies are the focus of histocompatibility risk assessment in the pretransplant setting.
  - Antibody testing results can be used in conjunction with donor typing to determine the presence of DSA in a **virtual crossmatch**, which facilitates organ allocation and predicts the physical crossmatch result and transplant outcome; the DSA information also **supports the diagnosis of AMR** in the posttransplant setting (see following sections).
- Anti-HLA antibody testing methods have evolved significantly over time, from CDC and enzyme-linked immunosorbent assay assays to multiplexed solid-phase immunoassays (SPI) on the Luminex platform or flow cytometers; multiplexed SPIs are the current standard care and will be described in detail in this section.
  - The technical advancement to multiplexed SPIs has been driven by the need to detect and identify clinically relevant anti-HLA antibodies to facilitate virtual crossmatch, organ allocation, and DSA interpretation.
  - Multiplexed SPIs analyze multiplexed antigen-coated Luminex beads or microparticles simultaneously to detect and identify HLA-specific antibodies using a PE-conjugated secondary antibody.
  - Different antigen-coated Luminex beads are distinguished by discrete amounts of red, infra-red, and extended infra-red dyes impregnated in the beads.
  - The binding of PE-conjugated secondary antibody is detected by a different laser in a separate channel.
- Bead configuration and assay modification: SPIs can be configured to include beads carrying a single recombinant antigen or multiple different antigens per bead; SPIs can be further modified to characterize the potential of complement activation or IgG subclasses of anti-HLA antibodies by using different detecting reagents.

Single-Antigen Bead Assays

Workflow

- Commonly used single-antigen bead (SAB) assays (**Figure 3-2**, **left panel**) use Luminex beads coated with a single purified recombinant HLA antigen per bead group; antibodies to class I and class II HLA are tested separately using class I and II panels, each offering over 100 antigen-coated bead groups.

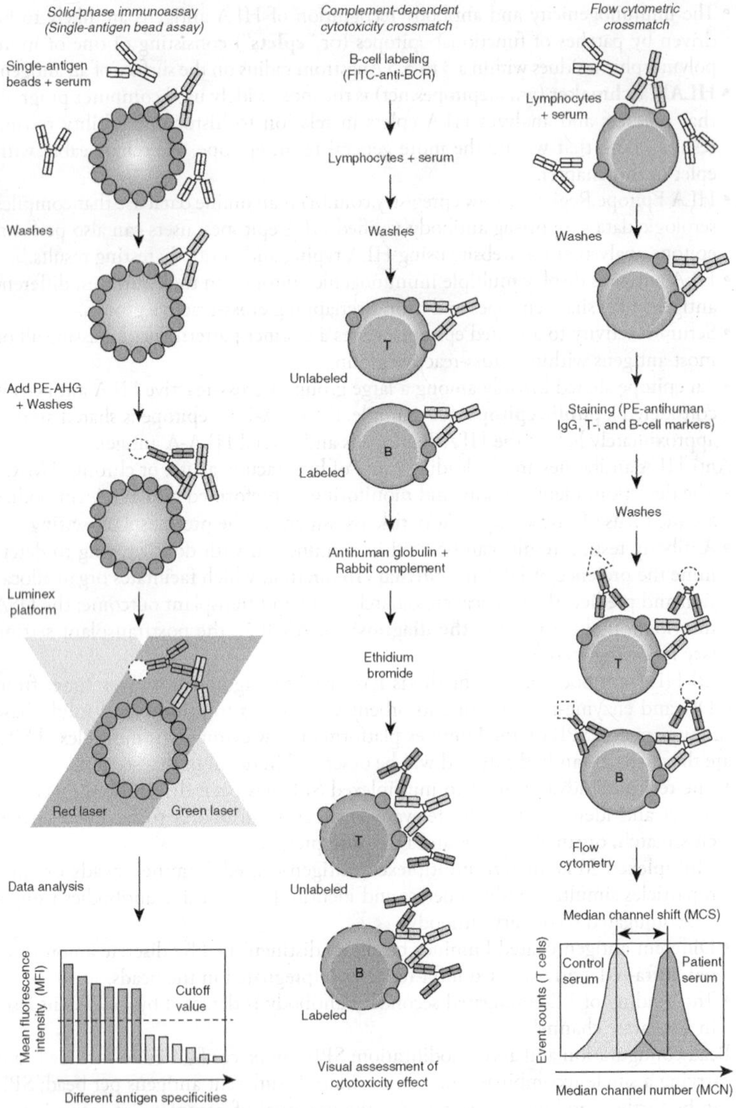

Figure 3-2. Anti-HLA antibody testing.

- Serum samples are incubated with antigen-coated beads, followed by washing and detection of anti-HLA IgG by PE-conjugated secondary antibody (antihuman IgG) on the Luminex platform.
- **Mean fluorescence intensity (MFI)** is acquired from each antigen-specific bead group on the Luminex platform, and background-normalized MFI values are

generated by subtracting signals from the negative control (NC) beads and NC serum; **note that MFI values do not quantify the concentration** or the binding affinity of anti-HLA antibodies.

Interpretation and Application of SAB Assay Results

- MFI values are converted to positive/negative or various risk categories for reporting based on laboratory-defined cutoff values.
  - These cutoff values should be correlated with physical crossmatch results or clinical outcomes such as graft rejection.
  - While cutoff values vary significantly among different centers, a cutoff value between 1,000 to 1,500 MFI may serve as a harmonized cutoff for multicenter clinical trials, as stated in the STAR (Sensitization in Transplantation: Assessment of Risk) 2017 Working Group Meeting Report.[11]
  - The following cutoff MFI values are used to define three risk categories at our center:
    - 1,000 to 2,000 MFI: low risk
    - 2,000 to 5,000 MFI: moderate risk (good correlation with positive FCXM results; antibodies with MFI above 2,000 are generally avoided)
    - >5,000 MFI: increased risk (expected to reliably predict positive FCXM results)
- Detection of any reactivity above center-defined cutoff values indicates that a patient is sensitized to HLA; this information should be interpreted together with the patient's sensitization history.
- **Unacceptable antigens (UAs):** SAB assays identify a list of antigens to which a serum specimen is reactive; these specificities can be listed at the United Network of Organ Sharing (UNOS) as antigens to avoid (i.e., "avoids" or UAs) to inform organ allocation.
  - For example, reactivities to multiple HLA-A2 beads (HLA-A*02:01, A*02:03, A*02:06) are detected in a candidate with MFI values between 5,000 and 10,000; HLA-A2 should be listed as a UA to avoid donors positive for HLA-A2.
  - Transplant centers may use a default MFI cutoff value such as 2,000 to identify and list UAs, which can be customized for individual patients to balance the risk of rejection and donor availability.
- **Calculated panel reactive antibody (cPRA)** is calculated based on the frequencies of listed UAs and indicates the percentage of donors expected to be incompatible with the candidate.
  - For example, listing HLA-A2 results in a cPRA of 47.9%; listing HLA-A2, DQ7, DQ8, and DQ9 results in a cPRA of 76.5%.
  - Candidates with a high cPRA face an increased immunological barrier and diminished donor pool to receive compatible kidney transplantations.
  - Caveat of cPRA: the current OPTN cPRA calculator does not consider allelic antibodies (see below) or reactivities to HLA-DQA1 and DP; therefore, cPRA underestimates the transplant barrier for candidates with these reactivities.
- **Epitope analysis: SAB results frequently demonstrate cross-reactive patterns**, with multiple positive beads carrying antigens that share one or more epitopes.
  - Two examples are shown in **Figure 3-3**.
  - Epitope analysis provides mechanistic explanations for reactivity patterns observed by the SAB assay, supports the clinical significance of the antibodies detected, provides clues to the origin of alloimmunization, and helps detect false-positive (FP) or underestimated reactivities.
  - Epitope analysis remains a largely manual process and may not be conclusive in high-cPRA samples reactive with multiple epitopes; the low throughput and lack of standardization hinder its clinical application.

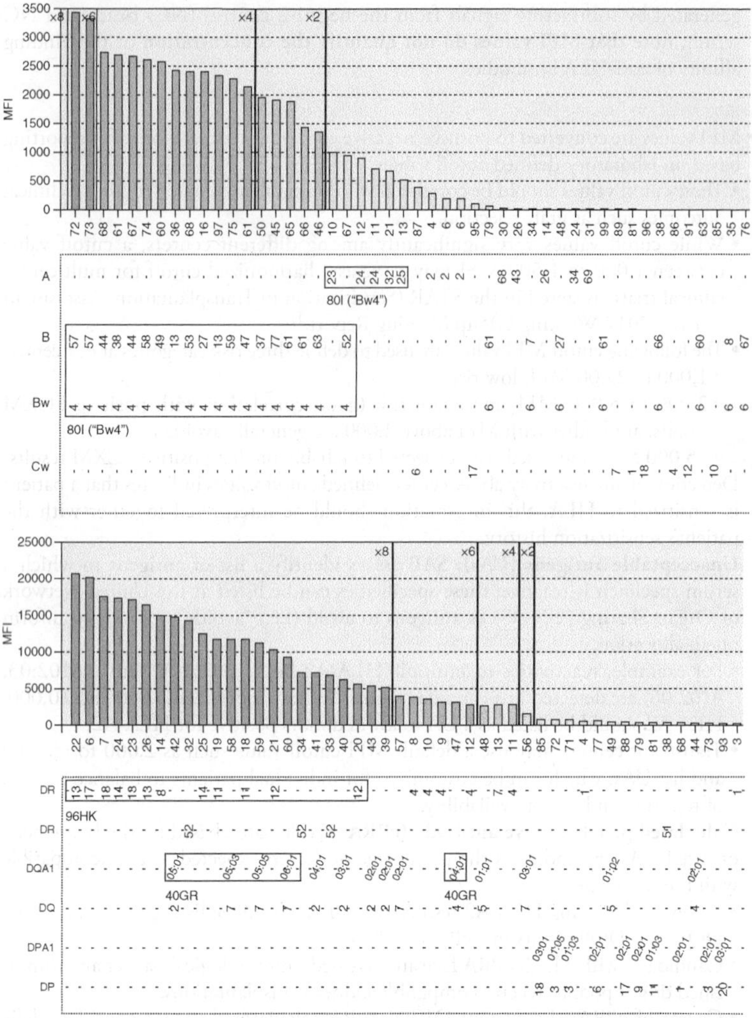

Figure 3-3. Examples of cross-reactive antibodies seen on the single-antigen bead (SAB) assay. The upper panel shows a pattern consistent with the 80I ("Bw4") epitope shared among boxed HLA-A and -B antigens; the lower panel shows a pattern consistent with the 96HK epitope shared among boxed HLA-DR antigens and the 40GR epitope shared among boxed HLA-DQA1 antigens.

- **Allelic antibodies** react with some but not all antigens within the same antigen group.
  - For example, HLA-A24 is represented by two different beads expressing HLA-A*24:02 and A*24:03 on the SAB panel; when a serum is reactive with HLA-A*24:02 but not A*24:03, an allelic antibody to HLA-A*24:02 should be considered.

  - The mechanism of allelic antibodies is that they only recognize epitopes present in a subset of antigens within an antigen group.
  - To extend the example above, the allelic antibody to HLA-A*24:02 is most likely explained by reactivity to the 166DG epitope, which is present in HLA-A*24:02 but not HLA-A*24:03; because 166DG is also present in most HLA-A*01 and A*23 antigens, the allelic antibody to HLA-A*24:02 is expected to react with HLA-A*01 and A*23 beads in the SAB panel.
- **Reactivity to the α or β chain or combinatorial epitopes of HLA-DQ and DP antigens**
  - SAB panels include multiple HLA-DQ and DP beads with various combinations of α and β chains, both chains being polymorphic.
  - Reactivity to a specific β chain, e.g., HLA-DQB1*03:03 (or DQ7), should cause all beads with DQB1*03:03 to be positive regardless of the α chain specificity in the heterodimers.
  - Reactivity to a specific α chain, e.g., HLA-DQA1*01, should cause all beads with DQA1*01 to be positive regardless of the β chain specificity in the heterodimers.
  - Reactivity to a specific α-β heterodimer, e.g., HLA-DQB1*03:03 paired with DQA1*05, should only cause beads with the specific heterodimer to be positive.
  - In our center, we sequentially evaluate the presence of antibodies to the β chain and then the α chain; if neither can explain the reactivity pattern, antibodies to individual heterodimers are assigned.

Limitations of the SAB Assays

- **SAB assays do not directly quantify the concentration or affinity of anti-HLA antibodies**; MFI values serve as a surrogate for the strength of anti-HLA reactivities and should be interpreted together with other laboratory and clinical data.
- **False-negative results** or falsely low MFI values due to complement interference:
  - Complement interference is more often observed in, but not limited to, serum samples with high levels of anti-HLA reactivity.
  - **Mechanism:** anti-HLA antibodies bind to SAB and activate the complement cascade on the bead surface; the accumulation of complement products sterically hinders the binding of PE-conjugated human IgG.
  - **Several methods can remove the complement interference**, including serum pretreatment with EDTA (to chelate calcium required for complement activation) or dithiothreitol (DTT), heat inactivation of complement factors in the serum, and dilution.
  - Because it is unpredictable which serum sample will be affected by complement interference, our center preemptively pretreats all serum samples with EDTA before SAB testing to prevent false-negative results.[12]
- Other interfering substances in serum samples may cause false-negative results by increasing the MFI values on the NC beads; when NC MFI values exceed 1,500, affected samples should be treated with DTT or adsorbed using Adsorb Out beads to remove the interference.
- Another type of false-negative result has been attributed to **the "spreading" of antibodies on multiple cross-reactive beads sharing the same epitope**, causing an underestimation of the true MFI values (**Figure 3-3, upper panel**).[13]
  - Summation of MFI values from cross-reactive beads sharing the relevant epitope has been proposed to better approximate the true antibody strength.
  - **However, the "spreading" theory was questioned by recent experimental findings:** increasing the number of beads carrying specific epitopes when testing serum

samples with known epitope-specific reactivities did not significantly lower the MFI values, suggesting that anti-HLA antibodies are typically in excess relative to the number of epitopes on beads.[14]

- The MFI values of anti-HLA antibodies may be high after recent sensitization events but wane over time to below the assay cutoffs; thus, in the absence of a longitudinal antibody history, SAB assays only provide **a snapshot of antibody levels without assessing the potential of memory (or recall) response** upon re-exposure to a previously encountered antigen.
- SAB assays may also produce FP **results** in various situations.
  - FP (with a 500 MFI cutoff value) results were frequently found on some beads after testing a panel of sera from nonsensitized males; the top three "hot" beads were: DP1 (DPB1*01:01/DPA1*02:01; FP in 18.6% of results; mean MFI: 1,253), DP5 (DPB1*05:01/DPA1*02:02; FP in 16.8% of results; mean MFI: 1,285), and DR53 (DRB4*01:01; FP in 15.4% of results; mean MFI: 855).[15]
  - Certain beads are thought to contain **denatured antigens** and produce spurious results that lack clinical significance; these FP reactivities will persist when testing the affected serum using acid-treated beads.
  - Certain SABs may carry recombinant HLA proteins with polyhistidine affinity tags; **antipolyhistidine antibodies**, if present in a patient, will produce FP results affecting these beads; pretreating affected sera using polyhistidine-coated beads can remove the FP reactivity.
  - **Intravenous immunoglobulin products** contain naturally occurring anti-HLA-E or nonspecific antibodies and have been shown to produce low to moderate MFI values with a broad range of beads when diluted and tested in vitro.[16]
  - **Antithymocyte globulin (ATG)** can cause FP results with beads coated with class I and II antigens due to the presence of anti-HLA reactivities in thymocyte-immunized animals and the cross-reactivity of PE-labeled antihuman IgG with animal-derived antibodies.
- **Table 3-3** summarizes FP and false-negative results from SAB assays.
- **Interassay variations**
  - When testing a panel of well-characterized reference sera, SAB assays from two different vendors showed good agreement, as reported in a multicenter study.
  - However, when testing a collection of sera with suspected FP reactivities, SAB assays from two different vendors produce divergent results in 55% of cases, as reported in an observational study.
- **Interlaboratory variations:** Even with the same assay and protocol, the interlaboratory variations may be as high as 25%, suggesting a need for more standardization or automation of the assay.[18]
- In addition to the limitations of the SAB assay itself, other quality issues such as misidentified samples and carry-over contaminations during the testing process may also lead to spurious screen results; these errors should be identified through a comparison of current and historical results and investigated promptly.

SPIs Assessing the Complement-Fixing Potential of Anti-HLA Antibodies

- The C1q assay differs from the SAB assay in several key aspects.
  - Heat-inactivated serum is tested, removing potential interference from endogenous complement factors.
  - HLA-coated beads and recombinant C1q beads (positive control) are incubated with test serum and human C1q.

TABLE 3-3 False-Negative and -Positive Results From SAB Assays

Typical Patterns	Potential Causes	Follow-Up Testing
False-Negative Results		
Falsely negative beads inconsistent with expected cross-reactive patterns; mostly affecting high cPRA sera	Complement interference	EDTA or DTT pretreatment, or dilution
Falsely low MFI values across all beads with high NC bead signal	Nonspecific interfering antibodies	DTT or Adsorb Out pretreatment
Falsely low MFI values across all beads with low PC bead signal	Nonspecific IgM interfering antibodies	DTT pretreatment
Low MFI values across multiple beads sharing a public epitope, e.g., Bw4 or Bw6[a]	Antigens on beads in excess compared with antibodies in sera	PRA assay or surrogate flow crossmatch
Significantly lower MFI values in current screen than previous screens	Waning humoral immunity or desensitization	Include historical reactivity in the risk assessment
False-Positive Results		
Positive reactivities on known "hot beads" or unexplained by epitope analysis; negative sensitization history	Denatured antigens or affinity tags on beads	PRA assay or surrogate FCXM
Positive reactivities on beads carrying autologous antigens	Denatured antigens or affinity tags on beads	PRA assay, autologous FCXM
Low-level reactivity across multiple beads	IVIG interference	PRA or C1q assay, or surrogate flow crossmatch
New reactivity in sera collected after ATG induction	PE-antihuman IgG cross-reacting with ATG	Repeat testing later

ATG, Antithymocyte globulin; cPRA, calculated panel reactive antibody; DTT, dithiothreitol; EDTA, ethylenediaminetetraacetic acid; FCXM, flow cytometric crossmatch; IVIG, intravenous immune globulin; MFI, Mean fluorescence intensity; NC, negative control; PC, positive control; PE, phycoerythrin; PRA, panel reactive antibody.

[a]This observation may also be explained by lower concentrations or affinity of the antibody and, therefore, may not represent a false-negative result according to recent literature.[17]

- **PE-conjugated** antihuman C1q antibody is used to detect C1q bound to anti-HLA antibodies on the SABs.
- **The MFI cutoff values** for the C1q assay, as reported in the literature or used at many laboratories, may differ from commonly used cutoff values for SAB assays; a cutoff of 1,000 MFI is used for the C1q assay at our center.

- C1q assay results are influenced by the concentration or titer of anti-HLA antibodies and the C1q binding effector function of these antibodies.
- Some early studies showed a stronger correlation between C1q-positive DSAs and kidney graft outcomes compared to DSAs detected by regular SAB assays, indicating a role for the C1q assay in risk-stratifying DSAs in pre- and posttransplant settings; however, conflicting results have been reported in the literature.
- The C1q assay may not add value to the regular SAB assay using EDTA-pretreated serum samples and after accounting for the MFI values.
  - An MFI cutoff value of 10,000 on the SAB assay after EDTA pretreatment can successfully predict most C1q-positive antibodies.
  - Most C1q-positive anti-HLA antibodies also showed a titer above 32 or 64 in dilution studies.
- Additional complement-fixing antibody screen assays have been developed that detect the complement pathway product, C3d or C4d, deposited on the SABs to estimate the risk of complement-mediate graft injury.
  - Like the C1q assay, studies have shown a good correlation between C3d positivity and high MFI values (>10,000) from the regular SAB assay.
  - C3d positivity may further stratify antibodies of lower MFI values and identify those associated with inferior graft outcomes.
- The STAR 2019 Working Group Meeting Report acknowledged the wide use of complement binding assays but cautioned that anti-HLA antibodies, when detected by regular SAB assays but not these modified assays, may still carry risks of rejection.[19]

SPIs Assessing the Isotype and IgG Subclass of Anti-HLA Antibodies

- The PE-conjugated antihuman IgM is available to detect anti-HLA IgM antibodies bound to SABs; the clinical utility of this assay is yet to be established.
- The PE-conjugated antihuman IgG used in the regular SAB assay is pan-reactive with all IgG subclasses; replacing antihuman IgG with secondary antibodies specific to IgG subclasses (IgG1, IgG2, IgG3, and IgG4) may theoretically refine the attributes of anti-HLA antibodies for risk stratification.
- IgG1 and IgG3 anti-HLA antibodies are the predominant subclasses predictive of graft rejection and loss; however, the prognostic role of IgG2 and IgG4 antibodies has not been ruled out.
- Several technical challenges hinder the clinical application of IgG subclass evaluation:
  - Reagents with stringent specificity must be used to mitigate intersubclass cross reactivity.
  - Subclass-specific secondary antibodies may vary in their affinity and fail to quantify the relative abundance of subclass-specific antibodies.
  - Anti-HLA antibodies of different subclasses frequently coexist in a complex and polyclonal humoral response, and it is unknown whether distinct multisubclass patterns correlate with graft outcomes.

SPIs Using Beads Carrying Mixed Antigens

- The Panel Reactive Antibody (PRA) assay includes Luminex beads coated with a mixture of class I or class II antigens extracted from donor-derived cell lines.
  - Each bead group carries antigens from a distinct donor, and the percentage of positive beads in the panel predicts the proportions of donors incompatible with a candidate.
  - Depending on how diverse and representative the bead panel is configured, PRA values may only approximate the donor availability in the local donor pool.
  - The PRA assay provides an alternative screen method using nonrecombinant HLA proteins and can be used to discern FP reactivities observed in the SAB assay (**Figure 3-4**).

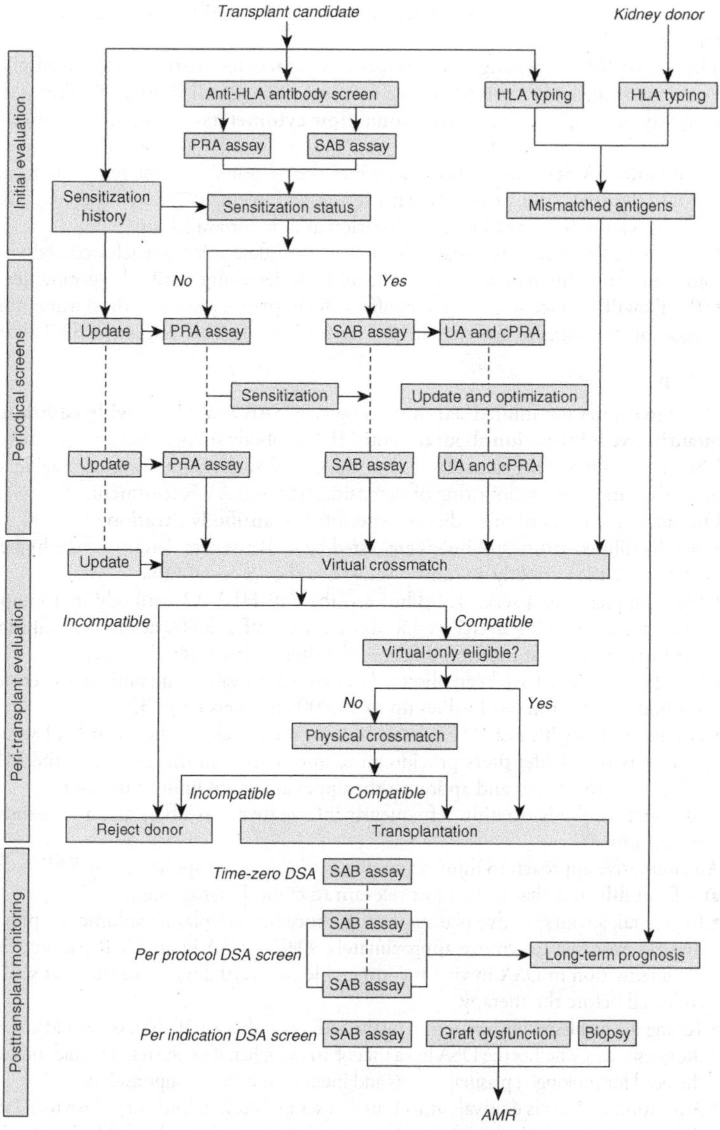

Figure 3-4. **Integrated histocompatibility testing for renal transplantation.**

- The PRA assay could not reliably determine the antigen- or epitope-level specificities, especially in highly sensitized patients; however, nonreactive beads may help identify acceptable antigens for such patients.

- **The mixed bead assay** differs from the PRA assay by using beads coated with class I or class II antigens from three donor-derived cell lines per bead; this assay has been used more often in blood donor screen to mitigate the risk of transfusion-related acute lung injury.

- **The FlowPRA Screening assay** offers microparticles coated with mixed class I or class II antigens derived from 30 donor-derived cell lines and collects the antibody binding data on **conventional flow cytometers** instead of the Luminex platform.
  - The FlowPRA Screening assay determines the percentage of antigen-coated microparticles that react positively with serum specimens to generate percent PRA values as an indicator of HLA sensitization and donor availability.
  - The FlowPRA Screening assay does not differentiate microparticles coated with antigens from different cell lines and could not determine antibody specificities.
  - The FlowPRA Screening assay also offers an alternative screen method using nonrecombinant antigens and may help discern FP reactivities seen in the SAB assay.

Dilution Studies

- Dilution studies test diluted serum specimens by SAB assays to **provide additional quantitative information** about the anti-HLA antibody strength beyond the cutoff-based positivity or MFI values from the neat serum; such information is valuable for prognostication and monitoring of desensitization and AMR treatment.
- One approach to dilution studies is to perform an **antibody titration**.[20]
  - Serially diluted serum specimens are tested by SAB assays to determine the highest titer where the antibody remains positive based on a cutoff value.
  - For example: after a serial 1:2 dilutions, the anti-HLA-A2 antibody in a sample remains positive with an MFI value above the cutoff of 2,000 at the 1:32 dilution but turns negative at the 1:64 dilution; the titer of this antibody is 32.
  - Good correlations have been observed between MFI values and antibody titers for antibodies with neat MFI values up to 10,000 and titers up to 32.
  - For antibodies with neat MFI above 10,000, the correlation between MFI values and titers is variable; titers provide more information in this setting as the MFI values start to plateau and approach the upper analytical limit of the assay.
  - Although antibody titration is frequently informative, it is laborious and expensive to perform.
- An alternative approach to dilution studies is to test serum specimens by SAB assays **at a fixed dilution** that is the most relevant to clinical management.
  - In general, a course of five plasmapheresis procedures (1 plasma volume per procedure) is expected to remove approximately 90% of DSA in an AMR patient; this 90% reduction in DSA in vivo is comparable to a 1:10 dilution of the neat serum collected before the therapy.
  - Testing the preplasmapheresis serum by the SAB assay after a 1:10 dilution would answer the question of whether the DSA has a titer of 10 or higher; if so, the result would indicate the need for prolonged plasmapheresis and intensified immune suppression.
  - A dilution of 1:16 is equivalent to four 1:2 serial dilutions and very close to a 1:10 dilution; recent clinical trials have proposed to use a single 1:16 dilution to risk stratify preformed DSAs in kidney transplant candidates.

VIRTUAL CROSSMATCH

Rationales

- Virtual crossmatch compares a patient's anti-HLA antibody profile with the donor's HLA typing to assess the immunologic compatibility for the pair.

- Virtual crossmatch integrates HLA typing and serology results already available for donor-candidate pairs, without incubating the patient's serum with the donor's lymphocytes as required in physical crossmatch procedures (CDC crossmatch or FCXM, see below).
- Virtual crossmatch offers **several benefits** at the time of organ allocation.
  - Histocompatibility can be evaluated immediately based on existing laboratory results for donor-patient pairs regardless of their geographical location.
  - The procedure is **especially valuable in identifying suitable donors in regional and national pools for highly sensitized patients**.
  - Negative virtual crossmatch results may allow kidney transplantations to proceed without waiting for a prospective physical crossmatch, which reduces the cold ischemia time.
  - Virtual crossmatch is HLA focused and may circumvent FP results in physical crossmatches due to non-HLA antibodies of little clinical significance.

Workflow

- Patients awaiting kidney transplantation should be screened for anti-HLA antibodies periodically to monitor their sensitization status and changes in their antibody strengths.
- For **patients on the deceased donor kidney waitlist**, their UAs are listed at UNOS and updated regularly; some centers choose to list all historical UAs accumulatively regardless of whether they are showing on the current screen.
  - When a deceased donor becomes available, the UNOS match run automatically excludes patients whose UAs overlap with the donor typing at the serologic split resolution.
  - Patients with no UA specific to the donor are likely to receive an offer, and **virtual crossmatch is performed at local hospitals to evaluate and document the following** as applicable:
    - Whether the UA listed at UNOS is accurate and up to date per center policy.
    - Whether patients have had additional sensitization events since the most recent antibody screen.
    - Low-level DSAs below the MFI value for UA and, therefore, not listed at UNOS; for example, low-level DSAs with MFI between 1,000 and 2,000 are noted as potential risk factors at our center.
    - Historical DSAs only present on previous screens and not listed at UNOS.
    - Allelic antibodies that could not be listed at UNOS; for example, anti-HLA-DQB1*06:04 detected in a patient typed as HLA-DQB1*06.
    - Additional antibodies not listed at UNOS as part of a customized strategy to increase donor availability for certain highly sensitized patients.
- For **patients with potential living kidney donors**, virtual crossmatch is routinely performed at our center by comparing the current and historical antibody profiles to the donor typing to determine the presence of DSAs before the decision to perform physical crossmatches.
- For patients who received organ transplantations previously, **repeat mismatched antigens** refer to mismatched donor antigens present in both current and previous donors; the presence of repeat mismatched antigens is not a contraindication for accepting the current donor unless the patient made DSAs against these antigens previously.
- Examples of several different scenarios of virtual crossmatch are provided in **Table 3-4**.
- An increasing number of kidney transplantations are performed based on virtual crossmatch results alone before a physical crossmatch can be completed prospectively.

TABLE 3-4 Examples of Virtual Crossmatch

	Donor Data	Candidate Data	Virtual Crossmatch
Example 1			
HLA typing	A2, A3; B7, B45; Cw4, Cw16; DR1, DR11; DQ5, DQ6	A24, A30; B45, B53; Cw4, Cw6; DR11, DR13; DQ6, DQ6	A/B/DR mismatch: 2/1/1
UA listed	–	None	No DSA
UA not listed	–	None	No DSA
Repeat mismatch	–	None	No repeat mismatch
Example 2			
HLA typing	A2, A29; B44, B57; Cw6, Cw16; DR7, DR7; DQ2, DQ9	A1, A29; B62, B44; Cw7, Cw7; DR7, DR7; DQ2, DQ9	A/B/DR mismatch: 1/1/0
UA listed	–	DQ6, DQ7, DR4, DR8, DR13, DR14, DR15, DR16, DR17, DR18, DR103, DR51, DR52	No DSA in the current screen
UA not listed	–	B57 (historical MFI: 3,150, current MFI: 1,040)	Historical DSA of moderate risk
Repeat mismatch	–	Previous transplant mismatched for A2	Repeat mismatch: A2
Example 3			
HLA typing	A24, A24; B35, B39; Cw4, Cw7; DR103, DR13; DQ5, DQ6 (DQB1*06:03)	A1, A24; B8, B44; Cw5, Cw7; DR14, DR15; DQ5, DQ6 (DQB1*06:02)	A/B/DR mismatch: 0/2/2
UA listed	–	A2, A3, A11, A23, A25, A26, A29, A30, A31, A32, A33, A34, A36, A43, A66, A68, A69, A74, A80, B27, B54, B55, B57, B58, B63, B65, B67, B73, Cw1, DQ2, DQ4, DQ7, DQ8, DQ9	See allelic DSA below

TABLE 3-4 Examples of Virtual Crossmatch (Continued)

	Donor Data	Candidate Data	Virtual Crossmatch
UA not listed	–	Allelic DQB1*06:03 (MFI: 24,397; cannot be listed because patient was typed as DQ6)	Allelic DSA of increased risk in current and previous screens
Repeat mismatch	–	None	No repeat mismatch

DSA, donor-specific antibody; HLA, human leukocyte antigen; UA, unacceptable antigen.

- Such practice, if based on a rigorous virtual crossmatch workflow, can safely reduce the cold ischemia time.
- Per regulatory requirements, **eligibility criteria** must be established by transplant centers to identify candidates suitable for bypassing the physical crossmatch while mitigating the risk associated with erroneous virtual crossmatch results.

Result Interpretation

- **The absence of DSA** in the most recent and historical screens predicts a negative physical crossmatch and minimal risk of hyperacute or acute AMR.
- **Positive virtual crossmatch**
  - The presence of DSA in the most recent screen, depending on the antibody strength, may predict a positive physical crossmatch and increased risk of AMR.
  - The presence of historical DSA in previous screens is not a contraindication to transplantation but may carry a risk of memory response upon re-exposure to the corresponding antigen.
  - The risk of a positive virtual crossmatch should be balanced with a candidate's cPRA level, wait time, and resources available to manage such a risk.
  - High-risk cases should receive adequate immune suppression posttransplantation and be monitored closely for DSA trending.
- Whenever possible, virtual crossmatch results should be interpreted together with the sensitization history and physical crossmatch results.

Limitations

- Despite the benefits of virtual crossmatch, its accuracy may be affected due to the limitations of donor typing, patient antibody testing, and data integration.
- **A FP virtual crossmatch** may deny a compatible donor for the affected patient and can be caused by erroneous donor or patient testing results as follows:
  - Incorrect donor typing containing FP antigens.
  - Failure of a lower-resolution donor typing to exclude certain alleles, in the presence of allelic antibodies detected in the patient.
  - FP antibodies detected by "hot" beads on the SAB panel.
  - FP antibodies in patients whose sera contain intravenous immune globulin (IVIG), ATG, or other interfering substances.
  - FP antibodies from a misidentified or contaminated serum sample.

- **A false-negative virtual crossmatch** carries a risk of unexpected positive physical crossmatch and AMR if transplanted; possible causes include the following:
  - False-negative donor typing with allele dropout.
  - False-negative anti-HLA antibody screen due to complement interference or high background signals on NC beads.
  - Underestimation of certain antibodies against public epitopes on the SAB assay.
  - Outdated antibody screen followed by new sensitization events during the interval.
  - Undetected or undocumented historical anti-HLA antibodies in the remote past.
- The limitations of virtual crossmatch highlight the need for integrative interpretation of clinical and laboratory data; **physical crossmatch, performed either prospectively or retrospectively, continues to play a role in verifying the serologic compatibility of donor-recipient pairs**.

CDC CROSSMATCH

Rationales

- CDC crossmatch determines whether a serum specimen contains antibodies that cause CDC to donor lymphocytes.
- Many studies have established **preformed cytotoxic antibodies against the donor as a contraindication for transplantation**[21]; one frequently referenced study by Patel and Terasaki in 1969 demonstrated that 80% of transplantations with positive CDC crossmatch (24 of 30) had immediate graft failure, while 14.8% of transplantations with negative CDC crossmatch (4 of 27) failed immediately.[22]
- CDC crossmatch has been replaced by FCXM in most histocompatibility laboratories including our center (see Limitations of CDC crossmatch below).

Workflow

- See **Figure 3-2, middle panel**.
- CDC crossmatch is a laboratory-developed test with many modifications to reagents and protocols at individual laboratories; the workflow historically performed at our center is briefly described here.
- Donor T and B lymphocytes are enriched from peripheral blood by a gradient centrifugation-based method or released from lymph nodes or spleens by needle flushing.
- A fluorescence labeling technique was used to distinguish B cells, which develop distinct "fluorescent caps" with fluorescein isothiocyanate (FITC)-conjugated anti-immunoglobulin (or B-cell receptor; BCR), from unlabeled T cells.
- Donor lymphocytes are dispensed to Terasaki microtiter trays to be incubated with preloaded positive/negative controls and patient sera; both neat and serial diluted patient's serum, with and without DTT treatment for IgM removal, are included on the tray.
- Following the initial incubation, two protocols are performed in parallel.
  - In the default **"four-wash" protocol**, cells are washed in Hank's balanced salt solution four times to remove unbound antibodies before adding exogenous complement from the rabbit; an enhanced sensitivity has been reported with this practice due to the removal of unbound nonspecific antibodies.
  - In the **antihuman globulin protocol**, antihuman κ light chain is added to washed cells, followed by rabbit complement; this practice further enhances the sensitivity of the assay.

  - After the incubation with complement, ethidium bromide is added to stain nonviable cells red.
- The percentage of cell death is assessed under a fluorescent inverted microscope and scored:
  - Scores of 1, 2, 4, 6, and 8 correspond to 0% to 10%, 11% to 25%, 26% to 50%, 51% to 75%, and 76% to 100% cell death.
  - A score of 1 is considered negative; 2 and 4 are considered doubtful or weak positive depending on the cell viability; 6 and 8 are considered positive.

Result Interpretation

- Quality controls
  - The lymphocyte purity and viability must be satisfactory to ensure reliable scoring.
  - Positive and negative control wells and other reagent control wells must generate expected results for the test to be valid.
  - All conditions are tested in triplicate wells, the scores of which must be within 1 different level (e.g., 1-2, 2-4, 4-6, or 6-8) to ensure reproducibility.
- **T- and B-cell crossmatch results and DSA to class I or II HLA**
  - Negative T- and B-cell crossmatch results indicate the absence of any DSA.
  - Negative T-cell crossmatch and positive B-cell crossmatch results indicate the presence of class II DSA.
  - Positive T- and B-cell crossmatch results indicate the presence of class I DSA, with or without class II DSA.
  - Positive T-cell crossmatch and negative B-cell crossmatch results may indicate the presence of non-HLA antibodies of questionable significance.
- Clinically significant antibodies are frequently positive at neat and multiple titers tested.
  - Exceptions may occur in serum with strong DSA, where the prozone effect may cause negative results at neat but positive results with dilutions.
  - When titering samples with strong DSA, neat and serial diluted sera are crossmatched, and the endpoint titer is reported for the last dilution that remains positive.
- Positive reactions that become negative with DTT treatment indicate the presence of IgM antibodies, which are generally not considered a contraindication to transplantation; the sensitization history is important in these cases to rule out newly developed DSA.

Limitations

- Despite the enhanced sensitivity with multiple washes and the antihuman globulin protocol, CDC crossmatch may miss weaker but clinically significant DSA detected by FCXM or SAB assays.
- The assay also lacks specificity and may detect non-HLA antibodies (e.g., autoantibodies of unknown specificity) or therapeutic antibodies (e.g., ATG, rituximab, Campath, etc.).
- **The CDC scores represent the operator's visual estimation, which can be subjective and may vary among different operators**; in external proficiency testing programs, CDC crossmatch results from different laboratories frequently failed to achieve consensus, while the FCXM results do.
- The procedure requires high-quality reagents and extensive reagent quality control to determine the optimal titers at which these reagents should be used.

- Although CDC crossmatch is widely considered the most physiological assay for assessing donor-recipient serologic compatibility, the procedure is laborious, technically demanding, and unsustainable with the staffing levels in many histocompatibility laboratories

FLOW CYTOMETRIC CROSSMATCH

Rationales

- Contemporary multicolor FCXM procedures enable rapid measurement of antibodies in the patient serum that can bind to donor T and B lymphocytes; FCXM has become the preferred crossmatch approach in most histocompatibility laboratories.
- The sensitivity of FCXM may approach that of SPIs, depending on the cutoff values, and FCXM can also detect clinically significant antibodies missed by CDC crossmatch.

Workflow

- See **Figure 3-2, right panel**.
- FCXM is a laboratory-developed test with many modifications to reagents and protocols at individual laboratories; our center uses a modified workflow based on the "Halifaster protocol" described by Liwski et al. in 2018.[23]
- Donor T and B lymphocytes are enriched from peripheral blood by negative selection using a magnetic bead-based method to remove all blood cells other than lymphocytes; alternatively, lymphocytes are released from lymph nodes (preferred) or spleens by needle flushing.
- Lymphocytes are **treated with pronase to reduce FP binding** and DNase to remove free DNA and dead cells.
- Donor lymphocytes are incubated with the following sera in a routine crossmatch run:
  - The pooled-negative serum (with no anti-HLA antibody to measure the background binding signal).
  - Two NC sera (expected to be negative in a valid run).
  - EDTA-pretreated patient sera to be tested in the run.
  - The pooled-positive serum (expected to be positive in a valid run).
- Lymphocytes are washed and then stained with a cocktail containing the following antibodies:
  - FITC-conjugated antihuman IgG to detect patients' IgG bound to donor lymphocytes.
  - PE-conjugated anti-CD19 to label B cells.
  - PE/Cy7-conjugated anti-CD3 to label T cells.
- Washed lymphocytes are stained with the viability dye, 7-AAD, to label nonviable cells, followed by data acquisition on a flow cytometer.
- Data analysis
  - Viable cells in the lymphocyte gate are separated into $CD3^+$ T cells and $CD19^+$ B-cell populations.
  - Median channel numbers (MCNs) of both cell populations in the FITC channel (antihuman IgG) are recorded for all samples.
  - Median channel shifts (MCS) are calculated for the NC sera, patient sera, and the pooled-positive serum, relative to the MCN of pooled-negative serum.

Result Interpretation

- The cutoff values for FCXM are determined statistically based on at least 50 crossmatches that are expected to be negative:
  - Sera confirmed to have no anti-HLA antibodies by the SAB assay are crossmatched against surrogate donor lymphocytes isolated from a variety of samples from deceased and living donors, including both peripheral blood and lymph nodes.
  - The MCS are calculated for T- and B-cell crossmatches relative to the pooled-negative serum.
  - The cutoff values for positive T and B cell crossmatches are defined as the mean MCS + the standard deviation of the MCS multiplied by 3.
  - The positive T- and B-cell cutoff values enable the detection of most class I and II DSA with MFI of 3,000 or higher.
- **Quality controls**
  - The lymphocyte purity and viability must be documented; poor purity or viability may be associated with spurious results.
  - At least one of the NC sera must be negative, and the pooled positive control serum must be positive, for the crossmatch run to be valid.
- **T- and B-cell crossmatch results and DSA to class I and II HLA**
  - Negative T- and B-cell crossmatch results indicate the absence of any DSA.
  - Negative T-cell crossmatch and positive B-cell crossmatch results indicate the presence of class II DSA.
  - Positive T- and B-cell crossmatch results indicate the presence of class I DSA, with or without class II DSA.
  - Positive T-cell crossmatch and negative B-cell crossmatch results have been observed for weak class I DSA at our center and described in the literature.

Limitations

- FCXM may have limited sensitivity and produce negative results in the presence of DSA detected on the SAB assay (i.e., positive virtual crossmatch):
  - The DSA should be considered clinically significant if there is a clear sensitization history and a cross-reactive pattern consistent with a known epitope.
  - On the other hand, the DSA detected by the SAB assay may lack significance if there is no sensitization history or a supportive cross-reactive pattern, or if the DSA cannot be detected on an alternative SPI such as the PRA assay.
- **Unexpected positive FCXM results** in the absence of DSA should be investigated promptly:
  - FP FCXM results in the absence DSA are infrequent with pronase-treated lymphocytes, affecting only about 2% of all FCXM at our center.
  - Factors causing false-negative virtual crossmatch, as outlined previously, should also be considered.
  - Non-HLA antibodies in the patient's serum, either autoantibodies or alloantibodies, can bind to donor lymphocytes, and it is important to differentiate these two types of antibodies by performing an autologous crossmatch.
  - Interfering substances such as immune complexes or therapeutic antibodies such as rituximab, Campath, ATG, IVIG, etc., can cause FP FCXM results.
  - Antibodies to cryptic antigens on T cells in HIV+ patients have been reported to cause FP T-cell crossmatch results with pronase-treated cells; these antibodies are not contraindications to transplantation.[24]

POST-TRANSPLANT MONITORING OF DSA

Rationales

- The presence of circulating anti-HLA DSA, in kidney recipients with graft dysfunction and characteristic histologic findings, **supports the diagnosis of AMR**; non-HLA allo- or autoantibodies have also been described in AMR cases.
- DSA detected in recipients with normal graft function is not diagnostic of AMR but **portends an increased probability of graft loss** in 5 years.
- Two types of DSA have distinct times of onset.
  - **Pre-existing or preformed DSA** is already detectable by SAB assays or physical crossmatches before transplantation; undetected preformed DSA may manifest as a memory response in some cases with a rapid increase in DSA levels within 2 to 3 weeks posttransplantation.
  - **De novo DSA** develops in the posttransplantation setting due to alloimmunization to donor antigens for the first time and may precede the onset of graft dysfunction; increased HLA epitope mismatch load, especially for HLA-DR and DQ antigens, and noncompliance to immune suppression are risk factors for developing de novo DSA.[25]

Workflow

- Timing of DSA testing
  - Our center tests a recipient's serum collected right before transplantation to document the "**time-zero**" DSA information.
  - **Close monitoring of DSA** (e.g., weekly) in the first few weeks after transplantation was reserved for patients with risk factors such as historical DSA and positive virtual or flow crossmatch results.
  - Low-risk patients are tested for DSA after transplantation **by indication**, typically when AMR is suspected in the presence of graft dysfunction.
  - **Per protocol** DSA testing at prespecified time points (e.g., at 1 week, 1 month, 3 months, 6 months, and 12 months, and then annually) has been implemented in some centers to capture the development of de novo DSA; per protocol DSA testing may coincide with cell-free donor-specific DNA testing and biopsy to provide comprehensive monitoring of graft injury.
- Recipients' serum specimens are pretreated with EDTA and tested by the SAB assay; the antibody profile is compared with the donor typing to determine and report donor-specific reactivity.

Result Interpretation

- Some centers only report qualitative DSA results, "**positive**" or "**negative**," based on center-defined cutoff values and, if positive, the DSA **specificity**.
- Many centers, including our center, report **MFI values of DSA** that can be risk stratified based on center-defined cutoff values; because of the good correlation between titers and MFI values up to 10,000 MFI, the quantitative DSA results may provide additional information within this lower MFI range and allow comparison of longitudinal data.
- Laboratories may encounter **uncertainties in DSA interpretation** due to **various resolutions of donor HLA typing** available at the time of DSA interpretation and **the limited number of antigens included in the SAB assay:**
  - LR deceased donor typing is performed by OPO laboratories and used for DSA interpretation at "time-zero."

- HR typing is performed for all deceased and living donors at our center and used for subsequent DSA interpretations when the HR typing result becomes available.
- The SAB panel includes a limited number of antigens encoded by specific alleles that are relatively prevalent in the population; donors may carry antigens encoded by alleles not represented on the SAB panel.

- In some cases, our center reports **inferred or possible DSA** with a description of the uncertainties encountered (see below).
- With an LR donor typing (e.g., HLA-A*02) and multiple beads on the SAB panel carrying antigens in the same antigen group as the donor (e.g., HLA-A*02:01, 02:03, and 02:06).
  - **The averaged MFI values** from beads within the same antigen group are reported if the reactivity is comparable across these beads.
  - If the reactivity is heterogeneous across different beads and indicates the presence of an allelic antibody, we report **the MFI value from the bead matching the inferred HR donor allele**; if positive, the reactivity is reported as a possible DSA and should be correlated with biopsy and clinical data.
  - For example, if only the HLA-A*02:03 bead is positive with an MFI value of 5,130 while the HLA-A*02:01 and A*02:06 beads are well below 1,000 MFI, the donor LR typing will be further analyzed based on additional laboratory data or population genetics to determine the most likely HR typing; if the inferred HR typing is HLA-A*02:03, a possible DSA with 5,130 MFI will be reported.
- With an HR donor typing
  - The MFI values from beads matching each donor alleles are reported by default, without averaging among beads within the same antigen group.
  - If the donor has one or more alleles not represented on the SAB panel, we use bioinformatic tools such as HistoCheck (www.histocheck.org)[26] to **identify the closest bead in the SAB panel and report the MFI value from this bead**; if positive, the reactivity is reported a possible DSA and should be correlated with biopsy and clinical data.
  - For example, a donor allele encoding HLA-A*02:04 is not represented on the SAB panel; the HLA-A*02:01 bead closely resembles the donor antigen with only one amino acid residue difference, while HLA-A*02:03 and A*02:06 are different at four and two residues respectively; the MFI value from the HLA-A*02:01 bead is reported with a comment describing the context.
  - When the closest bead on the SAB panel is substantially different from the donor allele with multiple amino acid residue differences (e.g., ≥5 residues), additional epitope analysis may help mitigate the risk of FP or false-negative DSA assignment.
- For DSA against HLA-DQ and DP antigens, the reactivity against the α chain, β chain, or α-β chain heterodimer should be differentiated (see the SAB assay section above) and matched with the donor typing as appropriate.

Limitations

- Limitations of the SAB assays, as outlined previously, may lead to FP or false-negative DSA results.
- Limited donor typing resolution and SAB panel representation necessitate the reporting of possible DSA in uncertain cases, as discussed above.
- Due to these limitations, DSA results should be used in conjunction with other laboratory and clinical data; DSA results inconsistent with the pretest probability of AMR should trigger additional investigations.
- Intra- and interlaboratory variations of MFI values should be considered when interpreting the longitudinal change in DSA levels.

INTEGRATION OF HISTOCOMPATIBILITY ASSESSMENT

- The current paradigm of histocompatibility assessment emphasizes the integration of multiple tools to evaluate the immunologic risk of donor-recipient pairs at serologic and genetic levels (**Figure 3-4**).
  - These evaluations span the pre-, peri-, and posttransplantation periods and provide actionable results and prognostic information.
  - Since none of these tests is perfect, some redundancy (e.g., multiple crossmatch methods; see below) is beneficial in this system to confirm significant findings or trigger further work-up.
  - It is crucial to detail the specifics related to these laboratory evaluations in the agreement between the kidney transplantation program and histocompatibility laboratory as required by the OPTN Bylaws.
  - There are many variables in the testing framework (**Figure 3-4**) that may differ among transplant centers: assays of choice, cutoff values, frequency of testing, approach to data analysis and reporting, etc.; each center should carefully validate their assays as part of their testing framework to deliver a coherent histocompatibility risk assessment.
- Antibody screen and identification by SPIs are central to the immunologic risk assessment; multiple assays of different configurations and characteristics, such as SAB and PRA assays, can be used together and in conjunction with patients' sensitization history to determine their UAs.
- Patients' antibody testing results should be interpreted together with their sensitization history and HLA typing to ascertain the allogeneic nature of the anti-HLA reactivities detected; for example, an anti-Bw4 alloreactivity should not be detected in a patient typed as Bw4 positive.
- The integration of patients' antibody testing results by SPIs and the donor HLA typing defines the virtual crossmatch and DSA interpretation.
- Multiple physical crossmatch procedures can be performed to complement the SPI in the detection and characterization of DSA.
  - **The relative sensitivity of these assays**: SPI > FCXM > CDC crossmatch.
  - **The relative specificity in terms of detecting anti-HLA antibodies:** SPI > FCXM = CDC crossmatch; the latter two can detect non-HLA antibodies, most of which are not clinically significant.
  - **The relative physiological relevance**: SPI (artificial assays on the Luminex platform) < FCXM (assessing the binding of DSA to antigens of their native conformation and density on the lymphocyte surface) < CDC (assessing the CDC of the DSA on donor lymphocytes).
- **Quantification of HLA molecular mismatch** integrates our current understanding of genetic disparity and immunogenicity of functional epitopes; increased loads of epitope mismatch in DR and DQ molecules have been associated with worse de novo alloimmunization and graft outcomes, and such knowledge is being applied to prospective clinical trials to enable customized immunosuppression in risk-stratified patient populations.[17]
- **Table 3-5** summarizes different levels of immunologic risk indicated by various combinations of laboratory results and clinical data; whether to void a certain risk or to take and manage such a risk should be balanced with the urgency of and barrier to transplantation in individual patients.

TABLE 3-5 An Integrated Approach to Histocompatibility Risk Assessment

CDCXM	FCXM	VXM (SAB Assay)	Sensitization History	Increased HLA MM	HLA Identical	Histocompatibility Risk Assessment
Major risk categories adapted from the STAR 2017 Working Group Meeting Report						
+	+	+	+			Active memory; at risk for hyperacute rejection
−	+	+	+			Active memory; at risk for AMR and TCR
−	−	+	+			Active memory; at risk for AMR and TCR
−	−	−	+			Latent memory against repeat-mismatched antigen; at risk for recall T- and B-cell responses
−	−	−	−	+		At risk for de novo alloimmune response compared to low HLA molecular MM load
−	−	−	−	−	+	Low risk for de novo alloimmune response
Additional Patterns of Histocompatibility Testing Results						
+	−	−	−			Non-HLA autoantibody or interfering antibodies; clinical history and further evaluation by autologous crossmatch
−	+	−	−			
+	+	−	−			
+	−	−	+			Non-HLA autoantibody or alloantibody or interfering antibodies; clinical history and further evaluation by autologous crossmatch
−	+	−	+			
+	+	−	+			
−	−	+	−			Possible spurious SAB result; low risk for rejection

AMR, antibody-mediated rejection; CDCXM, complement-dependent cytotoxicity crossmatch; FCXM, flow cytometric crossmatch; HLA, human leukocyte antigen; MM, molecular mismatch; SAB, single-antigen bead; STAR, Assessment of risk; TCR, T-cell mediated rejection; VXM, virtual crossmatch.

EMERGING THEMES IN HISTOCOMPATIBILITY TESTING

- There is an increasing interest in non-HLA antibody testing for kidney transplantation.
  - Research or commercial assays have been developed to test antibodies to AT1R (angiotensin type 1 receptor), MICA (MHC class I-related chain A), perlecan, collagen IV, and fibronectin, among other non-HLA antigens.[27]
  - These antibodies in pre- and posttransplant settings have been associated with worsened graft outcomes in some studies, and conflicting results were reported in others; anti-HLA DSA may synergize with these antibodies in causing graft dysfunction but also confound the independent effect of non-HLA antibodies.
  - Non-HLA immunoassays are not readily available in many clinical laboratories, including our center, and the results from send-out laboratories may not be able to meet the turnaround time for clinical decision-making.
- Building on the existing knowledge on HLA molecular mismatch, it is imperative for future investigations to clarify **the impact of epitope mismatch and epitope-specific antibodies on graft outcomes** and **how such data may inform risk-stratified immunosuppression**. Some prominent challenges ahead include the following:
  - Determine how the quantity of epitope mismatch and the immunogenicity of individual epitopes interact and affect graft outcomes.
  - Refine current bioinformatic tools for B-cell (e.g., HLAMatchmaker) and T-cell (e.g., PIRCHE) epitope prediction and quantification; collect additional experimental and clinical data for the validation of these epitopes.
  - Standardize and automate the process of epitope analysis to gain insight from large and longitudinal datasets of patient antibody screens.
- The capability of detecting donor-specific T- and B-cell memories due to past sensitizing events will complement existing histocompatibility testing and further reduce the risk of graft rejection; sensitive, specific, and rapid assays are needed to detect antigen-specific T and B cells, ideally in patients' peripheral blood.

REFERENCES

1. Robinson J, Barker DJ, Georgiou X, Cooper MA, Flicek P, Marsh SGE. IPD-IMGT/HLA database. *Nucleic Acids Res.* 2020;48(D1):D948-D955.
2. Marsh SGE, Albert ED, Bodmer WF, et al. Nomenclature for factors of the HLA system, 2010. *Tissue Antigens.* 2010;75(4):291-455.
3. OPTN. *Organ Procurement and Transplantation Network (OPTN) Policies.* 2023.
4. Liu C. A long road/read to rapid high-resolution HLA typing: the nanopore perspective. *Hum Immunol.* 2021;82(7):488-95.
5. Shi X, Lv J, Han W, et al. What is the impact of human leukocyte antigen mismatching on graft survival and mortality in renal transplantation? A meta-analysis of 23 cohort studies involving 486,608 recipients. *BMC Nephrol.* 2018;19(1):116.
6. Shi X, Liu R, Xie X, et al. Effect of human leukocyte antigen mismatching on the outcomes of pediatric kidney transplantation: a systematic review and meta-analysis. *Nephrol Dial Transplant.* 2017;32(11):1939-48.
7. Zachary AA, Leffell MS. HLA mismatching strategies for solid organ transplantation: a balancing act. *Front Immunol.* 2016;7:575.
8. Gebel HM, Norin AJ, Bray RA. From antigens to eplets: the evolution of HLA. *Hum Immunol.* 2022;83(3):197-98.
9. Duquesnoy RJ. Reflections on HLA epitope-based matching for transplantation. *Front Immunol.* 2016;7:469.

10. Vassallo RR, Fung M, Rebulla P, et al. Utility of cross-matched platelet transfusions in patients with hypoproliferative thrombocytopenia: a systematic review. *Transfusion.* 2014;54(4):1180-91.
11. Tambur AR, Campbell P, Claas FH, et al. Sensitization in transplantation: assessment of risk (STAR) 2017 working group meeting report. *Am J Transplant.* 2018;18(7):1604-14.
12. Liu C, Pang S, Phelan D, Brennan DC, Mohanakumar T. Quantitative evaluation of the impact of ethylenediaminetetraacetic acid pretreatment on single-antigen bead assay. *Transplant Direct.* 2017;3(8):e194.
13. Gebel HM, Bray RA. HLA antibody detection with solid phase assays: great expectations or expectations too great? *Am J Transplant.* 2014;14(9):1964-75.
14. Claisse G, Devriese M, Lion J, et al. Relevance of Anti-HLA Antibody Strength Underestimation in Single Antigen Bead Assay for Shared Eplets. *Transplantation.* 2022;106:2456-61.
15. Wehmeier C, Hönger G, Schaub S. Caveats of HLA antibody detection by solid-phase assays. *Transpl Int.* 2020;33(1):18-29.
16. Ravindranath MH, Terasaki PI, Pham T, Jucaud V, Kawakita S. Therapeutic preparations of IVIg contain naturally occurring anti-HLA-E antibodies that react with HLA-Ia (HLA-A/-B/-Cw) alleles. *Blood.* 2013;121(11):2013-28.
17. Wiebe C, Nickerson PW. More precise donor-recipient matching: the role of eplet matching. *Curr Opin Nephrol Hypertens.* 2020;29(6):630-35.
18. Reed EF, Rao P, Zhang Z, et al. Comprehensive assessment and standardization of solid phase multiplex-bead arrays for the detection of antibodies to HLA. *Am J Transplant.* 2013;13(7):1859-70.
19. Tambur AR, Campbell P, Chong AS, et al. Sensitization in transplantation: assessment of risk (STAR) 2019 Working Group Meeting Report. *Am J Transplant.* 2020;20(10):2652-68.
20. Tambur AR, Wiebe C. HLA diagnostics: evaluating DSA strength by titration. *Transplantation.* 2018;102(suppl 1):S23-S30.
21. Peña JR, Fitzpatrick D, Saidman SL. Complement-dependent cytotoxicity crossmatch. *Methods Mol Biol.* 2013;1034:257-83.
22. Patel R, Terasaki PI. Significance of the positive crossmatch test in kidney transplantation. *N Engl J Med.* 1969;280(14):735-9.
23. Liwski RS, Greenshields AL, Conrad DM, et al. Rapid optimized flow cytometric crossmatch (FCXM) assays: the Halifax and Halifaster protocols. *Hum Immunol.* 2018;79(1):28-38.
24. Szewczyk K, Barrios K, Magas D, et al. Flow cytometry crossmatch reactivity with pronase-treated T cells induced by non-HLA autoantibodies in human immunodeficiency virus-infected patients. *Hum Immunol.* 2016;77(6):449-55.
25. Wiebe C, Gibson IW, Blydt-Hansen TD, et al. Rates and determinants of progression to graft failure in kidney allograft recipients with de novo donor-specific antibody. *Am J Transplant.* 2015;15(11):2921-30.
26. *HistoCheck-a HLA Sequence Interpreter.* Accessed March 3, 2023, https://www.histocheck.org/histocheck/
27. Zhang Q, Reed EF. The importance of non-HLA antibodies in transplantation. *Nat Rev Nephrol.* 2016;12(8):484-95.

4 Evaluation of Kidney Transplant Candidates

Karen Flores, Helen Wijeweera, and Tarek Alhamad

GENERAL PRINCIPLES

- The pretransplant evaluation process is paramount for optimal patient and transplant surgical outcomes.
- It is defined as a collaborative process by the clinical team through a comprehensive evaluation of the patients' medical history, risk factors (tobacco use), comorbid conditions (i.e., cardiac disease, diabetes), current health status, adherence, and psychosocial assessment. See **Table 4-1**.
- At the end of the evaluation, recommendations are made regarding the candidacy for kidney transplantation.
- All patients regardless of socioeconomic status, sex, gender identity, or race/ethnicity should be considered for transplant.[1]
- The clinical team encompasses the utilization of a multidisciplinary committee.

OVERVIEW OF EVALUATION

- Kidney transplantation has been shown to improve patient survival and quality of life. It is more cost effective compared to remaining on dialysis.[2]
- Early referral to kidney transplantation is important for better patient outcomes.
- Patients can be referred when they reach stage 4 chronic kidney disease (CKD) or have a glomerular filtration less than 30 mL/min
- Patients are eligible for transplant when glomerular filtration <20 mL/min
- American Society of Transplantation and Kidney Disease Improving Global Outcomes have published guidelines for referral and management of patients for kidney transplantation.[1]
- Not all patients are suitable for transplant. In the evaluation process, the potential risks of transplantation are weighed against the relative to the risks of not receiving a transplant.

Medical History

- The pretransplant evaluation includes an assessment of the patient's medical history, motivation, risk for nonadherence, and perioperative risk.
- It is important to discuss types of donors, waiting times, and outcomes.
- The initial evaluation should include a detailed past medical history.[3] **Table 4-2** has a summary of the major illnesses that need to be examined.

Laboratories and Imaging Studies

- **Tables 4-3** and **4-4** summarize the required laboratory and imaging studies.
- We do access frailty in elderly candidates who are over 65 years of age or in patients with limited functional status.
- Based on Washington University (WU) guidelines, patients who walk less than 1,000 ft in 6 minutes are considered marginal for kidney transplantation.[4]

TABLE 4-1	Multidisciplinary Committee for Evaluation of the Kidney Transplant Candidate
Transplant surgeons	
Transplant nephrologists	
Financial coordinators	
Health care professionals experienced in assessment of psycho-social aspects of transplant (transplant psychologist, social worker)	

TABLE 4-2	Evaluation of a Kidney Transplant Recipient
Risk of kidney disease recurrence	
Cardiac disease	
Vascular disease	
Infection	
Cancer	
Liver Disease	
Gastrointestinal Disease	
Obesity	
Diabetes Mellitus	
Coagulopathy	
Surgical history	
Psychiatric History	
Medical Compliance	
Psychosocial condition	

Contraindications to Transplantation

- Absolute contraindications include active untreated malignancy, active infection, and positive T-cell cytotoxic crossmatch.
- Relative contraindications include advanced cardiopulmonary disease, extensive peripheral vascular disease, and history of noncompliance. See **Table 4-5**.
- Advanced age is not a contraindication to transplant; however, comorbidities and frailty need to be evaluated carefully.[2]
- Despite the high risk of recurrence of certain glomerulonephritis, these should not exclude candidates from evaluation and kidney transplantation.
- Delaying pretransplant evaluation can be considered for the following:
  - Psychiatric instability
  - Substance abuse
  - Ongoing health-threatening noncompliance
  - Recent cerebral vascular accident
    - Functional status needs to be evaluated after a stroke
    - Based on the etiology, evaluation for recurrent stroke is needed

TABLE 4-3 Initial Workup of a Kidney Transplant Candidate

History and Physical Examination
Laboratory Evaluation
Complete blood count
Chemistry panel
Coagulation studies
Serologic testing: HIV, CMV, VZV, HSV, EBV, Hepatitis B and C, RPR
Blood group and cross-matching
Immunologic testing: human leukocyte antigens and panel reactive antibodies
Urinalysis
Diagnostic Imaging
ECG
Cardiac echo/stress test
Chest radiography
Renal ultrasound
Evaluation of abdominal vasculature (CT)
Panorex or dental evaluation
Frailty Assessment
6-min walk

CMV, cytomegalovirus; CT, computed tomography; EBV, Epstein-Barr virus; ECG, electrocardiogram; HIV, human immunodeficiency virus; HSV, herpes simplex virus; RPR, rapid plasma regain; VZV; varicella zoster virus.

TABLE 4-4 Age-Appropriate Cancer Screening

Colonoscopy	≥45 y of age
Pap Smear	Onset of sexual intercourse or 21-65 y of age
Mammogram	Women ≥ 40 y of age or with family history of breast cancer
Prostate-specific antigen (PSA)	Men ≥ 55 y of age, high risk ≥45 y of age
Low-dose chest computed tomography (CT)	20 pack-year smoking history with age ≥ 50

- Recent coronary artery stent placement: Patients are placed on hold for 3 to 6 months.
- Active symptomatic cardiac disease, peptic ulcer disease, diverticulitis, acute pancreatitis, gallstone or gallbladder disease, inflammatory bowel disease, or infections.
- Severe hyperparathyroidism until medically or surgically treated.

TABLE 4-5 Contraindications for Kidney Transplantation

Absolute	Relative
Active, untreated, or metastatic malignancy	Advanced cardiopulmonary disease
Acute untreated infections	Extensive peripheral vascular disease
Active substance abuse	Cirrhosis with portal hypertension
Positive T-cell cytotoxic crossmatch	Clinically active immunological disease leading to renal failure
Reversible renal disease	Severe cardiovascular disease
Uncontrolled psychiatric disorder affecting compliance	Morbid obesity with BMI > 40
Noncompliance	Severe malnutrition
	Estimated lifespan < 5 y

BMI, body mass index.

- **Malignancy**
  - Active malignancy is a contraindication to kidney transplantation.
  - A cancer-free period varies according to the type and stage of cancer, lymph node involvement, and the presence of metastases.[2,5,6] For overall guidance, see **Table 4-6**.
  - Metastatic cancer and/or lymph node involvement require careful evaluation of the risk of recurrence.
  - Kidney transplant patients should be advised about the higher risk for certain malignancy posttransplantation (please see Chapter 17 for more details).

Living Donation Education

- The pretransplant evaluation is an opportunity to discuss and answer questions about the living donation process.
- The benefits of a living donation include a longer life expectancy of the allograft, decreased waiting time, and the ability to schedule the surgery.
- If a potential living donor is available but is found to be incompatible due to differences in blood types (ABO) or histocompatibility, there are other options available including the following: ABO-incompatible transplantation, desensitization protocols, and paired exchange programs.[7]

Dual Organ Transplant Consideration

Patients with end-stage kidney disease and a concomitant failure of other organs may be candidates for combined organ transplantation. The following are some conditions that would benefit from combined organ transplantation:

- Type I diabetics: consider a combined kidney and pancreas transplantation.
- Severe cardiomyopathy: consider combined heart and kidney transplantation.
- Primary hyperoxaluria type I or cirrhosis: consider combined liver and kidney transplantation.
- Cystic fibrosis or severe lung disease: consider combined lung and kidney transplantation.

TABLE 4-6 Cancer-Free Waiting Periods Before Transplantation

Malignancy	Waiting Period
Bladder	
Superficial lesions—NMIBC low and intermediate risk	<2 y
Localized lesions—high risk, MIBC postradical cystectomy	2 y
All other lesions (MIBC, postchemoradiation)	5 y
Breast	
Ductal carcinoma in situ/stage I	None
Low-grade, small lesions, stage II	<2 y
Stage III	3-5 y
Stage IV	NAC
Cervical	
Superficial	None
Localized lesions (stage I/II)	2-3 y
Stage II/III squamous/adenocarcinoma cervix	5 y
Recurrent or metastatic	NAC
Colorectal	
Stage I (T1 or T2, N0, M0)	1-2 y
Stage II (T3 or T4, N0, M0)	3-5 y
Stage III (any T, N+, M0)	3-5 y
Stage IV (any T, Any N, M+)	5 y
Lung	
Stages I, II, IIIA	3-5 y
Other stages	Not typically a candidate
Prostate	
Gleason score ≤7	None
All other lesions with negative PSA	2 y
Renal cell carcinoma	
T1a (≤4 cm)	None
T1b (4 ≤ 7 cm) with Fuhrman grade 1-2	None
T1b (4 ≤ 7 cm) with Fuhrman grade 3-4	1-2 y
T2	2 y
T3, T4	2-5 y
Any node involvement of metastatic disease	At least 5 y (NAC in advanced cases)

(Continued)

TABLE 4-6 Cancer-Free Waiting Periods Before Transplantation (Continued)

Malignancy	Waiting Period
Skin	
Melanoma	None
In situ	2 y
Stage Ia	2-5 y
Stages Ib-II	Not a candidate
Stages III-IV	
Squamous cell–localized lesion after resection	None
Removed with clear margin	2-3 y
With perineural invasion	
Basal cell–localized lesion after resection	2 y
Uterus	
IA or IB without lymph or vascular involvement	None
Other I and II	2-3 y
Stage III	5 y
Stage IV	Not usually a candidate

MIBC, muscle-invasive bladder cancer; NAC, not a candidate; NMIBC, non–muscle-invasive bladder cancer.
Data from Al-Adra D, Hammel L, Roberts J, et al. Pretransplant solid organ malignancy and organ transplant candidacy: a consensus expert opinion statement. *Am J Transplant.* 2021;21:460-74. doi:10.1111/ajt.16318.

Recurrence of Kidney Disease

- During the pretransplant evaluation, there should be a discussion about the cause of CKD, the risk of recurrence of native kidney disease, and the subsequent risk of allograft failure (**Table 4-7**).[7]
- If the patient has prior graft failure from recurrent primary disease, the risk of graft failure is higher for a subsequent transplant.[1]
- It is important to evaluate the clinical quiescence of certain primary diseases prior to kidney transplantation.

Focal Glomerulosclerosis

- The risk of recurrence is 20% to 50%.[2]
- Focal glomerulosclerosis (FSGS) can clinically recur within hours to days after transplantation.
- Secondary FSGS (i.e., due to reflux nephropathy or obesity) does not recur.
- Plasma exchange before transplant and early posttransplant, as well as rituximab, abatacept, and belatacept, has been suggested to decrease the risk of disease recurrence.

IgA Nephropathy

- Associated with recurrence rate of around 30%.[8]
- Outcomes of recurrent IgA nephropathy are favorable compared to other glomerulonephritis.

TABLE 4-7 Risk of Recurrent Disease After Renal Transplantation

Recurrent Disease	Risk (%)
FSGS	20%-50%
IgA nephropathy	30%
MPGN	20%-48%
Membranous nephropathy	40%-50%
aHUS	50%-75%
Oxalosis	80%-100%
Systemic lupus erythematosus	3%-10%

aHUS, atypical hemolytic uremic syndrome; FSGF, focal glomerular global sclerosis; MPGN, membranoproliferative glomerulonephritis.
Data from Bunnapradist S, Abdalla B, Reddy U. Evaluation of adult kidney transplant candidates. In: Danovitch GM, ed. *Handbook of Kidney Transplantation*. 6th ed. Lippincott Williams & Wilkins; 2017:206-37.

Lupus Nephritis

- Clinically significant lupus nephritis recurrence occurs in 2% to 9% of cases.[9]
- The risk for allograft failure due to recurrent lupus nephritis is small.
- Patients with systemic lupus erythematosus (SLE) should be tested for antiphospholipid antibodies before transplantation.

Anti-Neutrophil Cytoplasmic Antibody Vasculitis

- Antineutrophil cytoplasmic antibody (ANCA) vasculitis is associated with elevated risk of recurrence.
- It is said that a positive ANCA titer is not predictive of recurrence of glomerulonephritis in the transplanted organ.

Immune Complex Membranoproliferative Glomerulonephritis

- The rate of recurrence of idiopathic membranoproliferative glomerulonephritis (MPGN) ranges from 20% to 48%.[10]
- For secondary MPGN, treatment is directed at the cause. Hence, it is important to evaluate possible infective, autoimmune, or paraprotein-mediated causes.

Atypical Hemolytic Uremic Syndrome

- The presence of a complement pathway abnormality increases recurrence risk.
- The perioperative use of eculizumab should be considered.

Amyloidosis and Plasma Cell Dyscrasias

- Stem cell transplantation, immunotherapy, and novel chemotherapeutic agents have improved the prognosis of patients with primary amyloidosis, multiple myeloma, and plasma cell dyscrasias.[7]
- It is important to ensure complete remission, reflected by a normal free light chain ratio and the absence of monoclonal proteins prior to transplantation since monoclonal gammopathy of renal significance can recur often and quickly.[11]

Antiphospholipid Antibody Syndrome

- Patients with SLE should have antiphospholipid antibody levels checked.
- This disease may lead to thrombotic events, ischemia, renal infarction, and thrombotic microangiopathy.

Membranous Nephropathy

- Autoantibodies against phospholipase A2 receptor (PLA2R) are positive in most patients with idiopathic but not secondary membranous nephropathy.
- The presence of PLA2R antibodies is a risk factor for the recurrence of membranous nephropathy.

Oxalosis/Hyperoxaluria

- Primary oxalosis is an autosomal recessive disorder caused by the deficiency of the liver enzyme alanine glyoxylate aminotransferase. This leads to increased levels of calcium oxalate in urine and nephrocalcinosis.
- Graft failure usually occurs due to rapid deposition of oxalate despite treatment modalities including dialysis and oral phosphates, which minimize oxalate deposition.
- The preferred treatment for patients with primary oxalosis is combined liver and kidney transplantation.
- Lumasiran is a promising medication that could be used with kidney transplant alone. More data are needed to support such practice.
- Secondary hyperoxaluria is commonly due to diseases of the gut including inflammatory bowel disease and surgical bypass of the intestines.

Fabry Disease

- Fabry disease is caused by a deficiency of α galactosidase enzyme leading to an accumulation of glycosphingolipid in the kidneys and other organs.
- Kidney transplantation is the preferred treatment for patients with Fabry disease who do not have severe systemic disease.[7]
- Fabrazyme is a recombinant form of a galactosidase used in the treatment of Fabry disease.

Alport Syndrome

- Alport syndrome is a condition wherein there is a genetic abnormality in type 4 collagen.
- After kidney transplantation, the presence of normal collagen may induce antiglomerular basement membrane (GBM) disease. Clinically significant anti-GBM disease is rare.
- Screening for the disease should be done for donation from a living related donor.

Cystinosis

- Cystinosis is a rare lysosomal disorder leading to end-stage renal disease (ESRD).
- Renal transplantation is safe with excellent long-term outcomes in patients with cystinosis.
- We recommend using cysteamine (long-acting) posttransplantation to reduce the complications of cystinosis and improve kidney transplant outcomes.

Extrarenal Organ Involvement

An evaluation of extrarenal organ involvement of various diseases should be done. If severe, it may preclude listing the following:

- Cystinosis
- Sarcoidosis
- Fabry disease
- Amyloidosis
- Sickle cell disease

CARDIOLOGY EVALUATION

- ESRD has multiple cardiac disease comorbidities and increased risk of coronary artery disease (CAD), impaired left ventricular function, pulmonary hypertension, and valvular heart disease.
- Cardiac disease increases the risk of death and cardiac events peri- and posttransplant.[12]
  - ECG for all patients
  - Noninvasive stress testing for kidney transplant candidates with three or more CAD risk factors regardless of functional status.[13]
  - Routine prophylactic coronary revascularization is NOT recommended in patients with stable CAD with no symptoms and no indication for revascularization.[13]
  - Echocardiogram for patients with dyspnea of unknown origin or heart failure.[1]
  - Impaired left ventricular function <30% is a strong predictor of mortality in both general population and kidney transplant candidates.[14] Our center excludes these patients.
  - CT coronary angiography +/− coronary artery calcium scoring preferred over stress imaging in most transplant candidates for assessment of CAD.[15]
  - Pulmonary systolic pressure >45 mm Hg by echocardiographic criteria should be assessed by a cardiologist
  - The history of myocardial infarction requires assessment by a cardiologist to assess if further testing is warranted
- Delayed transplantation is based on recommendations of cardiologist following placement of coronary stent.
- Patients with excellent functional capacity, >10 metabolic equivalents (METs), may forgo exercise stress test.
- Patients with poor functional capacity (<4 METs, e.g., unable to climb one flight of stairs) should undergo cardiac stress test.[12]
- WU cardiac guidelines are summarized in **Table 4-8**.

PERIPHERAL ARTERIAL DISEASE

- Screen all patients for peripheral arterial disease (PAD) through history and physical exam.
- If patient is high risk for PAD, perform noninvasive testing
- Noncontrast CT abdomen and pelvis to evaluate vasculature in patients with known or high risk for PAD or if abnormal noninvasive testing
- Evaluate aortic aneurysm if established risk factors
- Exclude any patient with nonhealing wound ulcer/infection

INFECTIONS

- Patients should undergo screening for viral, fungal, and bacterial infections (**Table 4-9**).
- Orthodontal disease screen with dental plain radiograph (or dental clearance).
- Evaluation for any open ulcers or wounds (i.e., foot exam for diabetic patients).
- HIV/AIDS—may consider eligibility for transplant if the following conditions are met[1]:
  - Maintained on effective antiviral regimen
  - Undetectable viral load (or <20 copies/mL)
  - Normal T-cell counts (≥299 cells/m^3)

TABLE 4-8 Washington University Cardiac Guidelines

Condition	Testing	Cardiology Referral
• LVEF < 35% • Severe and mod/severe valvular disease • Mod/large area of ischemia on resting echo • PASP > 60	No stress	Referral to cardiologist for need of catheterization/testing recommendations
Prior cardiac events/revascularization • Myocardial infarction • PCI • Coronary artery bypass graft	No stress	Cardiac catheterization within the last 24-36 mo
• Diabetes mellitus >10 y • Peripheral vascular disease (PAD) procedures/symptoms • Dialysis duration >10 y • > 70 y old • PASP 50-60 (after decrease in EDW) • LVEF 35%-40%	Standard workup	Routine referral to cardiology

EDW, estimated dry weight; LVEF, left ventricular ejection fraction; PASP, pulmonary artery systolic pressure; PCI, percutaneous coronary intervention.

TABLE 4-9 Pretransplant Screening for Infections

CMV, EBV, HSV, RPR
VZV, MMR—if negative, immunization ≥4 wk prior to transplant
HIV
Hepatitis B and hepatitis C
Tuberculosis screening; serum QuantiFERON
Diseases endemic (malaria, Chagas, strongyloidiasis, coccidioidomycosis)

ECG, electric cardiography; CMV, cytomegalovirus; CT; computed tomography; EBV, Epstein-Barr virus; HIV, human immunodeficiency virus; HSV, herpes simplex virus; MMR, measles, mumps, and rubella; RPR, rapid plasma regain; VZV, varicella zoster virus.

- Cytomegalovirus (CMV) IgG and Epstein-Barr virus (EBV) IgG antibodies are checked to evaluate the risk for CMV and EBV infection after kidney transplantation and to determine prophylaxis needed.[2]
- Patients with hepatitis B infection should be referred for a liver biopsy to evaluate the severity of liver disease.[2]
- Patients with hepatitis C infection are also evaluated. In general, our center prefers not to treat hepatitis C prior to kidney transplantation, since these patients may receive offers from hepatitis C–positive donors. After transplantation, treatment using hepatitis C virus direct-acting antivirals has proven to be highly effective.[2]
- Whenever possible, vaccination is recommended for transplant for transplant candidates.

VACCINATIONS

Vaccination recommendations in pretransplant adult patients are summarized in **Tables 4-10** and **4-11**.[16]

OTHER MEDICAL CONDITIONS

Obesity

- Associated with increased risk of delayed graft function (DGF), surgical complications, hospital readmission rates, posttransplant diabetes mellitus, and 5-year incidence of cardiovascular events.[17,18]
- Most transplant centers have body mass index cutoff of <40 kg/m^2 for transplant eligibility.
- Candidates are encouraged to lose weight and may be referred to a dietitian. Bariatric surgery may be considered for candidates who are unable to lose weight.

Hypotension

Transplant candidates with chronic hypotension, such as those who require therapy with midodrine, are at high risk for developing DGF, primary nonfunction, and recurrent acute kidney injury.

Hypercoagulability/Thrombosis

- Patients with hypercoagulability are at an increased risk for early graft loss.
- Transplant candidates should have coagulation studies done. Patients with a history of thrombosis or spontaneous abortions should undergo testing for activated protein C resistance, factor V and prothrombin gene mutations, anticardiolipin antibody, lupus anticoagulant, protein C and S, antithrombin III, and homocysteine levels.
- Perioperative anticoagulation and long-term anticoagulation may be considered for high-risk patients.

Secondary Hyperparathyroidism

- Secondary hyperparathyroidism correlates with higher parathyroid hormone levels and higher calcium levels posttransplant
- Cinacalcet is usually needed to treat hypercalcemia associated with secondary hyperparathyroidism in the posttransplant period.[19]
- Pretransplant parathyroidectomy may be needed for hyperparathyroidism that is unresponsive to medical therapy.

Frailty

- Frailty is "A measure of physiologic reserve and augmented vulnerability described and validated in the geriatric population."[7]
- A greater severity of frailty has been associated with mortality, prolonged hospitalization after transplant, increased rate of DGF, and increased rate of readmission.[19,20]
- We use 6-minute walk test to measure frailty. If candidates walk less than 1,000 feet in 6 minutes, we consider the applicant not fit to proceed with transplantation.
- An estimation of frailty can be made based on five components that are summarized in **Table 4-12**.[20,21]

TABLE 4-10 Vaccination Recommendations in Pretransplant Patients

Vaccination	For Whom	Dose/Timing	Comments
Influenza (inactivated)	All candidates	1 dose yearly	Patients should receive **inactivated** influenza vaccine.
Hepatitis B	Candidates seronegative for hepatitis B surface antibody (anti-HBs)	Dependent on vaccination	Serologic testing of anti-HBs titers recommended ≥4 wk after final dose of primary series. Another 3-dose series hepatitis B vaccine to be administered if titer is <10 mIU/mL Annual anti-HBs titers annually in patients on dialysis. Another 3-dose series hepatitis B vaccine should be administered if titer <10 mIU/mL High-dose vaccine should be used in dialysis patients.
Pneumococcal	Candidates who have not received recommended vaccine/vaccine series	Dependent on vaccination	Vaccination with any of the following is acceptable: • PCV20 (Prevnar 20) • PCV15 (Vaxneuvance) + PPSV23 (Pneumovax 23) • PCV13 (Prevnar 13) + PPSV23 (Pneumovax 23)
Varicella (Varivax)	Candidates VZV IgG seronegative and have not recently received IS	2-dose series	Varivax only PRE-transplant (live). Consult transplant MD or PharmD prior to administration if candidates meet criteria. Review med list prior to vaccine to assess for IS. Hold antizoster antivirals 24 h prior to vaccination and avoid use 14 d after vaccination.

TABLE 4-10 Vaccination Recommendations in Pretransplant Patients (Continued)

Vaccination	For Whom	Dose/Timing	Comments
Zoster (Shingrix)	VZV IgG positive and have not received 2-dose series	2-dose series	Shingrix even if previously received Zostavax Shingrix recommended >50 y of age Consider Shingrix in patients <50 y of age Consider Shingrix in candidates VZV IgG negative.
COVID-19	All candidates	1-dose or 2-dose series depending on vaccine	Patients should receive an FDA-approved COVID-19 vaccine or vaccine series Booster vaccination guidelines following latest CDC recommendations
Hepatitis A	Candidates who have not received the 2-dose series	2-dose series	Hepatitis A vaccination is particularly important in liver transplant candidates
Tetanus/Diphtheria/Pertussis (Tdap) or (Td)	Candidates who have not received dose within 10 y	Tetanus every 10 y	≥1 dose of Tdap in adulthood. Tdap for all patients not previously vaccinated in adulthood regardless of last tetanus shot
Human Papillomavirus	Candidates ≤45 y of age who have not completed the vaccination series	3-dose series	

anti-HB, antibody to hepatitis B surface antigen; CDC, Centers for Disease Control and Prevention; FDA, Food and Drug Administration; IgG, immunoglobulin G; IS, immunosuppression; VZV, varicella zoster virus.

Adapted from Centers for Disease Control and Prevention. *Vaccines Indicated Based on Medical Indications*; 2022. https://www.cdc.gov/vaccines/schedules/hcp/imz/adult-conditions.html

TABLE 4-11 Vaccination Recommendations in Adult Pretransplant Patients—Special Populations

Vaccination	For Whom	Dosing/ Timing	Comments
Hemophilus influenzae type b (Hib)	Candidates at risk (anatomic or functional asplenia, persistent complement deficiencies)	1 dose	Consult transplant MD or PharmD prior to vaccine if candidates meet criteria for vaccination
Quadrivalent meningococcal conjugate vaccine (Menactra or Menveo)	Candidates at risk (anatomic or functional asplenia, persistent complement deficiencies, first-year college students, military recruits) OR if on complement inhibitors such as eculizumab or ravulizumab	1 or more doses depending on indication	Consult transplant MD or PharmD prior to vaccine if candidates meet criteria for vaccination Vaccination series should be completed with the same product
Serogroup B meningococcal vaccine (Bexsero or Trumenba	I Vaccine (Bexsero or Trumenba) if at risk (anatomic or functional asplenia, persistent complement deficiencies, increased risk from serogroup B meningococcal disease outbreak) OR for individuals started on complement inhibitors such as eculizumab or ravulizumab	2-dose series or 3-dose series depending on vaccine	Consult transplant MD or PharmD prior to vaccine administration if candidates meet criteria for vaccination Vaccination series should be completed with the same product
Measles, mumps, rubella (MMR)	Candidates who have not previously received the 2-dose series or those who are known to be seronegative and have not recently received immunosuppression	1 or 2 doses depending on indication	MMR ONLY pretransplant (live) Consult transplant MD or PharmD prior to vaccine if candidates meet criteria Review medication list prior to vaccine administration to assess for use IS.

anti-HBs, antibody to hepatitis B surface antigen; IS, immunosuppression; MMR, measles, mumps, and rubella.

Adapted from Centers for Disease Control and Prevention. *Vaccines Indicated Based on Medical Indications*; 2022. Accessed February 17, 2022. https://www.cdc.gov/vaccines/*schedules/hcp/imz/adult-conditions.html*

TABLE 4-12 Major Components of Frailty

Unintentional weight loss
Weakness (grip strength below an established cutoff based on sex and BMI)
Exhaustion
Low activity (kilocalories per week below an established cutoff)
Slow walking speed

BMI, body mass index.

Older Patients

- There is no age limit for kidney transplant candidates.
- Studies have shown that older patients who are considered appropriate candidates and receive a kidney transplant have a survival benefit compared to those who remain on the waiting list.[20]

Social Issues

- The social worker evaluates psychosocial factors that could affect the outcome of the transplant. These include the assessment of social support, substance use, psychiatric well-being, and compliance with medications, regular follow-up, and laboratory testing.
- Compliance can be evaluated via examination of dialysis records. Phosphorus levels and glucose control are also suggestive of good compliance.
- Psychiatric, psychosocial, and neurocognitive referrals may be made as needed.
- The financial coordinator evaluates sources of income and other resources which will be needed for the transplant procedure and for future medical needs.

REFERENCES

1. Chadban SJ, Ahn C, Axelrod DA, et al. KDIGO clinical practice guideline on the evaluation and management of candidates for kidney transplantation. *Transplantation.* 2020;104(4S1 suppl 1):S11-S103.
2. Katari S. Evaluation of the kidney transplant candidate. In: Alhamad T, Cheng S, Vijayan A, eds. *The Washington Manual: Nephrology Subspecialty Consult.* 4th ed. Lippincott Williams & Wilkins; 2021:293-301.
3. Cheng XS, Myers JN, Chertow GM, et al. Prehabilitation for kidney transplant candidates: is it time? *Clin Transplant.* 2017;31(8):e13020.
4. Alhamad TL, Lentine K, Anwar S, et al. Functional capacity pre-transplantation measured by 6-minute walk test and clinical outcomes. *Am J Transplant.* 2016;16:447-8.
5. Al-Adra D, Hammel L, Roberts J, et al. Pretransplant solid organ malignancy and organ transplant candidacy: a consensus expert opinion statement. *Am J Transplant.* 2020;00:1-15.
6. Zwald F, Leitenberger J, Zeitouni N, et al. Recommendations for solid organ transplantation for transplant candidates with a pretransplant diagnosis of cutaneous squamous cell carcinoma, Merkel cell carcinoma and melanoma: a consensus opinion from the International Transplant Skin Cancer Collaborative (ITSCC). *Am J Transplant.* 2016;16(2):407-13.
7. Bunnapradist S, Abdalla B, Reddy U. Evaluation of adult kidney transplant candidates. In: Danovitch GM, ed. *Handbook of Kidney Transplantation.* 6th ed. Lippincott Williams & Wilkins; 2017:206-37.
8. Moroni G, Belingheri M, Frontini G, Tamborini F, Messa P. Immunoglobulin A nephropathy. Recurrence after renal transplantation. *Front Immunol.* 2019;10:1332.

9. Contreras G, Mattiazzi A, Guerra G, et al. Recurrence of lupus nephritis after kidney transplantation. *J Am Soc Nephrol.* 2010;21(7):1200-7.
10. Andresdottir MB, Assmann KJ, Hoitsma AJ, Koene RA, Wetzels JF. Recurrence of type I membranoproliferative glomerulonephritis after renal transplantation: analysis of the incidence, risk factors, and impact on graft survival. *Transplantation.* 1997;63(11):1628-33.
11. Czarnecki PG, Lager DJ, Leung N, Dispenzieri A, Cosio FG, Fervenza FC. Long-term outcome of kidney transplantation in patients with fibrillary glomerulonephritis or monoclonal gammopathy with fibrillary deposits. *Kidney Int.* 2009;75(4):420-7.
12. Fleisher LA, Fleischmann KE, Auerbach AD, et al. 2014 ACC/AHA guideline on perioperative cardiovascular evaluation and management of patients undergoing noncardiac surgery: a report of the American College of Cardiology/American Heart Association Task Force on practice guidelines. *J Am Coll Cardiol.* 2014;64(22):e77-e137.
13. Lentine KL, Costa SP, Weir MR, et al. Cardiac disease evaluation and management among kidney and liver transplantation candidates: a scientific statement from the American Heart Association and the American College of Cardiology Foundation—endorsed by the American Society of Transplant Surgeons, American Society of Transplantation, and National Kidney Foundation. *Circulation.* 2012;126(5):617-63.
14. De Mattos AM, Siedlecki A, Gaston RS, et al. Systolic dysfunction portends increased mortality among those waiting for renal transplant. *J Am Soc Nephrol.* 2008;19(6):1191-6.
15. Levy PE, Khan SS, VanWagner LB. Cardiac evaluation of the kidney or liver transplant candidate. *Curr Opin Organ Transplant.* 2021;26(1):77-84.
16. Centers for Disease Control and Prevention. *Vaccines Indicated Based on Medical Indications.* 2022. Accessed December 25, 2022. https://www.cdc.gov/vaccines/schedules/hcp/imz/adult-conditions.html
17. Aziz F, Ramadorai A, Parajuli S, et al. Obesity: an independent predictor of morbidity and graft loss after kidney transplantation. *Am J Nephrol.* 2020;51(8):615-23.
18. Kristensen SD, Knuuti J, Saraste A, et al. 2014 ESC/ESA Guidelines on non-cardiac surgery: cardiovascular assessment and management – the Joint Task Force on non-cardiac surgery—cardiovascular assessment and management of the European Society of Cardiology (ESC) and the European Society of Anaesthesiology (ESA). *Eur Heart J.* 2014;35:2383-431.
19. Tillmann FP, Wächtler C, Hansen A, Rump LC, Quack I. Vitamin D and cinacalcet administration pre-transplantation predict hypercalcaemic hyperparathyroidism post-transplantation: a case-control study of 355 deceased-donor renal transplant recipients over 3 years. *Transplant Res.* 2014;3(1):21.
20. Harhay MN, Rao MK, Woodside KJ, et al. An overview of frailty in kidney transplantation: measurement, management and future considerations. *Nephrol Dial Transplant.* 2020;35(7):1099-112.
21. Xie B, Larson JL, Gonzalez R, Pressler SJ, Lustig C, Arslanian-Engoren C. Components and indicators of frailty measures: a literature review. *J Frailty Aging.* 2017;6(2):76-82.

5 Living Donor Evaluation

Seth Goldberg

GENERAL PRINCIPLES

- Donation of a kidney from a living person was first performed in 1954 and remains an option for those in need of a kidney.[1]
- Living kidney donation is an elective procedure, requiring a rigorous evaluation of potential donors. Given that these donors must be in excellent health and that the ischemia time of the allograft can be minimized at the time of the operation, kidneys from living donors have better outcomes than those from deceased donors.
- Generally, recipients who have a living donor can receive a kidney transplant sooner than those on the waiting list, and in many cases are able to undergo a preemptive transplant without spending time on dialysis.
- Despite the advantages to the recipient of living kidney donation, the guiding principle of whether a donation is appropriate is centered on the **safety to the living donor**. A potential donor who is not suitable cannot donate, regardless of the urgency or need of the recipient.
- The evaluation of a potential living donor should be performed by a nephrologist who is not part of the transplant team to ensure impartiality. The nephrologist should not be involved in the care of the potential recipient to minimize the chance of a conflict of interest.

MEDICAL EVALUATION

- The medical evaluation of potential living donors is extensive and utilizes bloodwork, urine studies, imaging, and cardiac risk assessment.[2] Please see **Table 5-1** for a list of tests performed as part of the evaluation at Washington University.
- Human leukocyte antigen (HLA) typing is performed on the potential donor and recipient to determine the degree of match.
- The goals of the medical evaluation are to test the renal function, screen for common metabolic diseases which can affect the kidneys (e.g., hypertension and diabetes), assess for transmissible infectious diseases, to screen for potential malignancies, and to stratify perioperative cardiac risk.
- A thorough history and a complete physical examination are also part of the evaluation.
- Occasionally, minor abnormalities may be discovered through testing, such as mildly elevated liver enzymes or mild anemia. These do not necessarily preclude donation, as long as they are deemed to not pose a risk to a person with a solitary kidney or to significantly affect the quality of the organ being removed.

HISTORY AND PHYSICAL EXAMINATION

- A thorough history is required of all potential living donors. Some centers also use a standardized questionnaire as part of the initial step.

TABLE 5-1 Testing for Potential Donors

Standard blood tests
- Blood type and screen
- Human leukocyte antigen (HLA) typing
- Comprehensive metabolic panel
- Phosphorus
- Uric acid
- Gamma glutamyl transferase (GGT)
- Hemoglobin A1c
- Complete blood count with differential
- Protime, INR, aPTT
- Lipid panel
- HIV 1/2 antibody plus p24 antigen
- Hepatitis B panel (surface antigen, total core antibody, surface antibody)
- Hepatitis C antibody
- Rapid plasma reagin (RPR)
- Cytomegalovirus IgG
- Epstein-Barr virus viral capsid antigen (VCA) IgG
- Human chorionic gonadotropin (hCG), quantitative (women of childbearing potential)

Standard urine tests
- Urinalysis with microscopy
- Urine culture
- Albumin creatinine ratio
- Human chorionic gonadotropin (hCG), qualitative (women of childbearing potential)

Standard ancillary tests
- Chest radiograph
- 12-lead electrocardiogram
- CT scan, abdomen and pelvis, with and without contrast, with 3D reconstruction
- 24-h urine creatinine clearance (if eGFR ≥80 mL/min/1.73 m^2)
- ^{125}I-iothalamate GFR (if eGFR <80 mL/min/1.73 m^2)
- Pap smear in women

Additional testing, if indicated
- Mammography (women ≥ 40)
- Prostate-specific antigen, total (men ≥ 40)
- Colonoscopy (age ≥ 45 if average risk, see text for guidelines if increased risk)
- Stress echocardiography (age ≥ 60)
- 2-h glucose tolerance test (if fasting glucose >100 mg/dL)
- 24-h ambulatory blood pressure monitor (if history of hypertension or if screening blood pressure >140/90)
- 24-h urine stone battery (if history of nephrolithiasis or if kidney stone seen on imaging)
- Sickle cell screening (self-reported recent African ancestry)
- APOL-1 genotyping (age <40 with self-reported recent African ancestry)
- See text for additional infectious disease testing, based on travel history
- ^{99m}Tc-labeled split function assay (if kidney volumes differ by >20 mL)

aPTT, activated partial thromboplastin clotting time; eGFR, estimated glomerular filtration rate; GFR, glomerular filtration rate; INR, international normalized ratio.

- The evaluator should ask about the postdonation caregiving plan. The donor and recipient should not serve as each other's caregiver posttransplantation.
- A thorough physical examination is required. Abnormalities, particularly of the cardiovascular system and the skin, may prompt further investigations.

Medical Conditions

- Special attention is needed when inquiring as to a prior history of kidney disease, kidney stones, hypertension, diabetes, and cancer.
- A history of hypertension diagnosed at age ≥40 years does not necessarily preclude donation, though the blood pressure should be well-controlled on no more than a single antihypertensive agent.
- Gastrointestinal disorders that may predispose to volume depletion should be sought.
- A prior surgical history, particularly involving the abdomen, is relevant when considering the anticipated operative approach.
- A history of bariatric surgery may preclude donation given the potential for enteric hyperoxaluria and nephrolithiasis in a patient with a solitary kidney.

Medications

- A thorough medication and allergy history must be taken.
- Direct questioning should be performed regarding the use of over-the-counter medications such as NSAIDs; though not absolutely contraindicated after donation, potential donors should be informed about their risks on the remaining kidney with the recommendation to minimize or avoid their use, and to ensure adequate hydration if taken.
- The use of estrogen-containing compounds should be ascertained, and given their thrombotic risk, should be discontinued for at least 6 weeks prior to donation.

Family History

- Family history of renal disease is important to assess, as many potential donors are seeking to give the kidney to a relative who has renal disease.
- A person at risk for autosomal dominant polycystic kidney disease (ADPKD) (i.e., having an affected parent) may require additional screening.
  - Ultrasonography showing 0 to 1 renal cysts in a person ≥40 years of age carries a negative predictive value of 100%, sufficient to exclude the disease.
  - For at-risk potential donors younger than 40 years of age, or if the imaging is indeterminate, genetic testing would be required.
  - Typically, the affected relative would be tested first to locate the mutation, followed by directed testing of the potential donor to look for the same mutation.

Social History

- Social history should assess for recent travel in the past 3 years, smoking history, alcohol use, and recreational drugs, particularly IV drug use.
- Potential donors should be questioned on their willingness to accept blood products during the perioperative phase.
- As living donation is an elective procedure without a direct medical benefit to the donor, a potential donor unwilling to accept blood products may be rejected as an unsafe donor.
- High-risk sexual behaviors should be ascertained, and if present, would need to be disclosed to the recipient after obtaining consent from the potential donor.

ASSESSMENT OF KIDNEY FUNCTION

- A baseline creatinine is obtained from the complete metabolic panel. The chronic kidney disease (CKD)-EPI equation can be used to calculate the estimated glomerular filtration rate (eGFR), though it frequently underestimates renal function in healthy individuals. Those with a value <60 mL/min/1.73 m^2 should be excluded from donation.
- A measurement of the creatinine clearance or glomerular filtration also needs to be performed. This can be accomplished with a 24-hour urine collection for creatinine clearance or an ^{125}I-iothalamate clearance. At Washington University, potential donors with an eGFR ≥ 80 mL/min/1.73 m^2 can undergo the 24-hour urine collection for creatinine clearance; those with an eGFR <80 mL/min/1.73 m^2 or with an indeterminate 24-hour urine creatinine clearance would undergo iothalamate testing.
- Most centers would exclude potential donors with a value <60 mL/min/1.73 m^2 and accept otherwise suitable donors with a value >90 mL/min/1.73 m^2. An individualized approach is needed for potential donors with intermediate values. At Washington University, a cutoff of 80 mL/min/1.73 m^2 is typically used, though lower cutoffs may be considered for appropriate donors. See **Table 5-2**.
- Renal imaging is performed with a CT scan of the abdomen and pelvis, with and without contrast, with 3D reconstruction. Imaging must demonstrate the presence of two discrete kidneys, free of masses or obstructions. Incidental simple cysts (apart from ADPKD considerations above) would not typically preclude donation.
- A history of a single kidney stone with a noncomplicated course or the finding of a single kidney stone on imaging would not preclude donation, though the potential donor should undergo additional testing for lithogenic risk factors with a 24-hour urine stone battery.
- Significantly elevated urine calcium, oxalate, or uric acid levels on this collection may exclude donation. Also, a person with a history of more than one kidney stone or imaging revealing more than one stone should not donate; as a recurrent stone former, there would be an increased risk for obstruction of a solitary kidney in either the donor or the recipient.
- If there is asymmetry of the two kidneys, further testing with a split function assay should be performed.
  - At Washington University, a difference in volume of >20 mL between the two kidneys would prompt technetium-labeled testing to determine the relative contribution of each kidney to the total function.

TABLE 5-2 Acceptable eGFR Prior to Donation at Washington University in St. Louis. Other Donor Factors Could be Part of the Final Decision

Donor Age (years)	eGFR (mL/min/1.73 m^2)
Up to 59	80
60–64	75
≥65	65

eGFR, estimated glomerular filtration

- This test may help in deciding with the surgical team which kidney will be removed, where the higher-functioning kidney is typically left with the donor unless there is a compelling reason otherwise, such as technically challenging vascular anatomy.
- Infrequently, the split function assay reveals a wide difference (greater than 60/40 split) which may preclude donation when considered in the context of the overall glomerular filtration rate or absolute kidney sizes.

HYPERTENSION SCREENING

- A history of hypertension should be assessed, and if present, the age of diagnosis recorded.
- Three home blood pressure readings should be obtained by the patient. Additionally, a reading in the clinic should be taken. In the absence of renal disease, a blood pressure ≤140/90 would be acceptable.
- As noted above, a history of hypertension diagnosed at the age of 40 years or older does not necessarily preclude donation. The blood pressure should be well controlled on no more than a single antihypertensive agent.
- Testing with a 24-hour ambulatory blood pressure monitor should be performed for potential donors with a history of hypertension or for those with an elevated blood pressure (>140/90) on any of their home readings or the in-office reading. The average blood pressure on the 24-hour monitor should be ≤140/90 during the daytime, with nocturnal dipping of 10% to 15%.
- Much uncertainty currently surrounds the utility of testing for APOL-1 variants (G0, G1, G2). Two variants (G1 and G2) convey resistance to African trypanosomiasis and thus are found with increased frequency in sub-Saharan Africa. However, homozygosity (G1/G1, G2/G2) or compound heterozygosity (G1/G2) may increase the risk of CKD, end-stage kidney disease, the pattern of collapsing focal segmental glomerulosclerosis. This "high-risk" genotype is found in 13% of Americans with recent African ancestry (within the past 500 years).
- Emerging evidence from deceased kidney donation has found poorer outcomes from kidneys from donors with a high-risk genotype.[3] While receiving such a kidney still offers a survival advantage when compared to starting or remaining on dialysis, additional consideration is required when discussing living kidney donation; as opposed to the cadaveric donor, the living donor often has many decades of anticipated survival. Whether the life expectancy will be negatively impacted by donor nephrectomy remains an unanswered question.[4]
- While clinical studies are underway to provide more guidance, at Washington University the current recommendation is to offer genetic testing for APOL-1 for potential donors with self-reported recent African ancestry if they are under the age of 40. If a high-risk genotype is discovered, then counseling is provided as to what is known about the potential added risk of donation with the general recommendation to not go forward with donation, though still allowing the patient an opportunity to make as informed a decision as possible.
- There are no standardized guidelines regarding screening for sickle cell trait. Large prospective cohort studies found that the presence of sickle cell trait was associated with an increased risk of CKD and albuminuria.[5] At Washington University, potential donors with self-reported recent African ancestry are screened for sickle cell trait and if found to be present are recommended to not donate.

DIABETES MELLITUS SCREENING AND URINE TESTING

- A history of type 1 diabetes mellitus is a contraindication to donation.
- Type 2 diabetes mellitus is also traditionally considered a contraindication to donation, though some transplant centers consider donors deemed to have a low lifetime risk of renal complications on an individualized basis.
- A history of gestational diabetes would not preclude donation if the fasting glucose and hemoglobin A1c testing are normal at the time of evaluation.
- Screening is with a fasting blood sugar which should not exceed 100 mg/dL. Additionally, a hemoglobin A1c level should be obtained and be <5.7%.
- Overt diabetes mellitus with a fasting glucose ≥126 mg/dL or a hemoglobin A1c ≥ 6.5% on two separate tests should preclude donation.
- Potential donors in the intermediate ranges (fasting glucose 101-125 mg/dL or hemoglobin A1c 5.7%-6.4%) can be offered the option of glucose tolerance testing; those with a 2-hour glucose level <140 mg/dL may be acceptable donors.
- Ideally, potential donors would have a body mass index (BMI) ≤30 kg/m^2. The decision to approve donors beyond this threshold can be individualized based on the patient's health profile and wound healing risk in consultation with the surgical team. At Washington University, it is generally recommended for potential donors younger than 40 to have a BMI ≤ 32 kg/m^2 and for potential donors ≥40 to have a BMI ≤ 35 kg/m^2.
- Urine testing for all potential donors should include a urinalysis, urine microscopy, urine culture, and urine albumin-to-creatinine ratio.
- The urine dipstick should be negative for protein, blood, glucose, leukocyte esterase, and nitrite. A positive finding for protein should prompt further quantification.
- The finding of dipstick-positive blood is an insensitive marker, and should be confirmed on the urine microscopy.
  - If there is concern for contamination, a repeat specimen should be obtained.
  - A positive dipstick for blood without blood on microscopy would not typically preclude donation, as a retrospective study found equivalent outcomes for these donors.[6]
- The presence of persistent blood on urinary microscopy precludes donation, and the patient should undergo urologic examination outside of the transplant evaluation.
  - Isolated hematuria may represent thin basement membrane disease or IgA nephropathy, and while these may not require specific treatment at the time of evaluation, their presence would nonetheless prevent donation as they can be associated with a decline in renal function over time.[7]
  - At Washington University, biopsies of potential donors with persistent isolated hematuria are not typically performed, given the procedure's nontrivial complication risk and the inability to conclusively rule out early-stage focal glomerular disease.
- An albumin-to-creatinine ratio should be performed on at a urine specimen, with the normal range being <30 mg/g. Samples that are too dilute to assure a ratio <30 mg/g should be repeated with less aggressive hydration until a useable ratio can be obtained.
- Potential donors with a positive urine culture should be treated with standard antibiotics for urinary tract infections and testing repeated to ensure a sterile urine prior to donation.
- A urinary pregnancy test (qualitative human chorionic gonadotropin, hCG) should be obtained for women of childbearing potential; a serum quantitative hCG test is also typically performed.

INFECTIOUS DISEASE TESTING

- All potential donors should be tested for HIV, hepatitis B, hepatitis C, syphilis, and West Nile virus. Testing for cytomegalovirus (CMV) and Epstein-Barr virus (EBV) is also performed to determine the donor's status and guide posttransplant management of the recipient.
- A positive test for HIV, if confirmed, would preclude donation. Though there has been a push to expand the deceased donor pool by accepting HIV-positive donor kidney in select circumstances, this has not yet applied to living donation since antiretroviral therapy can affect the remaining kidney.
- Hepatitis B testing is with total core (IgG/IgM), surface antigen, and surface antibody. Results indicative of prior exposure should prompt DNA nucleic acid testing (NAT).
  - A potential donor who is core antibody positive (IgG), and surface antigen negative, with a negative nucleic acid test may be able to donate, needing to consent to disclosing this information to the recipient.
  - Potential donors who are surface antigen positive should not donate to hepatitis B negative recipients. However, donation to recipients with immunity may be acceptable with informed consent, though one must consider the potential risk of glomerulonephritis to the donor with chronic infection.
- Hepatitis C antibody testing can reveal prior or active infection. Potential donors with a positive test result should undergo RNA quantification, and if detectable, referred to a hepatologist for possible treatment with direct-acting antiviral agents. Given these recent advancements in available therapy, a patient who has successfully cleared the virus may be considered for living donation with close consultation of the recipient's team, though the donor would need to consent to disclosing this information to the recipient.
- HIV, hepatitis B, and hepatitis C testing should be within 28 days of donation.
- Potential donors are screened for syphilis (rapid plasma reagin test), and if positive a confirmatory test (fluorescent treponemal antibody absorption) should be performed. If also positive, the potential donor should complete treatment prior to further consideration.
- West Nile virus NAT is recommended for potential donors within 28 days of donation.
- All potential donors are tested for CMV (IgG) and EBV (viral capsid antigen IgG). Prior exposure with these viruses is common, with 80% of potential donors testing positive for each. A positive result does not preclude donation, though the information obtained from these tests is used to manage posttransplant viral prophylaxis in the case of CMV and for stratification of the risk for posttransplant lymphoproliferative disorders in the recipient in the case of EBV.
- Additional infectious disease testing is individualized based on the recent travel history of the potential donor, typically from the prior 3 years.[8] Suggested tests, along with the endemic areas of the infectious agents, are described in **Table 5-3**.

CANCER SCREENING

- Age-appropriate cancer screening is required for potential donors.
- All potential donors should undergo chest radiography.
- Women should have undergone cervical cancer screening with a pap smear within the prior 3 years.
- Women ≥40 years of age should have undergone mammography within the past year.

TABLE 5-3 Regional-specific Infectious Disease Testing

Tuberculosis (QuantiFERON-TB Gold)
• Most areas outside of the United States, Canada, Western Europe
Malaria (Plasmodium blood parasite evaluation)
• Most areas outside of the United States, Canada, Western Europe
Strongyloidiasis (IgG antibody)
• Tropical and subtropical regions
• Rural Appalachian region of the United States
Schistosomiasis (IgG antibody)
• Africa
• Brazil and northeastern part of South America
• Middle East
• South Asia, Southeast Asia, China, the Philippines, Indonesia
Chagas Disease (*Trypanosoma cruzi* total antibody)
• Mexico
• Central America
• South America
Human T-lymphotropic virus 1 (HTLV-1 qualitative antibodies)
• Caribbean area and parts of South America
• West/Central Africa
• Japan

- Men ≥40 years of age should have a prostate-specific antigen checked.
- Potential donors who are at least 45 years old and who are at average risk for colon cancer should have had a colonoscopy (with frequency determined by findings on prior testing). If there is a family history of colon cancer in a first-degree relative, then screening should have begun by age 40 or 10 years before the age of the affected relative.
- While stool DNA testing and other less-invasive screening tests are gaining popularity, they are not currently recommended for screening in potential donors, given their nontrivial false-negative rate and the risk of significant harm to the recipient should a malignancy be transmitted.
- All potential donors undergo a CT scan of the abdomen and pelvis with and without contrast, as noted above. Although this testing is primarily done to evaluate the kidney anatomy, it can pick up other abnormalities which may require further imaging or a waiting period followed by further imaging. Such testing is dictated by the specific abnormalities found.
- A history of malignancy typically excludes a potential donor, unless the cancer is of minimal risk of transmission to the recipient (<0.1% transmission). Few cancers fall into this category; examples include squamous cell or basal cell carcinoma of the skin, carcinoma in situ of the cervix or vocal cord, and several types of thyroid carcinomas.[9] A history of skin cancer should prompt a dermatology evaluation within the prior year to exclude melanoma.

CARDIAC RISK STRATIFICATION

- Assessment of cardiac risk plays several roles in determining candidacy for donation. Potential donors must be healthy enough to endure the surgical procedure and any underlying cardiovascular disease must not be expected to impair the function of the remaining kidney.

- A family history of cardiac disease is obtained, along with bloodwork for cholesterol panel, complete blood count, and coagulation parameters (protime, international normalized ratio, aPTT). Potential donors with significant cardiac risk factors or those aged 60 years or older should undergo a cardiac stress test, and if positive for ischemia, further testing as per standard cardiology guidelines.
- Patients with underlying structural heart disease are not recommended to donate given the risk of perioperative complications from an elective procedure which does not provide direct medical benefit to the patient.
- Major predictors (e.g., unstable coronary syndromes, decompensated heart failure, significant arrhythmias, and severe valvular disease) and intermediate predictors (e.g., angina and myocardial infarction) of increased perioperative cardiac risk typically contraindications to donation. Minor predictors (e.g., stroke and atrial fibrillation) require an individualized approach.
- A baseline electrocardiogram is required for all potential donors.

PSYCHOLOGIC EVALUATION

- Donors with psychiatric disease may still be able to donate as long as their underlying illness is well controlled. Patients should be on a stable dose of their usual medications under the guidance of a psychiatrist for at least 6 months prior to donation.
- At Washington University, it is recommended for potential donors with a significant history of psychiatric disease to be evaluated by a clinical psychologist who is part of the transplant team. Examples of significant disease include prior history of suicide attempt, psychotic disorders, and severe mood disorders.
- Additionally, potential donors who are between the ages of 18 to 21 or those not donating to someone they know ("altruistic" or nondirected donation) are referred to the clinical psychologist.
- Donors must be free of coercion and be able to provide informed consent. Payment for organ donation is not permitted, and suspicion for undisclosed financial remuneration would preclude donation.

POST-DONATION COUNSELING

- Potential donors who qualify meet with members of the surgical team for a thorough discussion of the planned operative procedure. However, it is important to review short-term and long-term postdonation expectations, and this can be done effectively as part of the donor evaluation process by the nephrologist.
- Most donations are performed laparoscopically with a 4 to 5 cm incision to remove the kidney as well as several smaller incisions for the surgical instruments. Should there be complicated vascular anatomy, the surgical team may consider an open procedure along the lateral flank sometimes necessitating the removal of part of a rib. The laparoscopic procedure is associated with less postoperative pain and shorter recovery times, with similar long-term outcomes, and is thus preferred if the anatomy is conducive to this approach.
- The risk of perioperative mortality is 3 out of 10,000. When deaths have occurred, the most common cause is a pulmonary embolism, and early ambulation is encouraged.
- The hospitalization has traditionally been for 3 days following the operation, though there is a trend toward earlier discharge after 1 to 2 days in uncomplicated cases.
- After returning home, recovery time is typically 4 to 6 weeks, with the recommendation to avoid heavy lifting during this time period. Once the incision site is healed,

donors can resume their regular activity, though contact sports putting at risk blunt trauma to the remaining kidney are generally discouraged.

- There is no expectation of dietary changes postdonation. Donors are advised to follow a healthy balanced diet, without specific restrictions related to having a solitary kidney.
- Aside from the typical medications offered in the postoperative period (pain control and stool-softeners), there are no expectations of new long-term medications.
- Pregnancy is discouraged for 6 months after donation. Women who complete the donor evaluation process are considered to be in the lowest risk group for obstetrical complications; following donation, they revert to the standard risk category.[10]
- Patients should be advised that their creatinine level will rise postdonation, by approximately 0.5 to 1 mg/dL. After 1 to 2 years, it is common to see a modest dip in the creatinine to an intermediate level as the remaining kidney enlarges to provide some degree of compensation.
- Long-term longitudinal follow-up studies found that up to one-third of donors develop hypertension, with a median time to diagnosis of slightly over 15 years.[11] This prevalence is comparable to the general population.
- The risk of a former donor requiring a kidney transplant is 4 to 10 out of 10,000 and oftentimes is unrelated to the prior donation. The United Network for Organ Sharing allocation policy does give priority to former donors who are listed for kidney transplantation.
- The life expectancy of donors is not shortened. Statistically, the life expectancy is increased as compared to the general population, though this is likely due to selection bias given the requirement to be healthy in order to donate.
- Donors should have follow-up laboratory studies performed for at least 2 years after donation. At Washington University, renal studies (comprehensive metabolic panel and panel and urinalysis) are assessed at 6 months, 12 months, and 24 months following donation.

REFERENCES

1. Harrison JH, Merrill JP, Murray JE. Renal homotransplantation in identical twins. *Surg Forum.* 1956;6:432-6.
2. Lentine KL, Kasiske BL, Levey AS, et al. KDIGO clinical practice guideline on the evaluation and care of living kidney donors. *Transplantation.* 2017;101(8S Suppl 1):S1-S109.
3. Freedman BI, Pastan SO, Israni AK, et al. APOL1 genotype and kidney transplantation outcomes from deceased African American donors. *Transplantation.* 2016;100(1):194-202.
4. Mohan S, Iltis AS, Sawinski D, DuBois JM. APOL1 genetic testing in living kidney transplant donors. *Am J Kidney Dis.* 2019;74(4):538-43.
5. Naik RP, Derebail VK, Grams ME, et al. Association of sickle cell trait with chronic kidney disease and albuminuria in African Americans. *JAMA.* 2014;312(20):2115-25.
6. Winn S, Rashid L, Talbot B, et al. Non-visible haematuria in living kidney donors. *Nephrol Dial Transplant.* 2015;30:349.
7. Voskarides K, Damianou L, Neocleous V, et al. COL4A3/COL4A4 mutations producing focal segmental glomerulosclerosis and renal failure in thin basement membrane nephropathy. *J Am Soc Nephrol.* 2007;18(11):3004-16.
8. Levi ME, Kumar D, Green M, et al. Considerations for screening live kidney donors for endemic infections: a viewpoint on the UNOS policy. *Am J Transplant.* 2014;14(5):1003-11.
9. Zhang S, Yuan J, Li W, Ye Q. Organ transplantation from donors (cadaveric or living) with a history of malignancy: review of the literature. *Transplant Rev.* 2014;28(4):169-75.
10. Ibrahim HN, Akkina SK, Leister E, et al. Pregnancy outcomes after kidney donation. *Am J Transplant.* 2009;9(4):825-34.
11. Sanchez OA, Ferrara LK, Rein S, Berglund D, Matas AJ, Ibrahim HN. Hypertension after kidney donation: incidence, predictors, and correlates. *Am J Transplant.* 2018;18(10):2534-43.

6 Allocation System and Organ Procurement Organization

Karen Flores, Mohamed M. Ibrahim, and Gary Marklin

GENERAL PRINCIPLES

- Organ Procurement and Transplant Network (OPTN) was first developed in Congress in 1984 through the National Organ Transplant Act (NOTA).[1]
- The OPTN links all professionals involved in the US donation and transplantation system.[2]
- The OPTN establishes transplant policies, laws, and guidelines that regulate organ transplantation in the US.
- The Health Resources and Service Administration is the government agency responsible for organ transplantation, and, per NOTA, is awarded the contract to United Network for Organ Sharing (UNOS), a private nonprofit organization, to administer, regulate, update, and change policy and provide oversight for organ transplantation.
- The members of UNOS are organ procurement organizations (OPOs), transplant centers, and HLA labs. One of the main functions of UNOS is to develop allocation policy and provide the infrastructure for allocating organs via the match run.
- UNOS operates OPTN.
- The OPTN ensures the ethical principles of justice, utility, respect for persons, and autonomy in the process of organ allocation.[3]
  - Justice: equal and fair distribution of organs
  - Utility: efficiency and matching
  - Respect for people: honesty
  - Respect for autonomy: right to self-determination

THE DEVELOPMENT OF UNOS REGIONS

- The US is divided into organ procurement regions and donation service areas (DSAs).
- OPOs are 57 nonprofit organizations, working under a federal contract, whose purpose is to identify potential donors, obtain authorization for donation, medically manage the donor, allocate organs per the national match list, arrange the procurement, and transport the organ to the transplant center.
- Each OPO is responsible for a federally donator service area.
- UNOS divided the US into 11 regions by contiguous states[4] (**Figure 6-1**).
- Previously, allocation of kidneys was based on DSAs first (local), then regionally, and finally nationally.
- The DSAs and regions are not evenly distributed and not equal in size; hence, there is less optimal allocation in some areas.[5]
- To avoid geographical disparity, since March 15, 2021, the OPTN has launched a policy based on a more consistent measure of distance between the donor hospital and the transplant hospital.[5]
- Kidney and pancreas donor offers will be made to candidates listed at transplant hospitals which are within 250 nautical miles of the donor hospital.[5] See example **Figure 6-2**.[6]

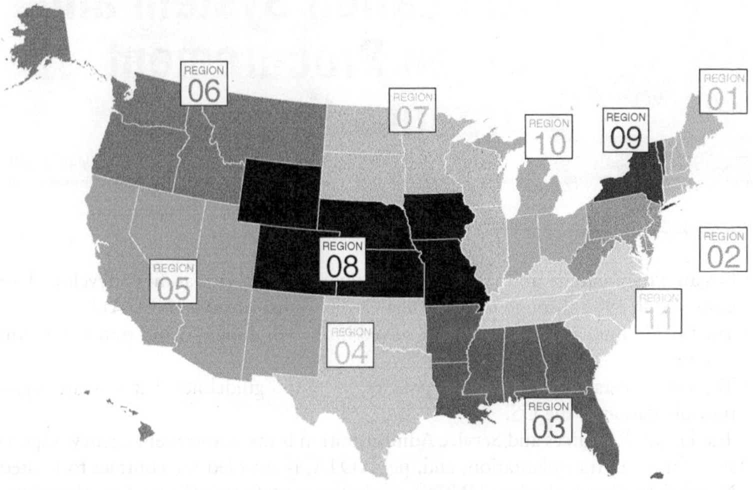

Figure 6-1. **The geographic boundaries of UNOS regions of the US.** (Reproduced from the Organ Procurement & Transplantation Network. Regions. Accessed April 12, 2023. Retrieved from https://optn.transplant.hrsa.gov/about/regions/.)

- If the offers are not accepted, then it will open to candidates beyond the 250 nautical mile distance (national offer).
- The policy change is projected to improve equity in the access of potential recipients nationwide.

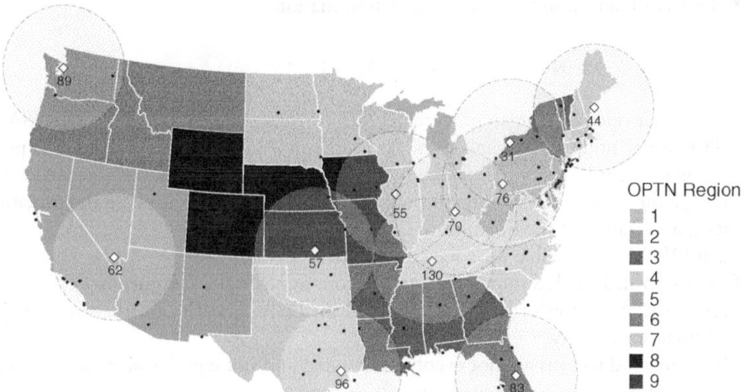

Figure 6-2. **An illustration of the 250-nautical mile circle that starts from the donor hospital.** (Reproduced from the Organ Procurement and Transplantation Network. Removal of DSA and Region from Kidney and Pancreas Distribution. Accessed April 12, 2023. Retrieved from https://optn.transplant.hrsa.gov/media/2802/kidney_pancreas_publiccomment_20190122.pdf.)

KIDNEY ALLOCATION SYSTEM

- The Kidney Allocation System (KAS) was introduced on December 4, 2014, in response to a high discard rate of kidneys and variability in the access of kidney transplant candidates.
- Each candidate receives a kidney allocation score, based on age, calculated panel reactive antibody (cPRA) score, waiting time, proximity to donor hospital, previous living donor, and HLA A, B, and DR matching.
- Each candidate also receives an estimated posttransplant survival (EPTS) score, based on age, current diabetes, history of a prior transplant, and dialysis.
- The EPTS score is a single number, ranging from 0 to 100, and represents the percentage of kidney candidates in the nation with a longer expected posttransplant survival time.
- The quality of the donor kidney is assessed by the Kidney Donor Profile Index (KDPI) and includes age, height/weight, ethnicity/race, hypertension history, diabetes history, cause of death, serum creatinine, hepatitis c status, and donation after circulatory death.
- The KDPI is a single number, ranging from 0% to 100%. It is based on 10 donor factors and estimates the potential risk of graft failure after a kidney transplant.
- A higher KDPI is associated with lower expected posttransplant longevity.
- **Figure 6-3**, from the OPTN, shows an analysis of data on kidney transplants from 2008 to 2018. Results showed that as the KDPI increased, there was a substantial decrease in the expected graft survival.[7]
- **Figure 6-4** from the OPTN shows the difference in expected longevity between low, medium, and high KDPI kidneys. The figure shows how deceased donor kidneys with a low KDPI (0%-20%) are expected to function for 11.5 years on average. On

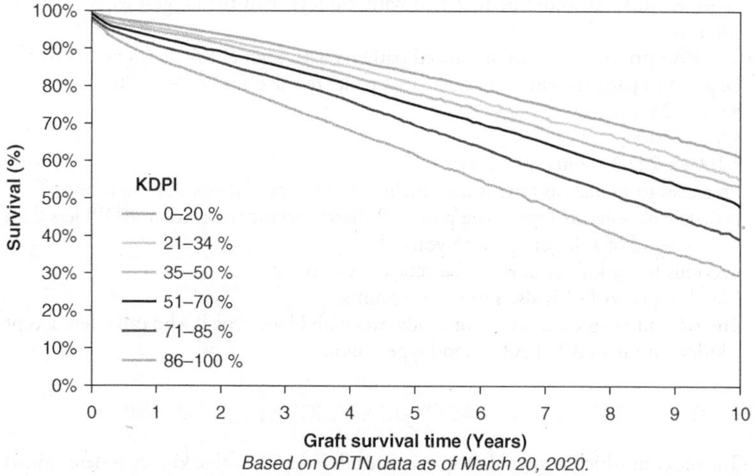

Figure 6-3. **Graft survival estimates of deceased donor kidney transplants between 2008 and 2018 according to Kidney Donor Profile Index (KDPI).** (Reproduced from Organ Procurement and Transplantation Network. A Guide to Calculating and Interpreting the Kidney Donor Profile Index. Accessed January 20, 2023. Retrieved from https://optn.transplant.hrsa.gov/media/1512/guide_to_calculating_interpreting_kdpi.pdf.)

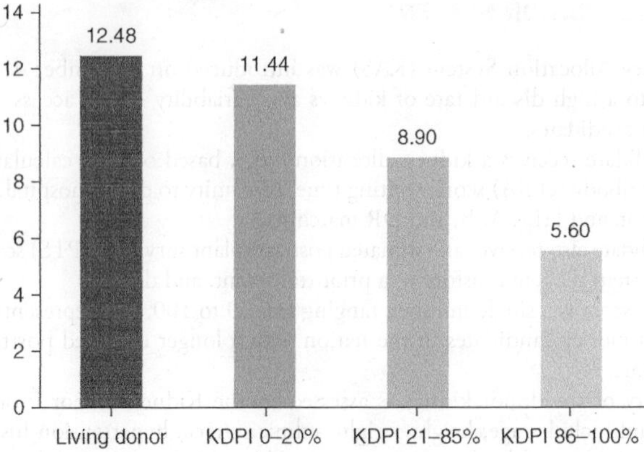

Figure 6-4. **Estimated kidney graft half-lives in years according to Kidney Donor Profile Index (KDPI).** (Reproduced from Organ Procurement and Transplantation Network. A Guide to Calculating and Interpreting the Kidney Donor Profile Index. Accessed January 20, 2023. Retrieved from https://optn.transplant.hrsa.gov/media/1512/guide_to_calculating_interpreting_kdpi.pdf.)

the other hand, kidneys with KDPI greater than 85% are expected to function for around 5.5 years.[7]

- The KAS promotes graft longevity by giving preference in matching kidneys with lower KDPI scores with recipients with lower EPTS scores. People with the longest expected survival would be matched with kidneys with the longest expected graft survival.
- The KAS prioritizes highly sensitized patients with high cPRA. Extra points would be given to patients with high calculated panel reactive antibodies (>20%):
  - 98%: 24.4 points
  - 99%: 50.1 points
  - 100%: 202.1 points
- Preregistration dialysis time is now included in the candidate's waiting time.
- Pediatric patients are given extra points. Pediatric priority is based on KDPI less than 35% instead of a donor age < 35 years old.
- Previous living kidney donors also receive extra points.
- Matching HLA DR is also given extra points.
- The KAS allows greater access for candidates with blood type B who can safely accept a kidney from an A2 or A2B blood type donor.

POINT SYSTEM FOR DECEASED DONOR KIDNEY ALLOCATION

- The order in which potential recipients are offered an available kidney is determined by a set algorithm.
- **Table 6-1** shows the point system used to rank potential kidney transplant recipients.[8]
- 0-A, B, and DR mismatch organs are part of a national mandatory sharing program if the recipient is highly sensitized.

TABLE 6-1 Point System for Ranking Potential Kidney Transplant Recipients

Factor	Points Awarded
Time waiting	1 for each year of waiting time. (1/365 per day)
Quality of HLA match	2 for zero DR mismatches
	1 for one DR mismatch
Degree of sensitization (cPRA)	0-202
Pediatric recipient	4—Pediatric candidate (age 0-10) with a zero-antigen mismatch offer
	3—Pediatric candidate (age 11-17) with a zero-antigen mismatch offer
Prior living organ donor	4
Proximity to donor hospital	0-4 depending on miles from donor hospital

cPRA, calculated panel reactive antibody; HLA, human leukocyte antigen.
Reproduced from Organ Procurement and Transplantation Network. OPTN Policies. https://optn.transplant.hrsa.gov/media/eavh5bf3/optn_policies.pdf.

- Medical judgment may be used by a patient's transplant physician to transplant a patient out of sequence due to medical urgency. The physician must contact other transplant programs within the DSA in order to arrive at an agreement to allocate the kidney out of sequence.[9]
- Expanded Criteria Donors (ECDs)
  - Term to describe the quality of a kidney. This term has already been discontinued. It was previously used to describe kidneys with the following characteristics:
    - From a deceased donor older than 60 years
    - From a deceased donor 50 to 59 years of age, with two of the following risk factors: history of hypertension, death as a result of cerebral vascular disease or elevated terminal creatinine >1.5.
  - The term *marginal kidney* is now preferred.
  - ECD was replaced with a more refined and continuous metric system: the Kidney Donor Profile Index or KDPI (see previous discussion).[9]
  - ECD kidneys are now similar to kidneys with KDPI scores ≥ 85%.

KIDNEY MATCH LIST

- The OPO generates a kidney match list.
- Kidneys must be allocated according to the multiorgan, liver-kidney, pancreas-kidney match list before offering a kidney to a single candidate.
- The match system eliminates candidates with an incompatible ABO blood type.
- Candidates are then ranked based on the allocation sequences found in the organ allocation policies.
- OPOs must first offer organs to potential transplant recipients (PTRs) in the order that the PTRs appear on a match run; the highest priority recipient receives the first organ offer.

- A transplant hospital has a total of 1 hour after receiving the **initial** organ offer notification to evaluate the deceased donor information and submit a provisional yes or an organ offer refusal.
- A transplant hospital has a total of 1 hour to accept or refuse a **primary** kidney offer; if the transplant hospital has already provided a provisional acceptance, then they have 30 minutes to accept or decline the kidney.
- The transplant hospital that received the offer for the candidate with higher priority on the waiting list will get to choose first which of the two kidneys it will receive (right vs. left).
- In candidates with 0-ABDR mismatch, cPRA > 99%, or a combined kidney and nonrenal organ transplant, the host OPO determines whether to offer the left or the right kidney.

DUAL KIDNEY ALLOCATION

- Both kidneys from donors with a KDPI > 35% and weight > 18 kg may be transplanted in the same candidate. Transplant centers must identify which candidates are willing to accept dual kidneys. Dual kidneys receive the lowest priority in the KDPI 35 to 85 sequence and the >85% sequence.
- In donors weighing <18 kg, both kidneys must be offered en bloc.
- The use of dual kidneys has been shown to improve survival.

TRENDS AFTER THE INTRODUCTION OF THE KAS[5]

- More patients with high cPRA are being transplanted. There was approximately a sixfold increase in transplantation for this group of patients.
- There is an increased number of transplants for younger patients.
- There is an increased number of transplants for African Americans.
- The discard rate of donor kidneys is 19%.
- More kidneys are shared across donor service area boundaries. There have been higher cold ischemia times, and higher rates of delayed graft function (DGF). The rate of DGF has increased from 25% to 29%.[8]
- A study analyzed the Scientific Registry of Transplant Recipients during the first 9 months of the implementation of the new KAS. Results showed a twofold increase in the number of kidneys imported from nonlocal OPOs. There was also an increase in the proportion of recipients with high cPRA ranging from 81% to 98% (12% vs. 8%). Furthermore, there was an increased cold ischemia time by a mean of 2 hours. Rates of DGF, however, were noted to be similar on adjusted analysis.[10]
- An early retrospective study in the East Coast showed that the new kidney allocation policy has led to an increase in KDPI of donors with longer cold ischemia time, and higher DGF rates. As a result, this has led to an increase in logistical and financial costs.[11]
- Our center conducted a retrospective, cross-sectional analysis of organ offers, kidney transplantation outcomes, and associated costs after the implementation of the new kidney allocation policy in March 2021. Results showed an increase in the percentage of imported kidneys from 14% to 60% ($P < .001$). There was also an increase in the percentage of DGF from 21% to 30% ($P < .05$), as well as an increase in the cold ischemia time from 15 to 20 hours ($P < .001$). The KDPI also increased from an

average of 40% to 50%. The percentage of KDPI ≥85% increased from 6% to 12% ($P < .001$). It was also noted that the number of organ offers significantly increased after the kidney allocation changes.[12]

REFERENCES

1. *History and NOTA.* Organ Procurement and Transplant Network. Accessed December 4, 2023. https://optn.transplant.hrsa.gov/about/history-nota/
2. *What Is the OPTN.* Accessed March 10, 2022. Optn.transplant.hrsa.gov
3. *Ethical Principles in the Allocation of Human Organs.* Organ Procurement and Transplant Network. Accessed December 4, 2023. https://optn.transplant.hrsa.gov/professionals/by-topic/ethical-considerations/ethical-principles-in-the-allocation-of-human-organs/
4. *OPTN Regional View.* UNOS. Accessed December 4, 2023. https://unos.org/community/regions/regional-review/
5. *New Kidney, Pancreas Allocation Policies in Effect.* 2021. Accessed December 4, 2023. https://optn.transplant.hrsa.gov/news/new-kidney-pancreas-allocation-policies-in-effect/
6. *Removal of DSA and Region from Kidney and Pancreas Distribution.* Organ Procurement and Transplant Network. Accessed December 4, 2023. https://slideplayer.com/slide/15638215/
7. *A Guide to Calculating and Interpreting the Kidney Donor Profile Index.* Accessed December 4, 2023. https://optn.transplant.hrsa.gov/media/1512/guide_to_calculating_interpreting_kdpi.pdf
8. *OPTN Policies Effective as of Mar 16 2023 [modify heart].* Organ Procurement and Transplant Network. Accessed December 4, 2023. https://optn.transplant.hrsa.gov/media/eavh5bf3/optn_policies.pdf
9. Mone T, Jandali R, Garimella P. Allocation of deceased donor kidneys. In: Danovitch GM, ed. *Handbook of Kidney Transplantation.* 6th ed. Lippincott Williams & Wilkins; 2017.
10. Puttarajappa C, Hariharan S, Zhang X, et al. Early effect of the circular model of kidney allocation in the United States. *J Am Soc Nephrol.* 2023;34(1):26-39.
11. Rohan VS, Pilch N, McGillicuddy J, et al. Early assessment of national kidney allocation policy change. *J Am Coll Surg.* 2022;234(4):565-70.
12. Alhamad T, Marklin G, Ji M, Rothweiler R, Chang SH, Wellen J. One-year experience with the new kidney allocation policy at a single center and an OPO in the midwestern United States. *Transpl Int.* 2022;35:10798.

7 The Art of Procurement

Abraham J. Matar and Ronald F. Parsons

GENERAL PRINCIPLES

- Deceased donors for a solid organ transplant are usually divided into two major categories: donation after brain death (DBD) and donation after cardiac death (DCD).
- DBD is defined based on neurological criteria, including the irreversible cessation of all clinical functions of the brain, including the brain stem.
- DCD is defined as a donor who has suffered a devastating and irreversible brain injury but does not meet formal neurological criteria for brain death. The donor is considered dead based on circulatory criteria after withdrawal of life support.
- Kidneys from DBD and DCD donors go through cold ischemia time after procurement. The likelihood of delayed graft function (DGF) increases with longer cold ischemia time.
- Kidneys from DCD donors go through warm ischemia time. The likelihood of DGF increases with longer warm ischemia time.
- Other differences between DBD and DCD kidneys are listed in **Table 7-1**.

EXPOSURE

Abdomen Exposure

- The abdomen is opened through a midline incision from xiphoid to the pubis symphysis (**Figure 7-1**).[1]
- Abdominal laparotomy incision can be extended to a cruciate incision at the level of the umbilicus, allowing greater exposure to the intraperitoneal contents.

Chest Exposure

- The chest is opened through a midline incision from sternal notch to the xiphoid.
- Sternotomy is performed to expose supradiaphragmatic inferior vena cava (IVC).

WARM DISSECTION

Distal Aortic Control

- A Cattell-Braasch maneuver (complete right medial visceral rotation) and Kocher maneuver (lateral mobilization of the duodenum) are performed to expose the intra-abdominal IVC and aorta.[2]
- The aorta is fully exposed to the level of the iliac bifurcation and encircled with two umbilical tapes proximal to the iliac bifurcation.
- The inferior mesenteric artery is identified and may be transected to improve exposure of the distal aorta.
- Identify inferior mesenteric vein (IMV) and isolate for future cannulation/perfusion.

TABLE 7-1 Comparison of Donation After Brain Death and Donation After Cardiac Death

	Donation After Brain Death	Donation After Cardiac Death
Diagnosis of death	Neurologic criteria	Circulatory criteria
% of deceased organ donors	~90% of all deceased organ donors	~10% of all decreased organ donors
Donor warm ischemia time	Absent or minimal	Present. Donor warm ischemia time cannot exceed 2 h
Kidney transplantation	Similar allograft and patient survival to DCD. Lower rate of DGF	Similar allograft and patient survival to DCD. Higher rate of DGF
Liver transplantation	Lower rate of graft failure and biliary complications	Higher rate of graft failure and biliary complications

DBD, donation after brain death; DCD, donation after cardiac death; DGF, delayed graft function.

Proximal Aortic Control

- If no planned procurement of heart or lungs, the left pleural cavity can be incised and the descending aorta can be identified and dissected for future cross-clamping.
- If planned procurement of heart or lungs, incise diaphragmatic fibers overlying the aorta to access and isolate the intra-abdominal supraceliac aorta.

Liver Mobilization and Portal Dissection

- The gastrohepatic ligament is incised, and the lesser omentum is entered and inspected.[3] Take note of replaced or accessory left hepatic artery arising from left gastric artery.
- The left triangular and coronary ligaments are incised.
- The portal triad is isolated by placing a finger through the foramen of Winslow. Take note of replaced or accessory right hepatic artery in the posterior portal hilum.
- The common bile duct (CBD) is identified and transected close to the duodenum.
- The gallbladder is incised and flushed with saline solution until the CBD is clear of bile.

Pancreas Mobilization

- The omentum is separated from the underlying transverse mesocolon along an avascular plane from the level of the duodenum to the spleen.[4]
- The pancreas is then dissected away from underlying retroperitoneal structures, along with the spleen.
- The duodenum is retracted cephalad and the superior mesenteric artery (SMA) is identified and encircled with a vessel loop.
- The SMA along with the superior mesenteric vein is transected, allowing the pancreas to be freed from the mesentery.

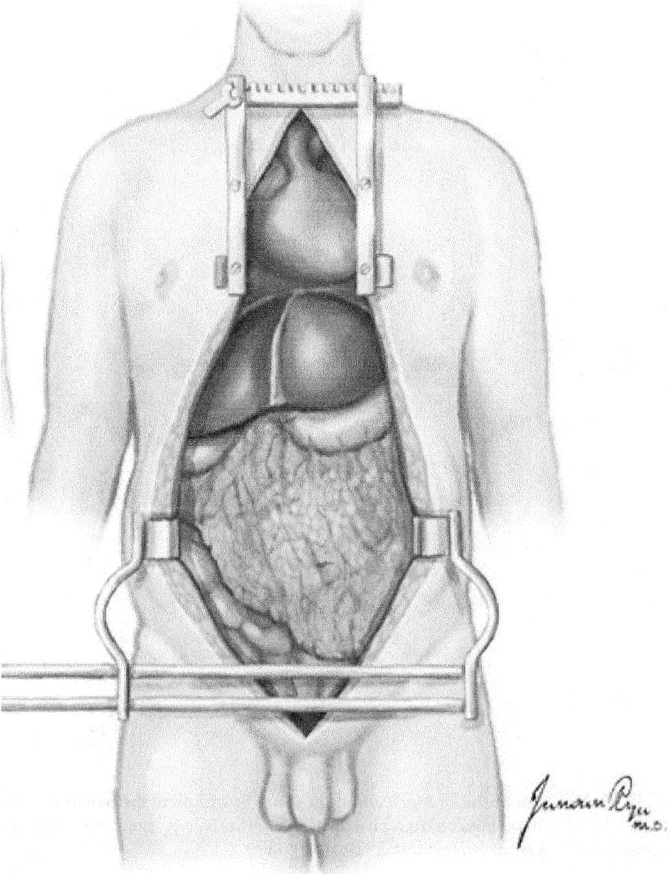

Figure 7-1. **The abdomen and chest exposure via a midline incision from sternal notch to the pubis symphysis exposing the thoracic and abdominal contents.** (Reproduced with permission from Hwang HP, Kim JM, Shin S, et al. Organ procurement in a deceased donor. *Korean J Transplant.* 2020;34:134-50.)

- The fourth portion of the duodenum and an area on the stomach proximal to the pylorus are selected for transection (**Figure 7-2**).

Perfusion

- 300 U/kg systemic heparin is administered and allowed to circulate for at least 3 minutes.
- Cannulas are inserted at the aortic bifurcation and the IMV, secured in place and connected to the tubing carrying preservation solution.
- Alternatively, the portal vein can be cannulated directly for portal flushing.

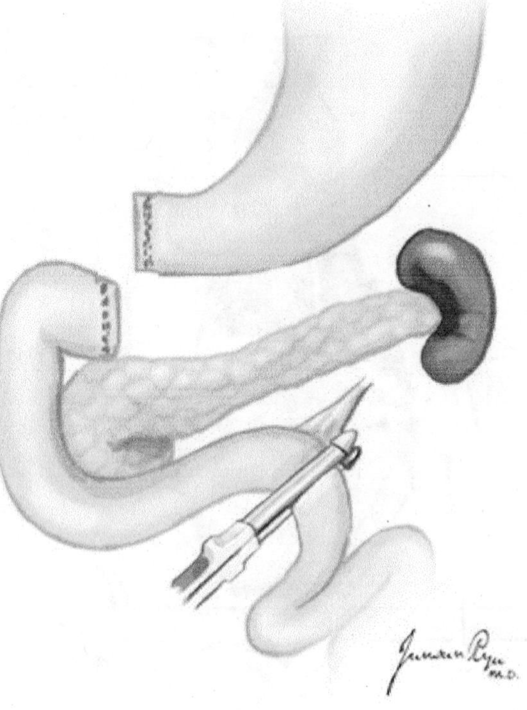

Figure 7-2. **Transection of the stomach and duodenum to complete the pancreas mobilization.** (Reproduced with permission from Hwang HP, Kim JM, Shin S, et al. Organ procurement in a deceased donor. *Korean J Transplant.* 2020;34:134-50.)

- Aorta is clamped, either at the intra-abdominal supraceliac location or in the chest.
- The intrapericardial suprahepatic IVC is transected to vent blood into the chest.
- Cold perfusate is infused via the aortic and IVC cannulas at 4 °C and the abdomen is packed with sterile ice.

COLD DISSECTION

- Following perfusion, the aorta is incised below the origin of the SMA and the orifice of the left and right renal arteries are identified.
- The aorta is transected proximal to the renal arteries, below the origin of the SMA.
- The liver is mobilized from its remaining inferior and lateral attachments as well as to the diaphragm.

- The supraceliac aorta is divided, followed by division of the infrahepatic IVC above the level of the renal veins.
- Portal structures are divided, and the liver, pancreas, duodenum, and spleen are removed en bloc.
- To procure the kidneys, the ureters are divided close to their insertion into the bladder.
  - The left renal vein can then be incised from the IVC.
  - Both the aorta and IVC are transected close to their bifurcation into the iliac vessels.
  - The ureters are then protected with clamps at the ends and not given unnecessary stretch as the dissection moves cranially from the pelvis.
  - The kidneys can be removed en bloc through division of the attachments along a plane on anterior to the psoas muscle, as well as from any superior and lateral attachments.
  - The kidneys can then be placed on ice for separating right and left.
  - The posterior aorta is divided in its midline ensuring an adequate aortic cuff for each renal artery.
  - The aorta is incised along the anterior aspect until the orifice of the left and right renal arteries is identified (**Figure 7-3**).
  - Some surgeons may remove the kidneys separately from the abdomen.
- Iliac vessels are harvested which may be required as vascular conduits during the recipient procedure, especially pancreas and/liver transplants.

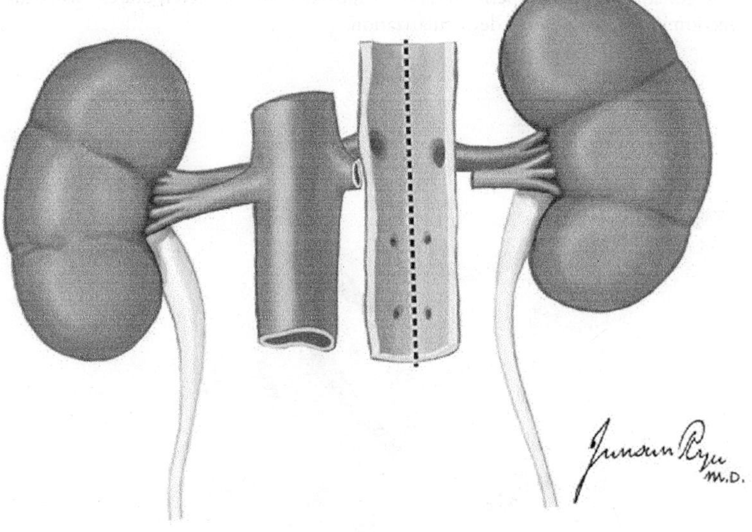

Figure 7-3. **The exposure of the aorta orifice of the left and right renal artery.** (Reproduced with permission from Hwang HP, Kim JM, Shin S, et al. Organ procurement in a deceased donor. *Korean J Transplant.* 2020;34:134-50.)

BACKTABLE PREPARATION

Pancreas Preparation

- The segment of donor duodenum is shortened.
- Donor spleen and retroperitoneal tissue are removed.
- Creation of Y-graft—The arterial supply via the donor superior mesenteric and splenic arteries is attached to a Y graft, usually the bifurcation of the donor common iliac artery in order to provide a single arterial inflow (**Figure 7-4**).

Liver Preparation

- The suprahepatic IVC is freed from is diaphragmatic attachments.
- Phrenic vein insertions are identified and ligated.
- The entire length of the IVC is then cleared of retroperitoneal connective tissue.
- The portal vein is cleared of peritoneal tissue until the bifurcation is exposed to simplify orientation of the portal vein during implantation.
- Arterial dissection begins at the celiac trunk proximally until the common hepatic is identified.
  - Once aberrant anatomy is excluded, branches along the celiac and common hepatic that terminate outside the liver are ligated, including the left gastric artery.
  - The aortic cuff is fashioned into a Carrel patch for implantation.

Kidney Preparation

- The kidney is cleared of its perinephric tissue, including the adrenal gland, but dissection is limited in the triangle of tissue near the ureter.
- Branches of the renal vein (gonadal, lumbar, and suprarenal) are ligated.
- The gonadal vein and superficial fat are removed from the ureter, but extensive dissection is avoided to limit devascularization.

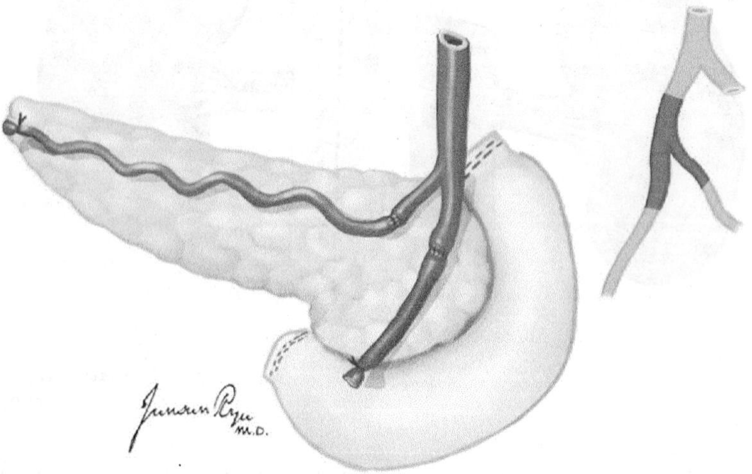

Figure 7-4. **Creation of superior mesenteric artery and splenic artery as a "Y-graft."** (Reproduced with permission from Hwang HP, Kim JM, Shin S, et al. Organ procurement in a deceased donor. *Korean J Transplant.* 2020;34:134-50.)

- The right renal vein may need a caval extension graft created to increase vein length.
- The aortic cuff is fashioned into a Carrel patch for implantation.
- Multiple arteries may be prepped for separate anastomoses or reconstructed for creation of a single anastomosis.

ORGAN PRESERVATION

Preservation Solutions

- University of Wisconsin (UW) solution with an osmolarity of 330 mOsm/L
  - It is considered the gold standard preservation solution
  - Osmotic concentration of UW solution is achieved through metabolically inert substances including lactobionic acid and raffinose.
  - It utilizes hydroxyethyl starch as a colloid carrier, oxygen radical scavengers, glutathione, allopurinol, and adenosine.
- Histidine-tryptophan-ketoglutarate solution with an osmolarity of 310 mOsm/L
  - It is originally developed as a cardioplegia solution.
  - It utilizes mannitol as both a colloid carrier and antioxidant, histidine as a buffer, and contains lower concentrations of Na^+, K^+, and Mg^{2+} compared to UW solution.
- Celsior solution with an osmolarity of 320 mOsm/L is a modified UW solution with a lower concentration of potassium and decreased viscosity due to elimination of hydroxyethyl starch.

Machine Preservation

- Hypothermic machine perfusion (HMP)
  - HMP provides a continuous flushing of kidney allograft with cold preservation solution to provide nutrients and minimize accumulation of lactic acid and toxic metabolites.
  - The measured parameters of HMP include perfusion pressure (25-30 mm Hg), perfusion flow (>0.4 mL/min/mm Hg), and renal resistance (<0.3 mm Hg/mL/min).[5]
  - Benefits of HMP preservation of renal allografts include the following:
    - Reduced rates of DGF.
    - Appraisal of organ quality based on pump parameters (i.e., machine measured real resistance).
    - Extension of cold ischemic time without additional damage to allograft.
- Normothermic machine perfusion (NMP)
  - NMP preserves the graft at near-physiological condition through perfusion of warm, oxygenated blood and supplied with nutrients.
  - NMP is shown to reduce early allograft dysfunction and ischemic biliary complications in liver transplantation compared to ischemic cold storage.[6]
  - NMP has the potential to serve as a platform for pharmacologic organ treatment and graft optimization.

REFERENCES

1. Hwang HP, Kim JM, Shin S, et al. Organ procurement in a deceased donor. *Korean J Transplant.* 2020;34(3):134-50.
2. Abu-Elmagd K, Fung J, Bueno J, et al. Logistics and technique for procurement of intestinal, pancreatic, and hepatic grafts from the same donor. *Ann Surg.* 2000;232(5):680-7.

3. Yersiz JFRa.H. The donor operation. In: Busuttil R, Klintmalm G, eds. *Transplantation of the Liver*. 3rd ed. Elsevier; 2015:Ch. 43.
4. Boggi U, Vistoli F, Del Chiaro M, et al. A simplified technique for the en bloc procurement of abdominal organs that is suitable for pancreas and small-bowel transplantation. *Surgery*. 2004;135(6):629-41.
5. Parikh CR, Hall IE, Bhangoo RS, et al. Associations of perfusate biomarkers and pump parameters with delayed graft function and deceased donor kidney allograft function. *Am J Transplant*. 2016;16(5):1526-39.
6. Dingfelder J, Rauter L, Berlakovich GA, Kollmann D. Biliary viability assessment and treatment options of biliary injury during normothermic liver perfusion—a systematic review. *Transpl Int*. 2022;35:10398. doi:10.3389/ti.2022.10398

8 Transplant Surgery and Surgical Complications

Jessica Lindemann, Jennifer Yu, and Jason R. Wellen

GENERAL PRINCIPLES

- Given the significant number of candidates on the transplant waiting list, living donation is an important means for increasing the donor pool and has become an integral part of the kidney transplant practice.
- The advantages of kidney transplantation from living donors are improved short- and long-term graft survival (1-year survival >95%), immediate allograft function, planned operative timing to allow for medical optimization, and, often, avoidance of dialysis.[1]
- Deceased donations are categorized into:
  - **Donation after brain death (DBD)**
    - To be qualified for DBD, donors have to meet strict criteria for brain death including irreversible coma and the absence of brain stem reflexes (i.e., pupillary, corneal, vestibulo-ocular, and gag reflexes).
    - Other useful diagnostic tests include blood flow scan, arteriography, and an apnea test.
  - **Donation after cardiac death (DCD)**
    - Potential organ donors that do not meet the strict brain death criteria are considered to have nonrecoverable devastating neurologic insults.
    - In DCD donors, life support is discontinued in the operating room, and organ procurement is initiated after a specified interval following cardiac asystole.
    - While effectively increasing the donor pool, 16% to 28% of DCD livers have biliary complications, including ischemic cholangiopathy.[2]
    - However, there is a growing body of evidence to suggest that in high volume centers and selected recipients, comparable outcomes can be achieved.[3]

SUITABILITY FOR ORGAN DONATION

- There are certain conditions where kidney donation is considered not appropriate such as TB and active cancer.
- Donors with localized infections such as urinary tract infections or pneumonia are routinely considered for donation.
- In the presence of bacteremia, a donation could still be appropriate with early initiation of antibiotic therapy.
- With the exception of primary central nervous system (CNS) tumors, active cancer, whether treated or not, is an absolute contraindication to organ donation.
- The blood-brain barrier protects CNS tumor cells from widespread dissemination in the heavily immunosuppressed patient.

Age

- As experience with marginal donors has grown, it has become apparent that arbitrary limits on donor age are unnecessary.

- Good allograft function has been achieved with kidney and liver donors with advanced age.
- We have accepted living donors who are more than 80 years old in Washington University Kidney Transplant Program.

Overall Health

- As the donor pool ages, systemic diseases that can affect specific organ function must be taken into consideration.
- Hypertension and diabetes can hinder the suitability of kidney allografts, while obesity with hepatic steatosis limits the suitability of liver allografts.

Social Behaviors

- All donors are tested for HIV, hepatitis, and other viral infections.
- Donors who engage in high-risk behaviors may still transmit an infection if donation were to occur within the window period prior to seroconversion.
- Potential recipients are counseled regarding socially high-risk donors and given the option of whether to consider organs allocated from this group.

RECIPIENT PROCEDURE

- In deceased donor kidneys, the kidney is removed from cold storage (either static or dynamic), and the graft is prepared on the back table by trimming excess soft tissue and ligating extraneous vein and arterial branches (**Figure 8-1**).[4]
- A Foley catheter is inserted, and the bladder is irrigated with antibiotic-containing solution, commonly gentamicin.
- A curvilinear paramedian (Gibson, "hockey-stick") incision is made in the right lower quadrant, and the SC fat is divided down to the external oblique fascia.
  - Fascia is incised, and the rectus muscle is mobilized from the posterior aspect of the rectus sheath.
  - At the lateral border of the rectus muscle, the retroperitoneal space is entered, and the lateral abdominal wall muscles are divided superiorly to develop the space further, while retracting the intraperitoneal contents medially.

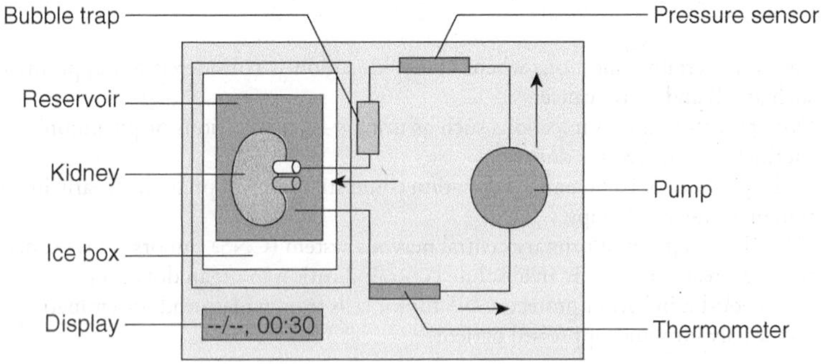

Figure 8-1. **Schematic representation of hypothermic machine perfusion in kidney transplantation.** (Reproduced with permission from O'Callaghan JM, Morgan RD, Knight SR Morris PJ. Systematic review and meta-analysis of hypothermic machine perfusion versus static cold storage of kidney allografts on transplant outcomes. *Br J Surg.* 2013;100:991-1001.)

    - The inferior epigastric vessels may be ligated and divided, or they may be retracted medially.
    - The spermatic cord should be retracted medially in males, and the round ligament can be ligated and divided in females.
- The recipient external iliac artery and vein are identified and isolated, resecting and/or ligating adherent surrounding lymphatic tissue.
- Caution in this area is critical to preserve as much lymphatic tissue and the crossing nerves (including the genitofemoral nerve along the medial edge of the psoas muscle).
- An end-to-side donor renal vein to recipient external iliac vein anastomosis is performed using nonabsorbable suture.
- The arterial anastomosis is created in a similar fashion, most often using a Carrel patch, which involves utilizing a cuff of donor aorta (**Figure 8-2**).[5]
- Mannitol and furosemide are administered intravenously prior to reperfusion. Care is taken to maintain the patient's systolic blood pressure (BP) above 120 mm Hg to ensure optimal perfusion of the transplanted kidney.
- The neoureterocystostomy is performed with imbrication of the bladder muscularis over the anastomosis to create an antireflux valve. Alternatively, the surgeon can anastomose the donor ureter to the recipient ipsilateral ureter. Both are fashioned over a double-J ureteral stent.

INTRAOPERATIVE CONSIDERATIONS

- Vascular assessment—Critical importance should be placed on preoperative evaluation of the quality of the patient's vasculature, with particular focus on the aortoiliac system.
- Advanced atherosclerotic disease may increase the patient's risk of arterial dissection during the transplant.
- Major atherosclerotic disease or symptomatic peripheral vascular disease may preclude transplant entirely.
- Left-sided placement may also be utilized for first-time kidney transplants based on surgeon preference or anatomical concerns, or more commonly for subsequent transplants.
- Intra-abdominal placement is necessitated if the patient has had two or more prior transplants with transplant kidneys still in place.
- Vascular anastomoses can be performed to the vena cava and either common iliac artery, and ureteral anastomosis is performed to the dome of the bladder.
- Ureteral anastomosis is most commonly performed via neoureterocystostomy as noted above. It can also be performed via ureteroureterostomy between the transplant and the native ureters.
- The ureter is spatulated to decrease the risk of stricture, and absorbable sutures are used to construct the anastomosis to avoid stone formation.

POSTOPERATIVE CONSIDERATIONS

IV Fluid Replacement

- Patients should be kept euvolemic or mildly hypervolemic in the early posttransplantation period with a goal of 120 mm Hg systolic BP to ensure adequate perfusion to the new allograft.
- Hourly urine output is usually replaced with one-half normal saline on a milliliter-for-milliliter basis.

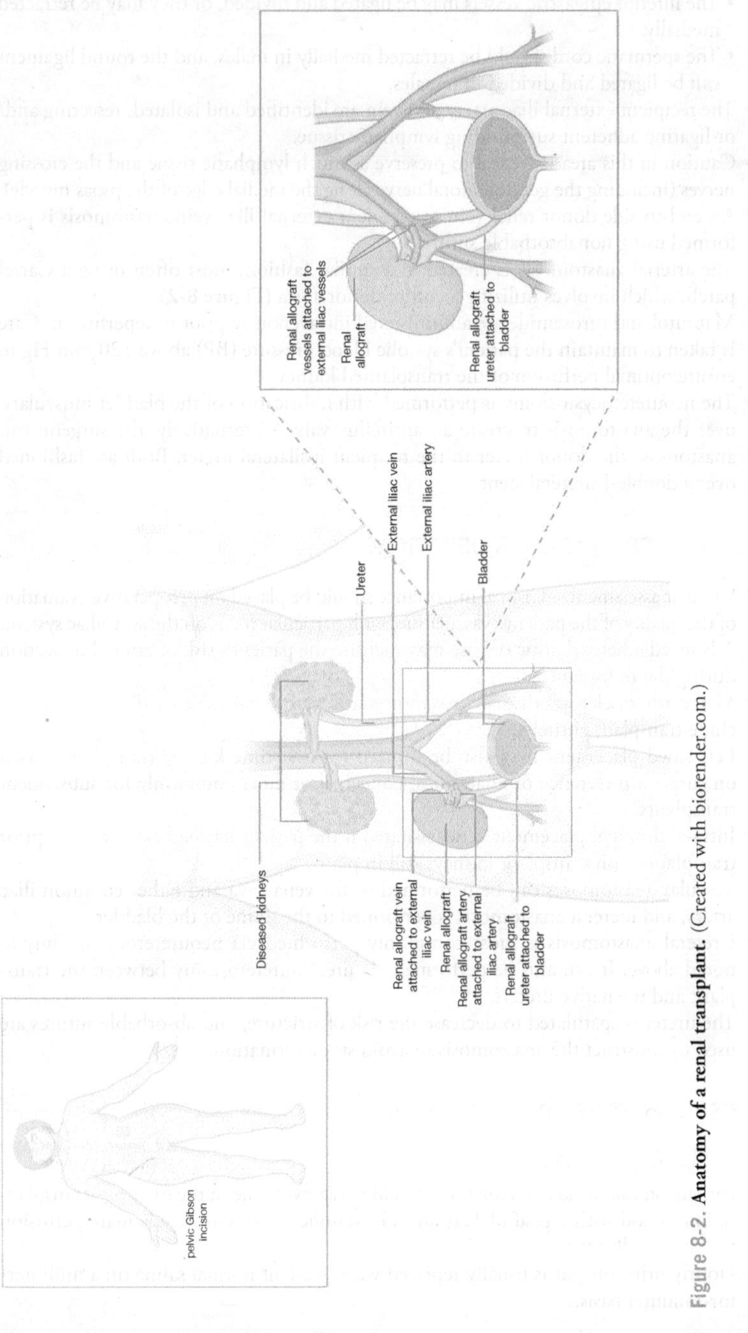

Figure 8-2. Anatomy of a renal transplant (Created with biorender.com.)

Renal Allograft Function or Nonfunction

- If the patient's urine output is low in the early postoperative period (<50 mL/h), perfusion to the new allograft must be assessed.
- After adequate volume resuscitation, low-dose (≤5 mg/h) dopamine infusion may be added to augment vasomotor tone and perfusion pressure.
- Early poor function of a transplanted kidney is most commonly due to reversible acute tubular necrosis (ATN) secondary to reperfusion injury.
- Before the diagnosis of ATN can be made, noninvasive studies (renal Doppler ultrasonography [US] or technetium-99m renal scan) demonstrating vascular patency and good renal blood flow in the absence of hydronephrosis or urinary leak must be obtained.
- If adequate renal blood flow is confirmed, dialysis can be continued until allograft function recovers.

SURGICAL COMPLICATIONS

A summary of the surgical complications is listed in **Table 8-1**.[6-8]

Lymphoceles

- Collections due to lymphatic leaks in the retroperitoneum.
- Present one to several weeks after transplantation.
- Generally asymptomatic and identified incidentally
- Diagnosis is done by ultrasound
- Treatment is indicated for symptomatic lymphoceles
- Treatment is done by drainage into the peritoneum, via laparoscopic, or open methods.

Renal Artery and Vein Thrombosis

- Arterial and venous thromboses most often occur in the first 1 to 3 days after transplantation.
- Signs and symptoms: Sudden cessation of urine output, rapid rise in serum creatinine, graft swelling, and local pain.
- Diagnosis: Technetium-99m renal scan or Doppler US.
- Treatment: Immediate operative exploration and repair to prevent graft loss.

Urine Leak

- Generally due to anastomotic leak or ureteral sloughing secondary to ureteral blood supply disruption.
- Signs and symptoms: pain, rising creatinine, and possibly urine draining from the wound.
- Diagnosis: Renal scan demonstrates radioisotope outside the urinary tract.
- Treatment: Placement of a bladder catheter to reduce intravesical pressure and subsequent surgical exploration.

TRANSPLANT NEPHRECTOMY

- Removal of the transplant kidney is a rare consequence but may be required in the setting of acute nonsalvageable graft thrombosis, chronic rejection with persistent clinical symptoms, recurrent infection, and cancer in the transplant kidney.

TABLE 8-1 Postoperative Complications Following Kidney Transplant[6-8]

Complication	Frequency	Key Points
Renal vein thrombosis	0.1%-5%	• Usually occurs within the first week after transplant • Frequently leads to graft loss and need for nephrectomy
Renal artery thrombosis	0.1%-3%	
Renal artery stenosis	2%-10%	• More common in deceased donor grafts • May be asymptomatic or present with new or progressive hypertension
Ureteral obstruction	3%-8%	• Lasix renal scan is a diagnostic exam of choice • Consider cystoscopic stent placement vs. percutaneous nephrostomy tube
Urinary leak	1%-5%	• Requires urinary catheter replacement for bladder decompression • Renal scan will demonstrate radiotracer outside of the urinary tract
Lymphocele	2%-40%	• Percutaneous drainage and lymphangiogram with sclerotherapy if amenable vs. surgical intervention (e.g. open or laparoscopic peritoneal window creation)
Surgical site infection	4%-20%	• Associated with higher body mass index (>30), diabetes, and return to operation room during index admission • Most commonly gram-positive organisms

Data from Eufrásio P, Parado B, Moreira P, et al. Surgical complications in 2000 renal transplants. *Transplant Proc.* 2011;43:142-4; Reyna-Sepúlveda F, Ponce-Escobedo A, Guevara-Charles A, et al. Outcomes and surgical complications in kidney transplantation. *Int J Organ Transplant Med.* 2017;8:78-84; and Kayler L, Kang D, Molmenti E, et al. Kidney transplant ureteroneocystostomy techniques and complications: review of the literature. *Transplant Proc.* 2010;42:1413-20.

- Transplant nephrectomy should only be performed by experienced surgeons given the high morbidity of the procedure and increased risk of uncontrolled devastating hemorrhage.
- In the early posttransplant period, the graft may be removed more easily through identification and isolation of the transplant renal vessels and ligation of this vasculature.

- Later (months to years) removal of the transplant kidney is generally performed in the subcapsular space given the intense retroperitoneal scarring that usually occurs after the initial transplant, making it more difficult to separate the kidney from the surrounding tissues.
- The renal parenchyma is bluntly dissected free from the capsule and isolated on the renal pedicle, in which it is frequently impossible to discern individual vessels. The pedicle is clamped en masse, and the external iliac artery is checked to ensure that the iliac vasculature has not been inadvertently caught in the clamp.
- The kidney tissue is then resected, and the vascular pedicle is oversewn with permanent suture. The ureter is identified and tracked to the bladder, and the ureter should be ligated as well.

PANCREAS TRANSPLANTATION

Indications

- Most patients who are evaluated for a pancreas transplant in conjunction with kidney transplantation are patients with type I diabetes who have concomitant nephropathy.
- Ninety-five percent of all pancreas transplants are performed in conjunction with renal transplant.[9]

Graft Selection

- **Simultaneous kidney-pancreas transplantation** is considered in insulin-dependent diabetic patients who are dialysis dependent (or imminent) and have a creatinine clearance <30 mL/min.
- **Pancreas after kidney transplantation**—Patients with living kidney donors can be listed separately for deceased pancreas transplantation.
- **Pancreas alone transplantation is** reserved for with severe diabetes with life-threatening hypoglycemic episodes.

Recipient Operation

- The most widely accepted technique uses whole-organ pancreas with venous drainage into the systemic circulation and enteric exocrine drainage, although there is wide variation across transplant centers (**Figure 8-3**).[10]
- The pancreas transplant is typically placed in the right paracolic gutter, and if simultaneous kidney transplantation is performed, it can be done on either the left or the right side.
- A midline laparotomy incision is made, and a right medial visceral rotation is performed. The right colon is reflected superiorly and medially, and the distal vena cava and aorta are identified and dissected free from surrounding tissues.
- The right common iliac artery and vein are similarly identified and isolated.
- The donor portal vein is anastomosed to the recipient vena cava or common iliac vein in an end-to-side fashion.
- The donor splenic artery and superior mesenteric artery are reconstructed on the back table with a donor iliac artery Y-bifurcation autograft and anastomosed in an end-to-side fashion to the right common iliac artery.
- The second portion of the duodenum is used to create a duodenojejunostomy. Alternatively, the duodenal segment can be anastomosed to the bladder.

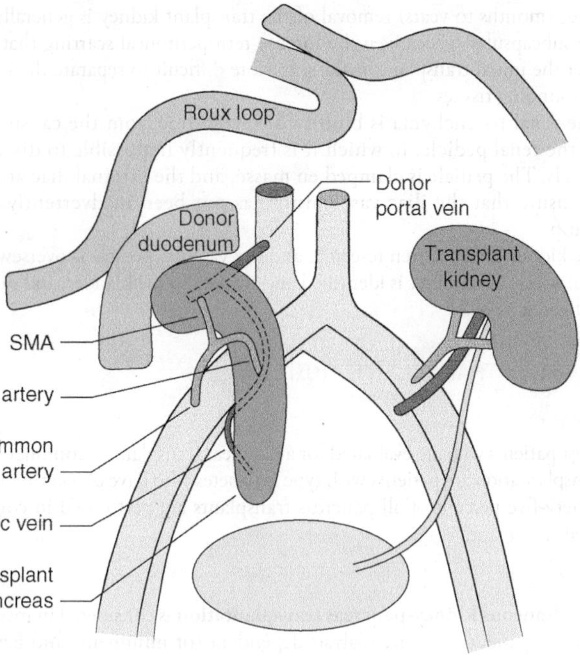

Figure 8-3. **Anatomy of a simultaneous kidney-pancreas transplant.** SMA, superior mesenteric artery. (Reproduced with permission from Hampson FA, Freeman SJ, Ertner J, Drage M, Butler A, Watson CJ, Shaw AS. Pancreatic trans plantation: surgical technique, normal radiological appearances and complications. *Insights Imaging*. 2010;1(5-6):339-47.)

Postoperative Considerations

Serum Glucose

- Followed closely during and after transplantation, usually checked every hour for the first 24 hours and then in decreasing frequency if appropriate.
- IV insulin infusions can generally be stopped intraoperatively or within the first few hours after pancreas transplantation.
- Serum glucose is expected to normalize almost immediately after the pancreas graft is reperfused, often with normal or near-normal glucose levels by the conclusion of the surgical procedure.
- Posttransplant elevations may indicate graft failure and should be investigated immediately.

Graft-Related Complications

- Graft thrombosis is the most common complication.
- Metabolic acidosis and dehydration due to loss of sodium and bicarbonate into the urine from the transplanted duodenum.
- Other common complications include pancreatitis, urinary tract infections, urethritis, and anastomotic leak from the duodenocystostomy.
- A summary of complications is listed in **Table 8-2.**[10-12]

TABLE 8-2 Postoperative Complications Following Pancreas Transplant[10-12]

Complication	Frequency	Key Points
Pancreatitis	10%-30%	• May range from asymptomatic to abdominal/pelvic pain, nausea, fever • Characterized by high amylase levels and graft edema on imaging • Can lead to abscess, pseudocyst, fistula, or pseudoaneurysm formation
Postoperative hemorrhage/hematoma	5%-15%	• Generally due to bleeding from site of mesenteric vessel ligation at the edge of the graft • Surgical re-exploration, if necessary, is often able to preserve graft
Graft thrombosis	2%-20%	• Most common cause of early graft failure • May see acute hyperglycemia • Venous thrombosis much more common than arterial thrombosis • Diagnosis by graft Doppler ultrasound or contrasted CT • Usually requires graft pancreatectomy though salvage may be possible with urgent percutaneous thrombectomy
Exocrine drainage issues	5%-30%	• Initial enteric drainage may be associated with higher intra-abdominal infection rates due to duodenal stump leak • Metabolic derangements or urologic symptoms/infections may require relaparotomy and conversion from bladder drainage to enteric drainage
Acute rejection	7%-25%	• Primary cause of graft loss within the first year after transplant • Doppler US helpful to rule out vascular causes of graft dysfunction • Requires tissue diagnosis, generally via percutaneous core biopsy
Posttransplant lymphoproliferative disorder	3%-12%	• Associated with higher levels of immunosuppression required in pancreatic transplant and donor-acquired EBV infection • Tissue diagnosis essential for treatment planning (i.e., decreased immunosuppression, chemotherapy)

CT, computed tomography; EBV, Epstein-Barr virus; US, ultrasound.
Data from Hampson FA, Freeman SJ, Ertner J, et al. Pancreatic transplantation: surgical technique, normal radiological appearances and complications. *Insights Imaging.* 2010;1:339-47; Dholakia S, Oskrochi Y, Easton G, Papalois V. Advances in pancreas transplantation. *J R Soc Med.* 2016;109:141-6; and Humar A, Kandaswamy R, Granger D, Gruessner RW, Gruessner AC, Sutherland DE. Decreased surgical risks of pancreas transplantation in the modern era. *Ann Surg.* 2000;231:269-75.

REFERENCES

1. Poggio ED, Augustine JJ, Arrigain S, Brennan DC, Schold JD. Long-term kidney transplant graft survival—making progress when most needed. *Am J Transplant.* 2021;21(8):2824-32.
2. Mourad MM, Algarni A, Liossis C, Bramhall SR. Aetiology and risk factors of ischaemic cholangiopathy after liver transplantation. *World J Gastroenterol.* 2014;20:6159-69.
3. Kollmann D, Sapisochin G, Goldaracena N, et al. Expanding the donor pool: donation after circulatory death and living liver donation do not compromise the results of liver transplantation. *Liver Transpl.* 2018;24(6):779-89.
4. O'Callaghan JM, Morgan RD, Knight SR, Morris PJ. Systematic review and meta-analysis of hypothermic machine perfusion versus static cold storage of kidney allografts on transplant outcomes. *Br J Surg.* 2013;100(8):991-1001.
5. Freise CE, Stock PG, Renal Transplantation. *Greenfield's Surgery: Scientific Principles and Practice.* Lippincott Williams and Wilkins; 2017.
6. Eufrásio P, Parada B, Moreira P, et al. Surgical complications in 2000 renal transplants. *Transplant Proc.* 2011;43(1):142-4.
7. Reyna-Sepúlveda F, Ponce-Escobedo A, Guevara-Charles A, et al. Outcomes and surgical complications in kidney transplantation. *Int J Organ Transplant Med.* 2017;8(2):78-84.
8. Kayler L, Kang D, Molmenti E, Howard R. Kidney transplant ureteroneocystostomy techniques and complications: review of the literature. *Transplant Proc.* 2010;42(5):1413-20.
9. Jiang AT, Rowe N, Rowe N, Sener A, Luke P. Simultaneous pancreas-kidney transplantation: the role in the treatment of type 1 diabetes and end-stage renal disease. *Can Urol Assoc J.* 2014;8(3-4):135-8.
10. Hampson FA, Freeman SJ, Ertner J, et al. Pancreatic transplantation: surgical technique, normal radiological appearances and complications. *Insights Imaging.* 2010;1(5-6):339-47.
11. Dholakia S, Oskrochi Y, Easton G, Papalois V. Advances in pancreas transplantation. *J R Soc Med.* 2016;109(4):141-6.
12. Humar A, Kandaswamy R, Granger D, Gruessner RW, Gruessner AC, Sutherland DE. Decreased surgical risks of pancreas transplantation in the modern era. *Ann Surg.* 2000;231(2):269-75.

9 Induction Therapy

Nicole Nesselhauf

GENERAL PRINCIPLES

- The goal of induction therapy is to avoid early acute rejection.
- Induction therapy is given prior to reperfusion and up to 1 week after transplant.
- Choice of therapy varies based on patient-specific factors, risks and benefit profile, and transplant center (**Table 9-1**).
- Induction immunosuppressive trends have changed over the years with more potent maintenance immunosuppression and availability of agents (**Figure 9-1**).
- In the early 1990s, most patients received no induction therapy and others received OKT3 (now off the market). Presently, only a small portion of patients receive no induction therapy (~less than 20%)[1] (**Figure 9-2**).
- Basiliximab use has increased in the late 1990s to 2000s and now remains around 20% of the US induction choice.[1]
- Rabbit antithymocyte globulin's (rATG) use has increased and continues to increase to about 50% of patients receiving rATG for induction immunosuppression.[2]

T-CELL-DEPLETING THERAPY

Anti-Thymocyte Globulin

- Equine antithymocyte globulin (eATG) was approved by the Food and Drug Administration (FDA) in 1981 for treatment of acute cellular rejection (ACR). At that time, it was also being used off label for induction immunosuppression for kidney transplant.[3]
- rATG was FDA approved in 1998 for treatment of ACR and 2017 for induction for kidney transplant.[4]
- eATG and rATG are prepared by immunizing horses or rabbits with human lymphoid tissue (thymocytes). The animal serum is harvested and immunoglobulins against T-cell surface markers are purified.[5]
- Antithymocyte globulin (ATG) has several mechanisms for causing lymphocyte depletion. It targets a broad range of T-cell surface antigens including CD2, CD3, CD4, CD5, CD8, CD28, CD45, and CD154. It causes T-cell depletion via complement-dependent lysis in the thymus and spleen as well as peripherally. It has action on natural killer (NK) cells (CD16 and CD56) and B cells (CD20) (**Figure 9-3**).
- ATG can cause opsonization and phagocytosis by macrophages and immunomodulation leading to long-term depletion via apoptosis and antibody-dependent T-cell-mediated cytotoxicity.
- ATG T-cell depletion occurs within 24 hours of administration and can last up to 6 months to 1 year.
- eATG is rarely used due to its lack of efficacy and side effect profile (see Induction Data below). eATG is dosed 15 mg/kg IV in operating room (OR) prior to

TABLE 9-1 Currently Available Options for Induction Immunosuppression for Kidney Transplantation

Induction Immunosuppression	
Monoclonal Antibodies • Basiliximab (Simulect) • Alemtuzumab (Campath)	T-Cell-Depleting Therapy • Alemtuzumab (Campath) • Equine antithymocyte globulin (Atgam) • Rabbit antithymocyte globulin (Thymoglobulin)
Polyclonal Antibodies • Equine antithymocyte globulin (Atgam) • Rabbit antithymocyte globulin (Thymoglobulin)	Non-T-Cell-Depleting Therapy • Basiliximab (Simulect)

reperfusion and for total of 3 to 14 days. It requires premedication and a skin test for hypersensitivity rejections prior to administration. It is given via central line only over 4 to 6 hours.[3]

- rATG is more commonly used for kidney transplant induction. It has several varying dosing strategies among transplant centers. FDA approval dosing is 1.5 mg/kg/d for 4 to 7 days. First dose is given in the OR prior to kidney reperfusion.[4]
- Premedication with acetaminophen, diphenhydramine, corticosteroid, and ± 5-HT3 antagonist have been shown to decrease infusion-related reactions.
- rATG is given via central or peripheral line over a minimum of 6 hours. Peripheral line rATG has heparin 1,000 units and hydrocortisone 20 mg added to the bag to help decrease incidence of phlebitis.[5]
- Bone marrow suppression with leukopenia (49%-57%) and thrombocytopenia (29%-37%) requires dose adjustments. Thrombocytopenia is thought to be caused by antiplatelet antibodies that cause cross reactivity of antibodies to nonlymphoid cells.[4]
  - Half the dose if white blood cells (WBCs) 2 to 3 or platelets 50 to 75.
  - Hold dose if WBC <2 or platelets <50.

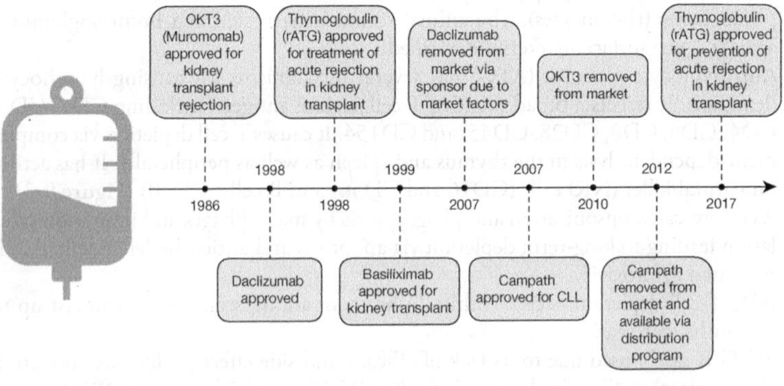

Figure 9-1. **Timeline of induction immunosuppression agents approved in the US used for prevention of rejection in kidney transplantation.**

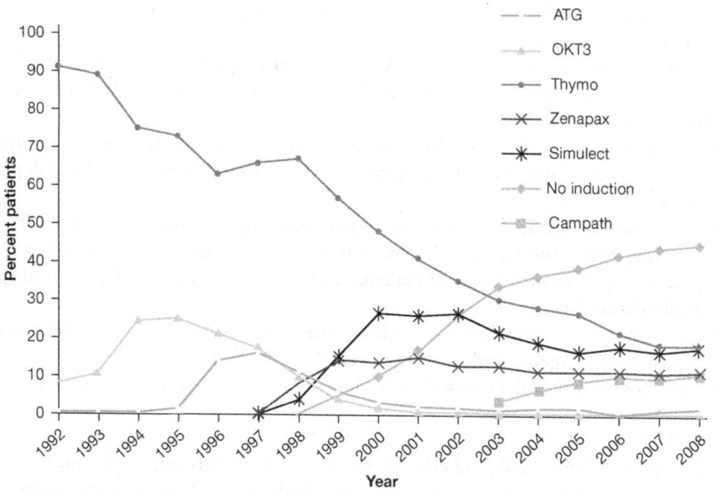

Figure 9-2. **Kidney induction therapy trends 1992–2008.** (Reproduced from Hardinger KL, Brennan DC, Kelin CL. Selection of induction therapy in kidney transplantation. *Transpl Int.* 2013;26:662-72.

- ATG can cause cytokine release syndrome (CRS) that can present as mild flu-like symptoms to severe shock reactions. This can include fever, chills, headache, nausea, diarrhea, pain, and pulmonary edema. This reaction is mediated by the production of tumor necrosis factor-α and production of interleukin (IL) 6. Management of CRS can include using premedications and slowing or stopping infusion rate.

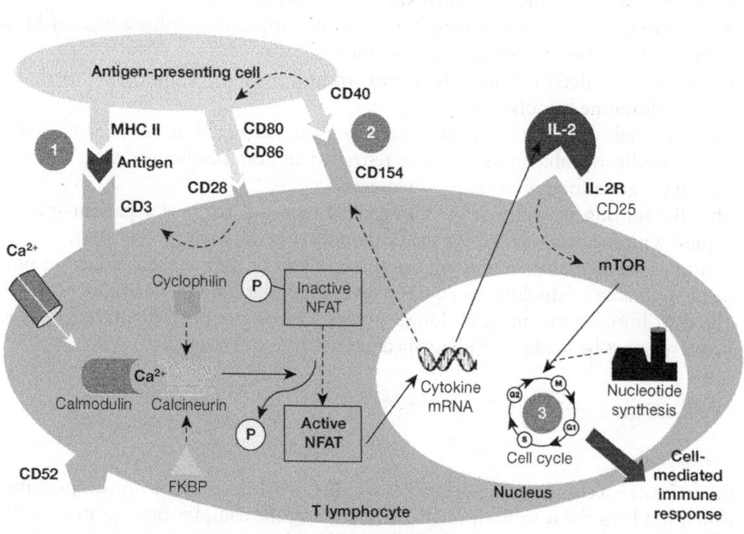

Figure 9-3. **Site of action for various induction immunosuppressions.**

- ATG can increase the risk of infection causing cytomegalovirus, herpes simplex virus, and other infections.
- A less common adverse reaction to ATG is serum sickness. It is reported in 7% to 27% of kidney transplants that receive ATG induction. Onset can be 7 to 14 days after administration of ATG.[5]
  - Serum sickness is caused by ATG (antigen) causes an antibody response resulting in activation of complement and formation of immune complexes that can deposit in tissues.
  - Serum sickness causes fever, arthralgias, lymphadenopathy, and rash. Usually affects multiple large joints (rarely the spine or temporomandibular joint). Presents as jaw pain with polyarthralgia's in all patients. Diagnosis supported by detection of IgG antibodies to horse or rabbit.
  - Risk factors of serum sickness included greater levels of heterologous protein, prior exposure to antigen (horse or rabbit), raised or ingested.
  - Treatment of serum sickness with high-dose steroids with or without plasmapheresis.

Alemtuzumab

- Alemtuzumab binds to CD52 cell surface glycoprotein on B and T cells, monocytes, macrophages, and NK cells to cause antibody-dependent and complement-dependent cell lysis.[6] See **Figure 9-3**.
- Alemtuzumab causes profound depletion of lymphocytes for up to 1 year. This is likely due to the CD52 antigen being one of the most abundant antigens presented on lymphocytes.
- Alemtuzumab is dosed in the OR prior to reperfusion at 30 mg IV for one dose. It can be given via central or peripheral line over 2 hours. It cannot be given via bolus or push.
- Premedications with acetaminophen, diphenhydramine, corticosteroid, and ±5-HT3 antagonist have been shown to decrease infusion-related reactions. Overall, it has less infusion-related side effects compared to ATG products.
- Alemtuzumab can cause profound bone marrow suppression. It has a high incident of neutropenia, thrombocytopenia, and anemia.
- Other adverse effects can include nausea, vomiting, diarrhea, headache, dizziness, and autoimmune hemolytic anemia.
- Alemtuzumab (Campath) was removed from the market in 2012. It is no longer commercially available in the US. It is restricted and can be obtained via a distribution in program for appropriate use patients.
- The distribution program is via Clinigen Direct and requires a patient-specific request with medical review. The medication usually ships within 24 hours.[7]
- Transplant centers that were using Campath as part of their regular induction protocol were able to disclose average use and stock that amount for induction use. The distribution program is no longer accepting new protocols for induction use. Requests must be made on patient-specific basis.

NON-T-CELL-DEPLETING THERAPY

Basiliximab

- Basiliximab is a chimeric monoclonal antibody (70% human, 30% murine proteins) which binds to the α subunit of IL-2/CD25 receptor complex on activated T-cells and inhibits IL-2 from binding and IL-2-mediated activation of lymphocytes.[8]

- Basiliximab prevents the T-cell activation and proliferation (signal 3) (**Figure 9-3**).
- Basiliximab was FDA approved in 1998 for prevention of acute rejection in kidney transplant.
- Dose used for renal transplant is 20 mg in OR prior to reperfusion and 20 mg IV postoperative day (POD) four. Basiliximab can be given via central or peripheral IV over 30 minutes. No premedications are required.
- Basiliximab has a limited side effect profile. Most commonly reported side effects include abdominal pain, vomiting, hyperglycemia, dizziness, and dyspnea. Hypersensitivity reactions, anaphylaxis can occur, but are rare.
- Overall, basiliximab is well tolerated with minimal side effects.
- KDIGO guidelines recommend basiliximab as the first-line therapy for induction immunosuppression for kidney transplant. This excludes those at higher immunologic risk.[9]

INDUCTION DATA

Equine Versus Rabbit Antithymocyte Globulin

- A randomized double blinded prospective trial of eATG versus rATG of adult kidney transplant recipient. Patients were randomized in a 2:1 fashion to rATG to eATG.[10]
- rATG group received 1.5 mg/kg/d for at least 7 days and eATG group received 15 mg/kg/d for at least 7 days.
  - Maintenance immunosuppression consisted of modified cyclosporine 4 mg/kg po bid dose adjusted on trough goals: months 0 to 3: 300 to 400 ng/mL; after month 3: 150 to 300 ng/mL.
  - Azathioprine at 5 mg/kg/d IV intraoperatively, then orally for 2 days, then at 2.5 mg/kg/d orally with adjustments for leukopenia.
  - Methylprednisolone at 7 mg/kg in OR, then prednisone 1 mg/kg/d orally, tapered over 9 months to .1 mg/kg/d.
- Primary endpoint of rate of rejection at 6 and 12 months. There were lower rejection rates in the rATG versus eATG at both 6 and 12 months, respectively, 2/48 (4%) versus 4/24 (17%) ($P = .038$) and 2/48 (4%) versus 6/24 (25%) ($P = .014$).[10]
- Patient survival was superior in rATG versus eATG, 98% versus 83% ($P = .02$) (**Figure 9-4**).[10]
- Event-free survival, defined as freedom from rejection, death, and allograft loss, was superior with rATG compared with eATG ($P = .0005$).[10]

Induction Versus No Induction

- A randomized, open-label, prospective, multicenter parallel-group study randomized kidney transplant recipients 1:1 to induction with rATG ($n = 151$) versus no induction ($n = 158$) with tacrolimus-based maintenance immunosuppression.[11]
  - rATG group received 1.5 mg/kg/d × 10 days (15 mg/kg total). Both groups had FK trough goals of day 1 to 42: 10 to 15 ng/mL; day 43 to 90: 5 to 10 ng/mL; day 91+: <10 ng/mL.
  - Steroid tapered to 5 mg/d at 3 months.
  - Azathioprine 1 to 2 mg/kg/d starting on POD 0.
- Primary endpoint was number of first biopsy-confirmed acuter rejection episodes (Banff 93). BPAR occurred in 15.2 % versus 30.4% of rATG versus no induction ($P = .002$).[11]

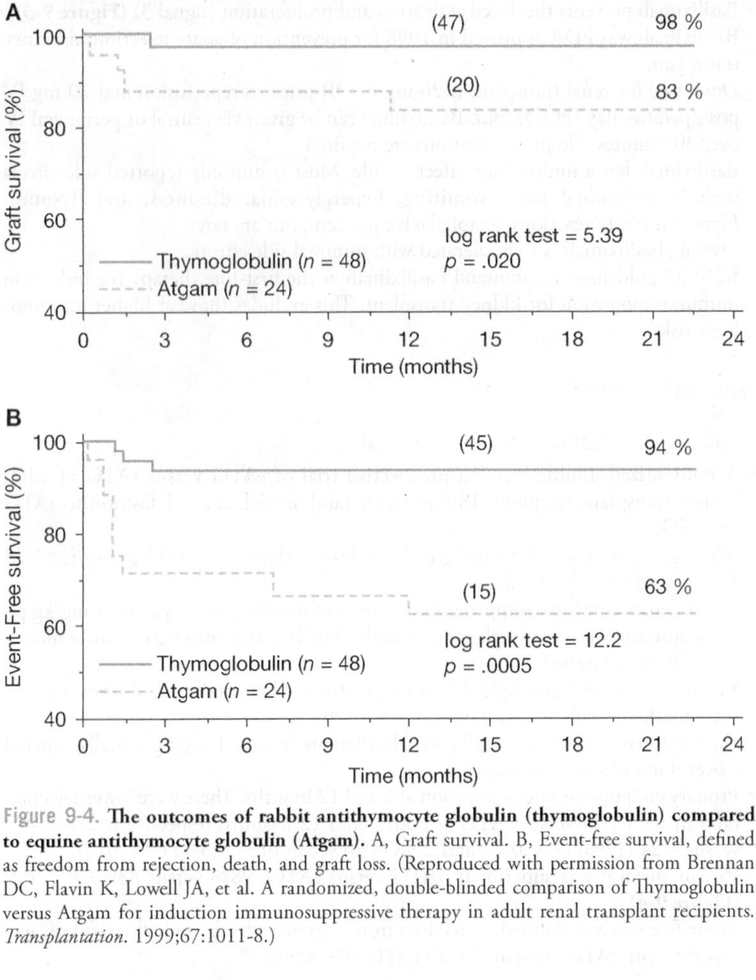

Figure 9-4. **The outcomes of rabbit antithymocyte globulin (thymoglobulin) compared to equine antithymocyte globulin (Atgam).** A, Graft survival. B, Event-free survival, defined as freedom from rejection, death, and graft loss. (Reproduced with permission from Brennan DC, Flavin K, Lowell JA, et al. A randomized, double-blinded comparison of Thymoglobulin versus Atgam for induction immunosuppressive therapy in adult renal transplant recipients. *Transplantation*. 1999;67:1011-8.)

Depleting Versus Nondepleting Therapy

Brennan and colleagues studied the safety and efficacy of basiliximab and ATG in patients at high risk for ACR or delayed graft function (DGF) undergoing a deceased donor kidney transplant[12]:

- It was a prospective, randomized, multicenter, international study where patients were randomized 1:1 to ATG or basiliximab according to variable-block randomization at each center.
- ATG group received a total dose of 7.5 mg/kg (1.5 mg/kg × 5 doses) and basiliximab group received 20 mg IV prior to reperfusion and 20 mg on POD 4. Maintenance immunosuppression consisted of cyclosporine, mycophenolate mofetil 1,000 mg BID, dose adjusted at investigators discretion and methylprednisolone 7 mg/kg in the OR, then tapered to prednisone 5 mg daily by 6 months.

- Composite primary endpoint of first biopsy-proven acute rejection, DGF, graft loss, or death occurred 71 (50.4%) in the ATG groups versus 77 (56.2%) in the basiliximab group (P = .3.34).
- Biopsy-proven acute rejection occurred in 15.6% of ATG and 25.5% of basiliximab (P = .02).
- Based on prior data, the average rate of rejection with ATG is 1.7 times less compared to basiliximab in the first-year posttransplant.
- No difference in DGF between ATG and basiliximab in patients at high risk for DGF. ATG was associated with reduced incidence of BPAR and reduced severity of rejection compared to basiliximab. There was higher incidence of infections in patients who received with ATG induction compared to basiliximab.
- Noel and colleagues also investigated the use of rATG versus daclizumab (IL2 inhibitor no longer on the market)[13]:
- A prospective, multicenter, randomized trial that compared BPAR in higher immunological risk kidney transplant recipients.
- ATG was dosed at 1.25 mg/kg/d on days 0 through 7.
- Daclizumab was dosed at 1 mg/kg on days 0, 14, 28, 42, and 56.
- Maintenance immunosuppression consisted of steroids tapered, mycophenolate mofetil, and tacrolimus was preferred. Trough goals were 10 to 15 ng/mL for the initial 3 months and then 8 to 12 ng/mL up to 1 year.
- The primary endpoint of the study was the proportion of patients with BPAR at 1 year. ATG group had lower BPAR compared to daclizumab (15% vs. 27.2%, P = .016).
- 12-month graft and patient survival rates had no difference between the two groups.

Antithymocyte Globulin Versus Alemtuzumab

A prospective, open-label, multicenter, randomized trial conducted at 30 centers compared the safety and efficacy of alemtuzumab versus basiliximab versus rATG for induction for deceased or living donor kidney transplant recipients[14]:

- Alemtuzumab: 30 mg at the time of transplant, basiliximab: 20 mg IV on POD 0 and POD 4, rATG: 4 doses of 1.5 mg/kg on POD 0, POD 1, POD 2, and POD 3 or 4.
- Maintenance immunosuppression consisted of tacrolimus, mycophenolate mofetil, and 1 g or less of prednisolone (or equivalent glucocorticoid) over a period of 5 days and discontinued. **Tacrolimus trough goal:** POD 0 to 90: 7 to 14 ng/mL; > POD 90: 4 to 12 ng/mL.
- Primary outcome was rate of BPAR at 6 and 12 months. The rate of BPAR was significantly lower in alemtuzumab group than conventional therapy both at 6 months (3% vs. 15%, P < .001) and 12 months (5% vs. 17% P < .001).
- BPAR for alemtuzumab versus basiliximab: 6 months: 2% versus 18%, P < .001; 12 months: 3% versus 20% P < .001; 36 months: 10% versus 22% P = .003.
- BPAR for alemtuzumab versus rATG: 6 months: 6% and 9%, P = .49; 12 months: 10% and 13%, P = .53; 36 months: 18% and 15%; P = .63.
- No difference in graft or patient survival between the three groups.

Pooled Analysis and Meta-Analysis of rATG Versus IL2

- A pooled analysis of the two larger international randomized controlled trials including rATG versus IL2 receptor antagonists were conducted to assess the noninferiority of rATG versus IL2 antagonists. The analysis included a total of 508 deceased donor kidney transplant recipients.[15]
  - The rATG dosing consisted of 1.5 mg/kg/d for 4 to 7 days or longer.
  - Patient level data were reanalyzed for this trial.

- The noninferiority of rATG versus IL2RAs with a noninferiority margin of 10%.
- The studies were also evaluated for superiority test for rATG versus basiliximab in the 1,010 study and a noninferiority test (with a margin of 15%) for rATG versus daclizumab in the TAXI study.
- The composite endpoint of the pooled analysis resulted in treatment failure in 25.1% of rATG and 36% of IL2RA, resulting in noninferiority of rATG to IL2RA.
- BPAR occurred at 11.8% and 20.9% (P = .0057) of rATG versus IL2.
- A meta-analysis was also conducted using a total of seven trials with rATG. The outcomes were BPAR, graft loss, death, and a composite of all of these at 12 months posttransplant.
- This included 1,293 kidney transplant recipients and overall incidence of BPAR at 12 months favored rATG versus control.

WASHINGTON UNIVERSITY SCHOOL OF MEDICINE IN ST. LOUIS GUIDELINES

Please see **Table 9-2** for Washington University and Barnes-Jewish Hospital induction guidelines. **Table 9-3** highlights glucocorticoid and rituximab schedules for kidney transplants.

TABLE 9-2 Guidelines for Induction Therapy at Washington University in St. Louis

Choice of Induction Therapy				
No Induction Therapy	Basiliximab (Simulect)	Rabbit Antithymocyte Globulin (Thymoglobulin)		
	20 mg POD 0 and POD 4	6 mg/kg	5 mg/kg	3 mg/kg
2-haplotype match white living donor recipients	• Per transplant team if not a candidate for antithymocyte globulin Possible rationales: • Hypotensive • Active or recent malignancy • On CNI-based immunosuppression • Prior nonkidney transplant • Baseline WBC <3 or platelets <120	• ABOi • SPK • PTA • PAK	• cPRA ≥30% • +flow crossmatch • ≤40 year old • Black • 2 DR mismatches • Prior kidney transplant • +DSA • Belatacept maintenance IS	If other criteria not met

ABOi, blood group incompatible; CNI, calcineurin; cPRA, calculated panel reactive antibody; DSA, donor-specific antibody; IS, immunosuppression; PAK, pancreas after kidney; POD, postoperative day; PLT, platelet; PTA, pancreas transplant alone; SPK, simultaneous pancreases kidney; WBC, white blood cell count.

TABLE 9-3 Guidelines for Glucocorticoids and Rituximab in Kidney Transplant Recipients

Glucocorticoids Schedule in All Recipients				
Steroids	Methylprednisolone (Solumedrol)	7 mg/kg IV (max 500 mg)	Intraoperative	
	Prednisone	1 mg/kg (max 80 mg)	POD 1-2	
	Prednisone	20 mg	POD 3-14	
	Prednisone	15 mg	POD 15-21	
	Prednisone	10 mg	POD 22-28	
	Prednisone	5 mg	POD > 28	
Rituximab in Selected Patients				
Monoclonal Ab	Rituximab (Rituxan)	200 mg IV	At time of discharge or outpatient	Given for primary FSGS or positive DSA

DSA, donor-specific antibody; FSGS; focal segmental glomerulosclerosis, POD, postoperative day.

REFERENCES

1. Hardinger KL, Brennan DC, Klein CL. Selection of induction therapy in kidney transplantation. *Transpl Int.* 2013;26(7):662-72.
2. Lentine KL, Smith JM, Hart A, et al. OPTN/SRTR 2020 annual data report: kidney. *Am J Transplant.* 2022;22(suppl 2):21-136.
3. ATGAM. Lymphocyte immune globulin, anti-thymocyte globulin [equine]. Package insert. Pfizer Injectables; 2021.
4. *Thymoglobulin®. Anti-thymocyte Globulin [rabbit].* Package insert. Genzyme Corporation; 2020.
5. Bowman LJ, Edwards A, Brennan DC. The role of rabbit antithymocyte globulin in renal transplantation. *Expert Opin Orphan Drugs.* 2014;2:971-87.
6. Campath. *Alemtuzumab.* Package insert. Genzyme Corporation; 2021.
7. Campath. Clinigen Direct; 2022. Accessed October 9, 2022. https://www.clinigengroup.com/direct/en/products/detail/087dd185-campath/
8. Simulect. *Basiliximab.* Package insert. Novartis Pharmaceuticals Corporation; 2003.
9. Kidney Disease: Improving Global Outcomes (KDIGO) Transplant Work Group. KDIGO clinical practice guideline for the care of kidney transplant recipients. *Am J Transplant.* 2009;9:S1-S155.
10. Brennan DC, Flavin K, Lowell JA, et al. A randomized, double-blinded comparison of Thymoglobulin versus Atgam for induction immunosuppressive therapy in adult renal transplant recipients. *Transplantation.* 1999;67(7):1011-8.
11. Mourad G, Garrigue V, Squifflet JP, et al. Induction versus noninduction in renal transplant recipients with tacrolimus-based immunosuppression. *Transplantation.* 2001;72(6):1050-5.

12. Brennan DC, Daller JA, Lake KD, Cibrik D, Del Castillo D; Thymoglobulin Induction Study Group. Rabbit antithymocyte globulin versus basiliximab in renal transplantation. *N Engl J Med.* 2006;355(19):1967-77.
13. Noel C, Abramowicz D, Durand D, et al. Daclizumab versus antithymocyte globulin in high-immunological-risk renal transplant recipients. *J Am Soc Nephrol.* 2009;20(6):1385-92.
14. Hanaway MJ, Woodle ES, Mulgaonkar S, et al. Alemtuzumab induction in renal transplantation. *N Engl J Med.* 2011;364(20):1909-19.
15. Alloway RR, Woodle ES, Aramowicz D, et al. Rabbit anti-thymocyte globulin for the prevention of acute rejection in kidney transplantation. *Am J Transplant.* 2019;19:2250-61.

10 Maintenance Immunosuppression in Kidney Transplantation

Kristin Progar

GENERAL PRINCIPLES

- The purpose of maintenance immunosuppression is to preserve graft function and protect the transplanted organ from rejection.
- Typically, maintenance immunosuppression consists of 2 to 3 agents in order to target different mechanisms of immune response and minimize toxicity of any 1 agent.
- The annual kidney transplant organ procurement transplant network report demonstrates that a majority of centers utilize a triple regimen including tacrolimus, mycophenolate, and prednisone (**Figure 10-1**).[1]
- Maintenance immunosuppression is a delicate balance between rejection, toxicity, infection, and malignancy and is often titrated to specific patient needs.
- All agents discussed in detail below are US Food and Drug Administration (FDA) approved for kidney transplantation.

CALCINEURIN INHIBITORS

- Calcineurin inhibitors (CNIs) are often considered the backbone of immunosuppressive therapy.
- Cyclosporine and tacrolimus are the currently available CNIs on the market.

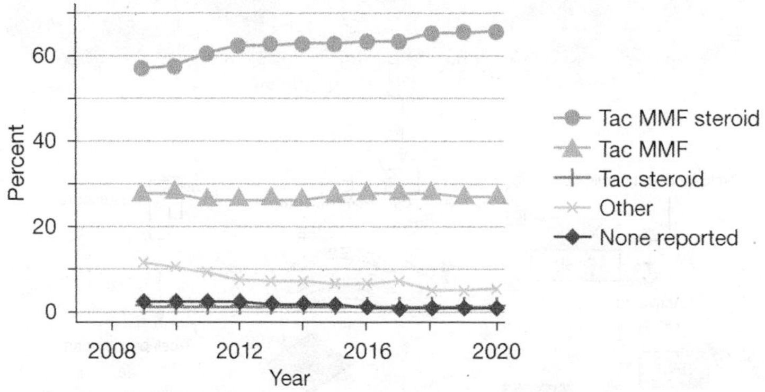

Figure 10-1. **Immunosuppression regimens among kidney transplant recipients between 2008 and 2020.** MMF, mycophenolate mofetil; Tac, tacrolimus. (Reproduced with permission from Lentine KL, Smith JM, Hart A, et al. OPTN/SRTR 2020 Annual Data Report: kidney. *Am J Transplant.* 2022;22(suppl 2):21-136. Figure KI 79.)

Mechanism of Action

- CNIs inhibit the first phase of intracellular T-cell activation by binding to either cyclophilin (where cyclosporine binds) or FK binding protein 12 (FKBP12) (while tacrolimus binds); this complex then binds to and inhibits calcineurin (**Figure 10-2**).
- Calcineurin is a phosphatase that normally dephosphorylates nuclear factors of activation, which facilitates their passage through the nuclear membrane.
- These regulatory proteins then promote gene transcription of several cytokines including interleukin (IL)-2, IL-3, IL-4, and interferon-γ (INF-γ). These are responsible for T-cell activation.
- Inhibition of calcineurin halts the production of key cytokines that are needed for T-cell activation resulting in an impaired T-lymphocyte proliferation response to foreign antigens.
- Calcineurin inhibitors are primarily metabolized and eliminated through cytochrome P (CYP) 3A4/5 and p-glycoprotein pump (PGP), which results in multiple concerns for drug interactions. In addition, genetic polymorphisms can also affect how well patients metabolize medications. Strong CYP3A4/5 or PGP inhibitors often require preemptive dose adjustment.
- Both tacrolimus and cyclosporine are predominantly eliminated via fecal route. No dose adjustment is required in renal dysfunction due to minimal renal elimination.[2,3]

Adverse Effects

- Adverse effects of CNIs include electrolyte abnormalities (hypomagnesemia, hyperkalemia), nephrotoxicity, hypertension, neurotoxicity (paresthesia, headache, tremor, posterior reversible encephalopathy syndrome), and posttransplant diabetes. Therapeutic windows are aimed to reduce toxicity but with cumulative exposure over time can also increase the risk.[4-7]

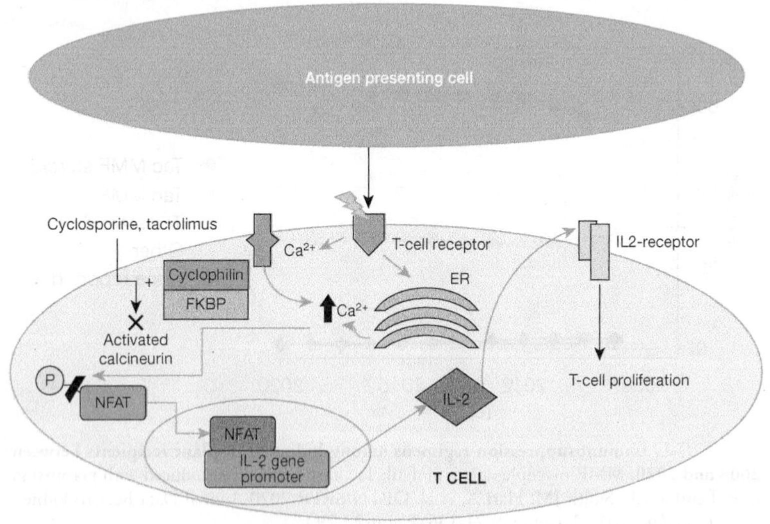

Figure 10-2. **Mechanism of action of calcineurin inhibitors.** Ca^{2+}, calcium; FKBP, FK binding protein; IL-2, interleukin-2; NFAT, nuclear factor of activated T cells.

- Tacrolimus can also cause alopecia and is more commonly associated with neurotoxicity and nephrotoxicity. There have been rare reports of myocardial hypertrophy with tacrolimus use.[5,8-10]
- Cyclosporine has been associated with gingival hyperplasia, hirsutism, and higher rates of hypertension, hyperuricemia, hyperlipidemia, and nephrotoxicity.[4,6,10,11]
- Toxicities are more commonly associated with higher levels and tend to be more common in the setting of CNI intravenous administration.[7]

- Both CNI agents carry a black box warning for increased risk of lymphomas and other malignancies and an increased risk of polyoma virus (BK, JC) and cytomegalovirus (CMV) infection.[8-10]
- Nephrotoxicity with CNIs makes them an unideal agent to utilize post kidney transplant despite superior results in preventing kidney allograft failure and rejection.
  - Acute nephrotoxicity is often prerenal and reversible driven by vasoconstriction of the afferent renal artery through an overall decrease in production of prostaglandins, cyclo-oxygenase-2, and nitric oxide with simultaneous upregulation of renin-angiotensin-aldosterone system, endothelin, and thromboxane.
  - In addition, CNIs increase sympathetic nerve activation as well as the potential to cause thrombotic microangiopathy.
  - Chronically, interstitial fibrosis and arteriolar thickening can cause permanent renal damage.[5]
  - CNI minimization through the use of belatacept or addition of a mammalian target of rapamycin inhibitor (mTORi) has been explored in the recent literature as a way to minimize nephrotoxicity.[11,12]
  - The vasodilatory properties of non-dihydropyridine calcium channel blockers have also been associated with improvement of nephrotoxicity in the setting of kidney transplantation and CNI use.

Safety and Efficacy in Trials

- Pirsch et al compared tacrolimus immediate release (IR) with cyclosporine demonstrating no differences in patient or graft survival but a significant decrease in biopsy-proven acute rejection at 1 year with tacrolimus versus cyclosporine (31% vs. 46%, $P = .001$). Five-year results published accounting for crossover between CNI groups showed improved graft survival with tacrolimus over cyclosporine. In addition, posttransplant diabetes was reported in 20% of patients in the tacrolimus group while cyclosporine was more commonly associated with hypertension and hyperlipidemia.[6,9]
- Maintenance immunosuppression consensus guidelines endorse tacrolimus as the CNI of choice due to efficacy and safety data from multiple randomized, controlled clinical trials. However, patients with intolerance to tacrolimus such as hyperglycemia or neurotoxicity may be switched to cyclosporine with improvement in side effects.[13]

Tacrolimus Dosing and Formulations

- A macrolide lactone antibiotic isolated from the fermentation broth of the soil microorganism *Streptomyces tsukubaensis*. It was first approved by the FDA in 1994. Tacrolimus is currently available in several forms.[2]
- Each tacrolimus formulation has a different pharmacokinetic profile depicted in **Figure 10-3**. However, there are currently no published studies to demonstrate differences in efficacy between the different formulations of tacrolimus.[8-10,13] However, the STRATO study published in 2015 demonstrated improved tremor in patients previously on tacrolimus IR switched to tacrolimus extended release (XR).[14]

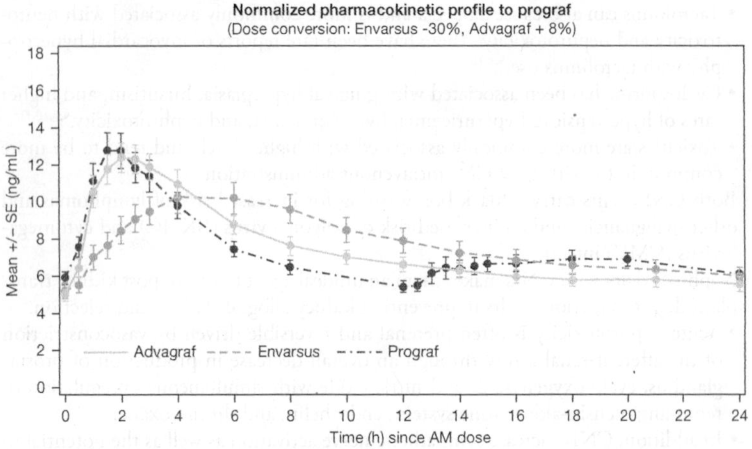

Figure 10-3. **Pharmacokinetic profile of envarsus XR, Astagraf/Advagraf XL, and Prograf.** (Reproduced with permission from Tremblay S, Nigro V, Weinberg J, Woodle ES, Alloway RR. A steady-state head-to-head pharmacokinetic comparison of all FK-506 (Tacrolimus) formulations (ASTCOFF): an open-label, prospective, randomized, two-arm, three-period crossover study. *Am J Transplant.* 2017;17(2):432-442. Figure 3B.)

- Tacrolimus extended-release dosing (XL, XR) has been shown to improve medication adherence in clinical trials.[9]
- Tacrolimus XR has also demonstrated less variability in pharmacokinetic profile in the setting of race or CYP3A5 genotypes based on the ASERTAA trial.
- Trough concentrations (C_0) have been found to correlate well with the area under the curve (AUC) despite variable intra- and interindividual blood concentration time curves. Target trough levels vary by transplant center and are usually between 3 and 15 ng/mL depending on patient risk for rejection, infection, and malignancy as well as time from transplant.[3,7,9,15] See **Table 10-1**.[8-10,12]

Tacrolimus Conversions

- Astagraf XL and Envarsus XR are **NOT interchangeable.**
- IR to XL: 100% of total daily dose (Tacrolimus IR 2 mg bid = Astragraf XL 4 mg daily)
- IR to XR: 75% of total daily dose (Tacrolimus IR 2 mg bid = Envarsus XR 3 mg daily)

Cyclosporine Dosing and Formulations

- Cyclosporine was first approved in 1983 and is currently available in 2 formulations: nonmodified or oil-in-water emulsion (Sandimmune) and modified or microemulsion (Neoral, Gengraf).[4,12,16]
- Cyclosporine is an aminopeptide first isolated from *Tolypocladium inflatum.*[2]
- Nonmodified cyclosporine is available in capsules, oral solution, and intravenous modalities.
- Nonmodified cyclosporine has highly variable pharmacokinetics due to poor bioavailability (~10%-90%) heavily dependent upon bile acid, fat content of meal, and

TABLE 10-1 Tacrolimus Formulations

Generic	Brand	Dosage Forms	Dosing/Pharmacokinetics
Tacrolimus IR	Prograf	PO capsule, granule packets for suspension, intravenous	• Dosing: 0.5 mg/kg twice daily • Dose adjustment required for sublingual (50% reduction) and intravenous administration (75% reduction) • Poor bioavailability 30%-40%
Tacrolimus XL	Astagraf XL	PO capsule	• Dosing: 0.15-0.2 mg/kg/d • Variable kinetics
Tacrolimus XR	Envarsus XR	PO tablet	• Dosing: 0.14 mg/kg/d • Melt Dose technology to increase bioavailability 50% higher than tacrolimus IR or XL • Lower C_{max} and similar AUC to both IR and XL

AUC, area under the curve; IR, immediate release; XL, extended release.
Data from Marcén R. Immunosuppressive drugs in kidney transplantation: impact on patient survival, and incidence of cardiovascular disease, malignancy and infection. *Drugs*. 2009;69:2227-43; Manjunatha TA, Chng R, Yau WP. Efficacy and safety of tacrolimus-based maintenance regimens in de novo kidney transplant recipients: a systematic review and network meta-analysis of randomized controlled trials. *Ann Transplant*. 2021;26:e933588; Karolin A, Genitsch V, Sidler D. Calcineurin inhibitor toxicity in solid organ transplantation. *Pharmacology*. 2021;106:347-55; and Nelson J, Alvey N, Bowman L, et al. Consensus recommendations for use of maintenance immunosuppression in solid organ transplantation: endorsed by the American College of Clinical Pharmacy, American Society of Transplantation, and the International Society for Heart and Lung Transplantation. *Pharmacotherapy*. 2022;42:599-633.

gastrointestinal motility. A nonlinear dose relationship also leads to difficulty with dose adjustment and response.[3,16]

- Shah et al. in a meta-analysis demonstrated that de novo use of nonmodified cyclosporine is associated with higher rates of acute rejection when compared with the modified formulation.[16]
- Modified cyclosporine is only available as solution and capsules with a more predictable pharmacokinetic profile less dependent on bile acid and high fat food for absorption with a bioavailability of ~30%.
- Initial dosing of cyclosporine is 9 ± 3 mg/kg/d given in 2 divided doses.[4,16]
- Cyclosporine trough levels correlate poorly with the AUC. CONCERT consensus guidelines recommend C_2 (2 hours post-dose or peak) levels as more accurately associated with AUC and rejection rates (correlation, $r^2 = 0.83$-0.85). However, C_2 levels are difficult to obtain in clinical practice.
- Target trough and C_2 level goals similarly to tacrolimus depend on patient risk for rejection, infection, and malignancy post transplant. The typical goal range for C_0 is 50 to 400 ng/mL and for C_2 400 to 1,200 ng/mL.[7,12,16]

ANTIMETABOLITES

Antimetabolites affect T-cell growth and proliferation through several different pathways often targeting DNA replication.

Azathioprine

- Azathioprine is an imidazolyl derivative of mercaptopurine (prodrug) converted to 6-mercaptopurine in peripheral blood via glutathione reduction.
- Active metabolites include 6-thioguanine nucleotide, which blocks purine incorporation into DNA and inhibits cell cycle progression, which disrupts the salvage pathway for purine synthesis, which a majority of cell lines rely.
- The 6-methylmercaptopurine metabolite causes inhibition of de novo purine synthesis and halting of DNA replication specific to pathways in T and B lymphocytes (**Figure 10-4**).
- Azathioprine is available as oral tablets and intravenous solution but can be compounded into a suspension.
- Initial dosing of 1 to 3 mg/kg dosed daily is recommended. Azathioprine is well absorbed and a 1:1 conversion is recommended from oral to intravenous formulation. Azathioprine is predominantly excreted in the urine (~50%) and thus requires dose modification with renal dysfunction.[2,17]
- Therapeutic drug monitoring has not been associated with improved outcomes and is not routinely done in clinical practice outside of potential concern for toxicity.[17]
- Adverse effects of azathioprine include pancytopenia (leukopenia, macrocytic anemia, and thrombocytopenia), alopecia, arthralgia, acute pancreatitis (rare), and hepatotoxicity (ranging from minor elevations in aspartate aminotransferase/alanine aminotransferase to cholestatic liver injury).[2,12,17]
  - Polymorphisms conferring reduced functionality in thiopurine methyltransferase are responsible for increased risk of myelotoxicity and hepatotoxicity.
  - Azathioprine carries a black box warning for malignancy. An increase in skin-related cancers is well documented with azathioprine in the solid organ transplant

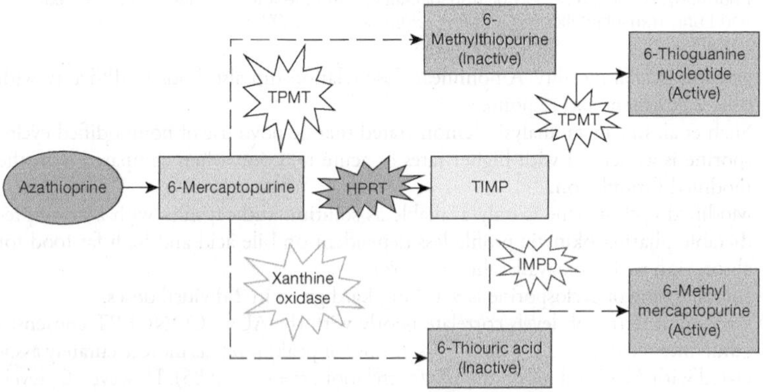

Figure 10-4. **Mechanism of action of azathioprine.** IMPD, Inosine monophosphate dehydrogenase; HPRT, hypoxanthine-guanine phosphoribosyltransferase; TIMP, tissue inhibitors of metalloproteinases; TPMT, thiopurine methyltransferase.

population. Azathioprine sensitizes skin cells to UV-induced damage through incorporation of 6-thioguanine into DNA affecting recovery or regeneration after reactive oxidative stress from UVA light.[18]

- Clinically relevant drug interactions requiring therapeutic modification are limited.
  - Xanthine oxidase inhibitors block inactivation of 6-mercaptopurine and increase potential for toxicity; a 75% dose reduction in azathioprine is recommended with concomitant use.[19]
  - A dose-dependent decrease in warfarin anticoagulant effect (reduction in international normalized ratio) is seen with azathioprine. The mechanism is unclear, potentially due to impaired warfarin absorption and/or enhanced warfarin metabolism via hepatic enzyme induction.[20]
  - Sulfamethoxazole and Trimethoprim can enhance myelotoxicity of azathioprine; no empiric dose reduction is recommended.[19]

Mycophenolate

- Mycophenolate (MPA) selectively and reversibly inhibits the rate-limiting enzyme inosine monophosphate dehydrogenase (IMDPH) type 2 effectively terminating the de novo purine synthesis on which T and B lymphocytes rely upon for growth and proliferation (**Figure 10-5**).[21]
- In addition, mycophenolate promotes B-lymphocyte apoptosis and suppressive antibody formation. Inhibition of IMDPH also interferes with recruitment, infiltration, and endothelial cell adhesion of leukocytes to sites of inflammation.[2]
- Dosing, formulation, and pharmacokinetic information can be found in **Table 10-2**.[22,23]
  - Higher doses of mycophenolate mofetil (MMF) of 3 g/d in African American patients have been associated with decreased rates of rejection, but pharmacokinetic studies cannot account for these differences.[24]

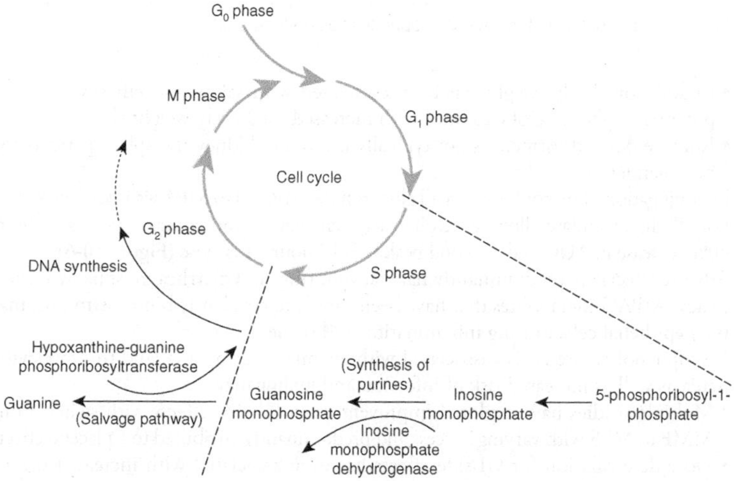

Figure 10-5. **Mechanism of action of mycophenolate.** (Reproduced with permission from Stepkowski SM. Molecular targets for existing and novel immunosuppressive drugs. *Expert Rev Mol Med.* 2000;21;2(4):1-23. Figure 1.)

TABLE 10-2 Mycophenolate Formulations, Dosing, and Pharmacokinetic Information

	Mycophenolate Mofetil (MMF)—CellCept	Mycophenolate Sodium (MPS)—Myfortic
Formulation	Esterified prodrug	Enteric-coated, delayed-release sodium salt
Dosing	500-1,000 mg twice daily	360-720 mg twice daily
	1:1:1 conversion between intravenous, suspension, and capsule/tablet formulations	360 mg of MPS equivalent to 500 mg MMF
Absorption	Hydrolyzed via plasma and tissue esterases in acidic environment of the stomach to MPA	Dissolves to ionized MPA in gastric acid of stomach
	MPA absorbed in stomach and proximal small intestine	Absorbed primarily in small intestine
Bioavailability	93%	72%
T_{max}	0.5-1 h	1.5-2.75 h
Metabolism	Glucuronidation of MPA occurs in the liver to MPAG. No recommended dose adjustment for hepatic impairment.	
Elimination and half-life (MPA)	Predominantly renal (~60%-80%) via inactive metabolite; no specific renal dose adjustment recommended	
	9-17 h for MPA, 13-17 h MPAG	
Available products	Capsule, tablet, oral suspension, intravenous solution	Tablet only

MPA, mycophenolic acid, MPAG, mycophenolic acid glucuronide.

  - In addition, body weight has been correlated with safety and efficacy due to a potential higher rate of clearance with increased total body weight.[25]
  - Routine dose adjustment is not typically utilized in kidney transplant patients for race, gender, or weight.
- Deconjugation of mycophenolic acid glucuronide (MPAG) to MPA via intestinal microflora β-glucuronidase allows enterohepatic recirculation and contributes to a 30% to 40% increase in AUC and a second peak 4 to 12 hours after dose (**Figure 10-6**).[26]
- Adverse effects are predominantly nausea, vomiting, and diarrhea most likely related to acyl-MPAG metabolites that have been shown to covalently bind gastrointestinal (GI) epithelial cells causing inflammation and tissue damage.[27]
- Mycophenolate use is also associated with anemia, neutropenia, and thrombocytopenia as well as increased risk of infection and malignancy.
  - Multiple studies have explored improvement in GI side effects with switch from MMF to MPS with varying success and predominantly attributed to a placebo effect.
  - Dose de-escalation for GI side effects has been associated with increased risk of rejection.[28,29]
- Mycophenolate has a voluntary risk evaluation and mitigation strategy program associated with potential for spontaneous abortion and fetal toxicity in pregnant patients. Use is contraindicated in patients who are or intend to be pregnant.

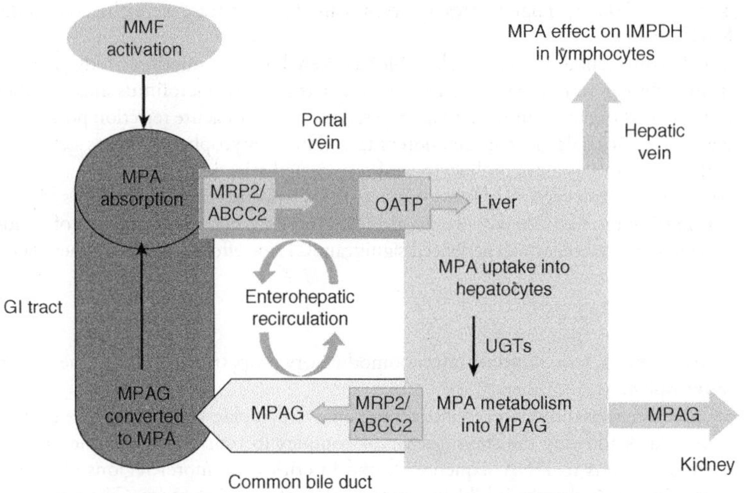

Figure 10-6. **Enterohepatic recirculation of mycophenolate.** ABCC2, adenosine triphosphate–binding cassette subfamily C member 2; IMPDH, inosine-5′-monophosphate dehydrogenase; MMF, mycophenolate mofetil; MPA, mycophenolic acid; MPAG, mycophenolic acid glucuronide; MRP2, multidrug resistance–associated protein 2; OATP, organic anion transporting polypeptide; UGT, uridine 5′-diphospho-glucuronosyltransferase. (Adapted from Sherwin CM, Fukuda T, Brunner HI, et al. The evolution of population pharmacokinetic models to describe the enterohepatic recycling of mycophenolic acid in solid organ transplantation and autoimmune disease. *Clin Pharmacokinet.* 2011;50(1):1-24.)

- Therapeutic drug monitoring is not routinely recommended in patients on mycophenolate due to burden of laboratory testing requiring 2 to 4 laboratory draws for AUC prediction and variable correlation with efficacy. Typical AUC targets for mycophenolate are 30 to 60 ng/mL.[7,30]
- Drug interactions
  - Cyclosporine inhibits the enterohepatic recirculation of MPAG via inhibition of biliary secretion by the MRP-2 transporter.[26]
  - Corticosteroids can increase glucuronidation of MPA, increasing conversion to inactive metabolite.
  - Cholestyramine, magnesium and aluminum-containing compounds, and antacids can decrease absorption of MPA when coadministered.
  - Levonorgestrel can decrease the AUC of MPA by up to 15%.
  - Antivirals such as valacyclovir, valganciclovir, and acyclovir compete for elimination in the renal tubules with MPAG and thus can result in increased MPAG concentrations.[19,23,24]

Efficacy of Azathioprine Versus Mycophenolate

- The US Renal Transplant Mycophenolate Mofetil Study, a multicenter, double-blind, randomized controlled trial in deceased donor kidney transplant recipients, demonstrated no difference in patient survival or graft loss when comparing azathioprine with mycophenolate. Lower rates of biopsy-proven acute rejection were observed with the MMF 2 g/daily group compared with the azathioprine group (31% vs.

47.6%, $P = .0015$). Higher rates of diarrhea and CMV disease were observed in the MMF groups.[31]

- The Tricontinental Mycophenolate Mofetil Renal Transplantation Study demonstrated similar results. However, more recent trials with tacrolimus and in other transplanted organs demonstrate no differences in rates of acute rejection post transplant. In these trials, the combination of tacrolimus + mycophenolate was associated with lower rates of antilymphocyte antibody treated rejection.[32,33]
- Based on scientific registry of transplant recipients reporting mycophenolate is still the antimetabolite of choice with azathioprine often being utilized in patients of childbearing potential or who experienced significant GI side effects with mycophenolate.[1]

CORTICOSTEROIDS

- Corticosteroids have multiple immunomodulatory properties relevant to the setting of transplant.
  - Corticosteroids diffuse intracellularly and bind to cytoplasmic receptors; the protein dissociates allowing the steroid-receptor complex to translocate into the nucleus where it binds to DNA sequences found in critical promoter regions of several cytokine genes thereby inhibiting transcription of cytokine genes. Corticosteroids also inhibit the translocation of transcription factor NF-κB inhibiting downstream production of IL-1, IL-2, IL-3, IL-6, TNF-α, and INF-γ.
  - Impair monocyte and macrophage function and decrease the number of circulating $CD4^+$ T lymphocytes.
  - Inhibition of the production and release of chemokines, permeability-increasing agents, and vasodilators preventing inflammatory damage to the allograft.
  - Redistribution of lymphocytes from the vascular compartment back into lymphoid tissue and inhibition of monocyte migration to sites of inflammation.[34,35]
- Prednisone is the corticosteroid of choice for most transplant recipients, but the use of methylprednisolone, prednisolone, and dexamethasone has also been explored. Dosing is often center, disease state, and patient specific. Weight-based and flat dose of steroids are utilized in clinical trials, and doses often taper to 5 to 10 mg daily or complete discontinuation.
- Adverse effects of steroids are discussed in several other chapters of this text and have been widely documented in patient populations both within and outside of the transplant population.
  - Immediate, dose-dependent effects of steroids include hyperglycemia, hyperlipidemia, delayed wound healing, hypertension, peptic ulcers, weight gain, insomnia, and psychosis.
  - Long-term effects include posttransplant diabetes, cataracts, glaucoma, osteoporosis, avascular necrosis, adrenal insufficiency, Cushing syndrome, growth impairment, acne, and hyperpigmentation.[36]
- Drug interactions
  - Prednisone is a substrate for CYP3A4; efficacy and toxicity can be affected by concomitant administration of CYP3A4 inhibitors or inducers.
  - Estrogen derivatives can increase levels of corticosteroids.
  - Coadministration with NSAIDs increases the risk of development of peptic ulcer disease.[19,34-36]
- Steroid avoidance versus maintenance strategies
  - The purpose of steroid avoidance/withdrawal strategies is to spare the long-term side effects and increased morbidity and mortality associated with cardiovascular

disease, malignancy, and infection. However, various success has been seen with a potential for increased risk of rejection.[11]

- Woodle et al explored differences in long-term outcomes in patients who remained on prednisone compared with those tapered off within 7 days of transplant. No differences were observed in patient death, graft loss, or moderate/severe rejection. Lower rates of hyperlipidemia, insulin use for treatment of diabetes, weight gain, and bone-related complications were seen in the steroid withdrawal group. However, there were higher rates of biopsy-proven acute rejection (BPAR) with steroid withdrawal and the patient population was at large at low risk for rejection.[37]
- Several other studies have shown significant increased risk of rejection in African American populations when a steroid withdrawal strategy was employed.
- Type of induction (depleting vs. nondepleting) does not seem to achieve a significant difference in outcomes in the context of steroid withdrawal.[38]

MAMMALIAN TARGET OF RAPAMYCIN INHIBITORS

- Sirolimus was FDA-approved in 1999, while everolimus was FDA approved in 2010. Structurally, both mTORi agents are macrolide antibiotics. Everolimus and sirolimus block signal 3 by binding to FKBP12 to inhibit the kinase activity of mTOR, which further inhibits the T-cell response to IL-2 (G1 to S phase) and stops cell growth (via reduction in protein synthesis) and proliferation.
- mTORis are also vascular endothelial growth factor (VEGF) inhibitors, block epidermal growth factor, and inhibit smooth muscle cell proliferation. These off-target effects are responsible for the adverse effect and unique antiproliferative properties compared with other maintenance immunosuppressive agents.
- Everolimus is a derivative of sirolimus with an added hydroxyethyl side chain that shortens the half-life and makes a loading dose unnecessary. Further dosing, formulation, and pharmacokinetic information are explored in **Table 10-3**.[2,12,39]
- Therapeutic drug monitoring is typically performed via C_0 monitoring similarly to that of CNIs. Goal ranges of sirolimus (5-15 ng/mL) and everolimus (3-10 ng/mL) are dependent on concomitant use of or use in place of CNI.[39,40]
- Similar concerns for drug interactions are observed with mTORis as CNIs have the same pathway of metabolism. Labeled recommendations for separation of cyclosporine and sirolimus administration by 4 hours due to increased absorption and potential for toxicity of sirolimus.[19]

Adverse Effects

- Both mTORis carry black box warnings for increased risk of infection and malignancy.[8]
- Of note, everolimus carries an increased risk of renal arterial and venous thrombosis when used within the first 30 days after transplant. However, this has not been noted in postapproval studies when used in de novo kidney transplant recipients.[39,40]
- Shared side effects of both agents include hypertension, anemia, leukopenia, thrombocytopenia, acne, hyperlipidemia, hypertriglyceridemia, mucositis/stomatitis, peripheral edema, pneumonitis, posttransplant diabetes, and angioedema (rare).
- mTORis have been linked to male infertility.
- Proteinuria with mTORis has been reported in 5% to 30% of patients with rare progression to nephrotic syndrome associated with chronic allograft injury and development of glomerular lesions. The cause of proteinuria is attributed to VEGF inhibition affecting podocyte activity increasing vascular wall permeability.[39-41]

TABLE 10-3 Dosing, Formulations, and Pharmacokinetic Profiles of mTORis

	Sirolimus (Rapamune)	Everolimus (Zortress)
Dosing	Loading dose of 6 mg on day followed by 2 mg daily	0.75 mg twice daily
Formulations	Oral tablet, solution	Oral tablet
$t_{1/2}$	62 ± 16 h	30 ± 11 h
F	15%	16%
C_{Max}	15 ng/mL	11.1 ± 4.6 ng/mL
T_{Max}	0.5 (solution) - 2 (tablets) hours	1-2 h
V_d	5.6-16.7 L/kg	107-342 L (Avg 110 L)
Metabolism	Substrate: 3A4, PGP	Substrate: 3A4, PGP
	Inhibit: 3A4	Inhibit: 3A4, 2D6
	Metabolites: make up 10% of activity	Metabolites: 100× less active
Excretion	91% feces, 2.2% urine	80% feces, 5% urine
	No renal or hepatic dose adjustment	No renal or hepatic dose adjustment

PGP, p-glycoprotein pump.

- Wound healing complications and acute tubular necrosis have been noted with mTORis in the setting of transplant surgery. Some centers elect to delay conversion until 1 month post transplant to ensure appropriate wound healing and resolution of delayed graft function.[12,39,41]
- Routine screening and monitoring for proteinuria, hyperlipidemia, and hypertriglyceridemia is recommended in patients on mTORi therapy.

Role of mTORi in Clinical Practice

- There are no randomized, controlled trials comparing everolimus with sirolimus in terms of rejection risk, graft function, and patient survival.
- De novo use of mTORi in kidney transplantation was explored in the RAD B201 and 251 study groups and several meta-analyses. Similar rates of BPAR were observed between everolimus + CNI reduction and antimetabolite + CNI with improvement of glomerular filtration rate (GFR) at 12 months post transplant. mTORis have been utilized as part of a regimen for CNI avoidance when given in combination with mycophenolate with or without prednisone. Higher rates of rejection and leukopenia were reported due to compounded side effect of mycophenolate with mTORi.[11,12,40,41]
- mTORi conversion from or minimization of CNI has been explored in multiple randomized, controlled trials such as ASCERTAIN, CONVERT, and ZEUS.[42-44] These trials show modest improvement in 12-month estimated GFR (eGFR) of kidney transplant recipients with no difference in patient and graft survival. In the long term, this improvement seems to narrow most likely due to natural decrease in CNI levels in the control arms. Studies where complete CNI elimination was utilized

showed higher rates of acute rejection.[40] eGFR improvement over time is more likely to occur in patients with eGFR > 40 to 50 mL/min at time of conversion.
- Higher rates of study drug discontinuation were seen in the mTORi groups in some studies predominantly due to proteinuria, impaired wound healing, stomatitis, and peripheral edema.[41]
- Posttransplant malignancies are addressed in another chapter, but mTORi-based regimens have been associated with fewer de novo and recurrent malignancies post transplant.[8,11]

BELATACEPT

- Belatacept is a fully humanized fusion protein that binds to the CD80/86 receptor on antigen-presenting cell inhibiting costimulation signal and preventing T-lymphocyte activation and proliferation leading to anergy and apoptosis (see **Figure 10-7**). Belatacept has 2 amino acid substitutions that distinguish it from its parent drug, abatacept, enhancing binding to CD80/86.[45]
- Belatacept replaces CNI in the immunosuppression regimen as a means to prevent long-term nephrotoxicity associated with CNIs. It has been explored for use in patients with delayed graft function or extended criteria/high kidney donor profile index donors.[11,46]
- Dosing of belatacept for de novo use is 10 mg/kg on day 1 (day of transplant, prior to implantation) and on day 5, followed by 10 mg/kg at the end of week 2, week 4, week 8, and week 12 following transplantation. Maintenance dosing of belatacept consists of 5 mg/kg every 4 weeks.[46] Every-8-week dosing has been explored with success in patients further out from transplant.[47]
- Therapeutic drug monitoring of belatacept is not routinely done or widely commercially available in a clinical setting.

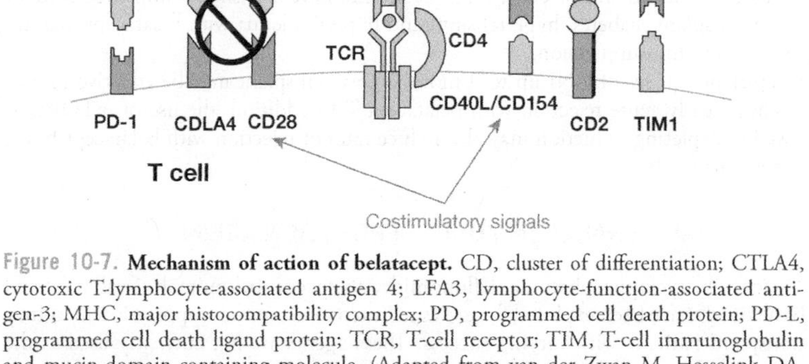

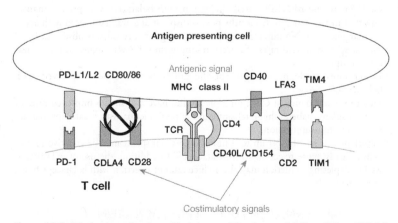

Figure 10-7. **Mechanism of action of belatacept.** CD, cluster of differentiation; CTLA4, cytotoxic T-lymphocyte-associated antigen 4; LFA3, lymphocyte-function-associated antigen-3; MHC, major histocompatibility complex; PD, programmed cell death protein; PD-L, programmed cell death ligand protein; TCR, T-cell receptor; TIM, T-cell immunoglobulin and mucin-domain-containing molecule. (Adapted from van der Zwan M, Hesselink DA, van den Hoogen MWF, et al. Costimulation blockade in kidney transplant recipients. *Drugs.* 2020;80(1):33-46.)

- There are no significant drug interactions reported with belatacept.
- Total body weight is utilized for dosing. There are no renal or hepatic dose adjustments for belatacept.
- Belatacept is only available for intravenous administration.
- Plasmapheresis has been shown to remove belatacept, and supplemental doses may be required.[48]
- Typically, studies with belatacept include coadministration of mycophenolate and prednisone taper/maintenance as part of the immunosuppression regimen.

Dose Conversion

- Multiple conversion dosing regimens exist for patients switched/tapered from CNI-based regimens to belatacept usually when patients are >6 months from time of transplant.[11]
- Conversion dosing is off-label; our center utilizes 5 mg/kg every 2 weeks (days 1, 15, 29, 43, and 57) and every 28 days thereafter in combination with CNI tapering over the first 3 doses of belatacept.[49]

Adverse Reactions

- Adverse reactions include an increased risk for posttransplant lymphoproliferative disease seen in Epstein-Barr virus seronegative recipients.
- Infusion-related reactions are rare.
- Increased risk of infection including increased rates of polyoma virus has been reported with use.[46]

Safety and Efficacy of Belatacept

- Belatacept use has been explored in low-risk kidney transplant recipients. Higher rates of acute rejection were observed with belatacept versus cyclosporine (19% vs. 10%) in the BENEFIT trial. Rejection with belatacept was predominantly reported in the first 3 to 6 months post transplant and was associated with acute cellular rejection. No difference in patient and graft survival was observed; however, despite increased rates of rejection long-term GFR was higher in the belatacept group.[46]
- Lower rates of de novo donor-specific antibodies have been observed with belatacept.[46]
- Due to the avoidance of CNI, multiple studies have also shown improved rates of posttransplant diabetes, hypertension, and hyperlipidemia with belatacept maintenance immunosuppression.[11]
- Transient courses of CNI up to 9 months post transplant may be effective in preventing early acute rejection with belatacept.[50] In addition, the use of mTORis as well as depleting induction may also reduce rates of rejection with belatacept-based regimens.[11,12,46]

OTHER MAINTENANCE IMMUNOSUPPRESSION AGENTS

Tofacitinib, cyclophosphamide, leflunomide, abatacept, belimumab, iscalimab, and basiliximab have been explored for use as maintenance immunosuppression in kidney transplant patients with varying success. These agents are not currently used as the standard of care and will not be discussed in this chapter.

IMMUNOSUPPRESSION SELECTION

- Selection of the appropriate maintenance immunosuppression regimen should account for some level of personalization between patients and provide a balance between rejection, graft survival, and toxicity.
- Center-specific protocols are often developed to account for each center's unique patient population as long-term outcomes with different immunosuppression combinations are similar and most differences are noted in acute rejection rates within 1 year.
- Current consensus guidelines recommend the use of tacrolimus and mycophenolate with or without long-term prednisone in kidney transplant recipients for prevention of rejection within the first year of transplant.
  - Azathioprine can be considered in the setting of toxicity with mycophenolate. Cyclosporine, belatacept, or mTORi can be utilized in the setting of toxicity with tacrolimus.
  - Belatacept can be considered for de novo use or conversion in low-risk kidney transplant recipients.
  - mTORis and belatacept can be utilized in the setting of CNI minimization or withdrawal to prevent long-term nephrotoxicity.
  - mTORi therapy has demonstrated potential benefit in the setting of malignancy and CMV infection. mTORis can be considered as part of a strategy to decrease overall immunosuppression in these settings.[12]

REFERENCES

1. Lentine KL, Smith JM, Hart A, et al. OPTN/SRTR 2020 annual data report: kidney. *Am J Transplant.* 2022;22(suppl 2):21-136.
2. Halloran PF. Immunosuppressive drugs for kidney transplantation. *N Engl J Med.* 2004;351(26):2715-29.
3. Srinivas TR, Meier-Kriesche HU, Kaplan B. Pharmacokinetic principles of immunosuppressive drugs. *Am J Transplant.* 2005;5(2):207-17.
4. Henry ML. Cyclosporine and tacrolimus (FK506): a comparison of efficacy and safety profiles. *Clin Transplant.* 1999;13(3):209-20.
5. Naesens M, Kuypers DR, Sarwal M. Calcineurin inhibitor nephrotoxicity. *Clin J Am Soc Nephrol.* 2009;4(2):481-508.
6. Vincenti F, Jensik SC, Filo RS, Miller J, Pirsch J. A long-term comparison of tacrolimus (FK506) and cyclosporine in kidney transplantation: evidence for improved allograft survival at five years. *Transplantation.* 2002;73(5):775-82.
7. Mohammadpour N, Elyasi S, Vahdati N, Mohammadpour AH, Shamsara J. A review on therapeutic drug monitoring of immunosuppressant drugs. *Iran J Basic Med Sci.* 2011;14(6):485-98.
8. Marcén R. Immunosuppressive drugs in kidney transplantation: impact on patient survival, and incidence of cardiovascular disease, malignancy and infection. *Drugs.* 2009;69(16):2227-43.
9. Manjunatha TA, Chng R, Yau WP. Efficacy and safety of tacrolimus-based maintenance regimens in de novo kidney transplant recipients: a systematic review and network meta-analysis of randomized controlled trials. *Ann Transplant.* 2021;26:e933588.
10. Karolin A, Genitsch V, Sidler D. Calcineurin inhibitor toxicity in solid organ transplantation. *Pharmacology.* 2021;106(7-8):347-55.
11. Wojciechowski D, Wiseman A. Long-term immunosuppression management: opportunities and uncertainties. *Clin J Am Soc Nephrol.* 2021;16(8):1264-71.

12. Nelson J, Alvey N, Bowman L, et al. Consensus recommendations for use of maintenance immunosuppression in solid organ transplantation: endorsed by the American College of Clinical Pharmacy, American Society of Transplantation, and the International Society for Heart and Lung Transplantation. *Pharmacotherapy*. 2022;42(8):599-633.
13. Tremblay S, Nigro V, Weinberg J, Woodle ES, Alloway RR. A steady-state head-to-head pharmacokinetic comparison of All FK-506 (tacrolimus) formulations (ASTCOFF): an open-label, prospective, randomized, two-arm, Three-Period Crossover study. *Am J Transplant*. 2017;17(2):432-42.
14. Langone A, Steinberg SM, Gedaly R, et al. Switching study of kidney transplant patients with tremor to LCP-TacrO (STRATO): an open-label, multicenter, prospective phase 3b study. *Clin Transplant*. 2015;29(9):796-805.
15. Oellerich M, Armstrong VW, Schütz E, Shaw LM. Therapeutic drug monitoring of cyclosporine and tacrolimus. Update on Lake Louise Consensus Conference on cyclosporin and tacrolimus. *Clin Biochem*. 1998;31(5):309-16.
16. Shah MB, Martin JE, Schroeder TJ, First MR. The evaluation of the safety and tolerability of two formulations of cyclosporine: neoral and sandimmune. A meta-analysis. *Transplantation*. 1999;67(11):1411-7.
17. Mardini HE, Arnold GL. Utility of measuring 6-methylmercaptopurine and 6-thioguanine nucleotide levels in managing inflammatory bowel disease patients treated with 6-mercaptopurine in a clinical practice setting. *J Clin Gastroenterol*. 2003;36:390-5.
18. Jiyad Z, Olsen CM, Burke MT, Isbel NM, Green AC. Azathioprine and risk of skin cancer in organ transplant recipients: systematic review and meta-analysis. *Am J Transplant*. 2016;16(12):3490-503.
19. Page RL II, Miller GG, Lindenfeld J. Drug therapy in the heart transplant recipient: part IV – drug-drug interactions. *Circulation*. 2005;111(2):230-9.
20. Vazquez SR, Rondina MT, Pendleton RC. Azathioprine-induced warfarin resistance. *Ann Pharmacother*. 2008;42(7):1118-23.
21. Stepkowski SM. Molecular targets for existing and novel immunosuppressive drugs. *Expert Rev Mol Med*. 2000;2(4):1-23.
22. Golshayan D, Pascual M, Vogt B. Mycophenolic acid formulations in adult renal transplantation—update on efficacy and tolerability. *Ther Clin Risk Manag*. 2009;5(4):341-51.
23. Ferreira PC, Thiesen FV, Pereira AG, et al. A short overview of mycophenolic acid pharmacology and pharmacokinetics. *Clin Transplant*. 2020;34:313997.
24. Neylan J. Immunosuppressive therapy in high-risk transplant patients: dose-dependent efficacy of mycophenolate mofetil in African-American renal allograft recipients. U.S. Renal Transplant Mycophenolate Mofetil Study Group. *Transplantation*. 1997;64(9):1277-82.
25. Kaplan B, Gaston RS, Meier-Kriesche H, Bloom RD, Shaw LM. Mycophenolic acid exposure in high- and low-weight renal transplant patients after dosing with mycophenolate mofetil in the opticept trial. *Ther Drug Monit*. 2010;32(2):224-7.
26. Sherwin CM, Fukuda T, Brunner HI, Goebel J, Vinks AA. The evolution of population pharmacokinetic models to describe the enterohepatic recycling of mycophenolic acid in solid organ transplantation and autoimmune disease. *Clin Pharmacokinet*. 2011;50:1-24.
27. Davies NM, Grinyó J, Heading R, Maes B, Meier-Kriesche HU, Oellerich M. Gastrointestinal side effects of mycophenolic acid in renal transplant patients: a reappraisal. *Nephrol Dial Transplant*. 2007;22(9):2440-8.
28. Langone AJ, Chan L, Bolin P, Cooper M. Enteric-coated mycophenolate sodium versus mycophenolate mofetil in renal transplant recipients experiencing gastrointestinal intolerance: a multicenter, double-blind, randomized study. *Transplantation*. 2011;91(4):470-8.
29. Sollinger HW, Sundberg AK, Leverson G, Voss BJ, Pirsch JD. Mycophenolate mofetil versus enteric-coated mycophenolate sodium: a large, single-center comparison of dose adjustments and outcomes in kidney transplant recipients. *Transplantation*. 2010;89(4):446-51.
30. Shaw LM, Figurski M, Milone MC, Trofe J, Bloom RD. Therapeutic drug monitoring of mycophenolic acid. *Clin J Am Soc Nephrol*. 2007;2(5):1062-72.
31. Sollinger HW. Mycophenolate mofetil for the prevention of acute rejection in primary cadaveric renal allograft recipients. U.S. Renal Transplant Mycophenolate Mofetil Study Group. *Transplantation*. 1995;60(3):225-32.

32. The Tricontinental Mycophenolate Mofetil Renal Transplantation Study Group. A blinded, randomized clinical trial of mycophenolate mofetil for the prevention of acute rejection in cadaveric renal transplantation. *Transplantation.* 1996;61:1029-37.
33. Remuzzi G, Cravedi P, Costantini M, et al. Mycophenolate mofetil versus azathioprine for prevention of chronic allograft dysfunction in renal transplantation: the MYSS follow-up randomized, controlled clinical trial. *J Am Soc Nephrol.* 2007;18(6):1973-85.
34. Fauci AS, Dale DC, Balow JE. Glucocorticosteroid therapy: mechanisms of action and clinical considerations. *Ann Intern Med.* 1976;84(3):304-15.
35. Smith L. Corticosteroids in solid organ transplantation: update and review of the literature. *J Pharm Pract.* 2003;16:380-7.
36. Stanbury RM, Graham EM. Systemic corticosteroid therapy—side effects and their management. *Br J Opthalmol.* 1998;82(6):704-8.
37. Woodle ES, First MR, Pirsch J, et al. A prospective, randomized, double-blind, placebo-controlled multicenter trial comparing early (7 day) corticosteroid cessation versus long-term, low-dose corticosteroid therapy. *Ann Surg.* 2008;248(4):564-77.
38. Thomusch O, Wiesener M, Opgenoorth M, et al. Rabbit-ATG or basiliximab induction for rapid steroid withdrawal after renal transplantation (Harmony): an open-label, multicentre, randomised controlled trial. *Lancet.* 2016;388(10063):3006-16.
39. Flechner SM. mTOR inhibition and clinical transplantation: kidney. *Transplantation.* 2018;102(2S suppl 1):S17-S18.
40. Mekki M, Bridson JM, Sharma A, et al. m-TOR inhibitors in kidney transplantation: a comprehensive review. *J Kidney.* 2017;3:146.
41. Sánchez-Fructuoso AI, Ruiz JC, Perez-Flores I, Gómez Alamillo C, Calvo Romero N, Arias M. Comparative analysis of adverse events requiring suspension of mTOR inhibitors: everolimus versus sirolimus. *Transplant Proc.* 2010;42(8):3050-52.
42. Holdaas H, Rostaing L, Serón D, et al. Conversion of long-term kidney transplant recipients from calcineurin inhibitor therapy to everolimus: a randomized, multicenter, 24-month study. *Transplantation.* 2011;92(4):410-8.
43. Schena F, Pascoe MD, Alberu J, et al. Conversion from calcineurin inhibitors to sirolimus maintenance therapy in renal allograft recipients: 24-month efficacy and safety results from the CONVERT trial. *Transplantation.* 2009;87(2):233-42.
44. Budde K, Becker T, Arns W, et al. Everolimus-based, calcineurin-inhibitor-free regimen in recipients of de-novo kidney transplants: an open-label, randomised, controlled trial. *Lancet.* 2011;377(9768):837-47.
45. van der Zwan M, Hesselink DA, van den Hoogen MWF, Baan CC. Costimulation blockade in kidney transplant recipients. *Drugs.* 2020;80(1):33-46.
46. Vincenti F, Charpentier B, Vanrenterghem Y, et al. A phase III study of belatacept-based immunosuppression regimens versus cyclosporine in renal transplant recipients (BENEFIT study). *Am J Transplant.* 2010;10(3):535-46.
47. Badell IR, Parsons RF, Karadkhele G, et al. Every 2-month belatacept maintenance therapy in kidney transplant recipients greater than 1-year posttransplant: a randomized, noninferiority trial. *Am J Transplant.* 2021;21(9):3066-76.
48. Jain A, Xu R, Venkataramanan R, et al. Plasmapheresis decreases belatacept exposure: requires consideration for dose and frequency adjustments. *Transplantation.* 2021;105(10):e152-3.
49. Budde K, Prashar R, Haller H, et al. Conversion from calcineurin inhibitor- to belatacept-based maintenance immunosuppression in renal transplant recipients: a randomized phase 3b trial. *J Am Soc Nephrol.* 2021;32(12):3252-64.
50. Adams AB, Goldstein J, Garrett C, et al. Belatacept combined with transient calcineurin inhibitor therapy prevents rejection and promotes improved long-term renal allograft function. *Am J Transplant.* 2017;17(11):2922-36.

11 Transplant Pathology

Nidia Messias and Joseph Gaut

GENERAL PRINCIPLES

- For the past 30 years, the kidney transplant pathology community has been united in accepting the Banff classification of kidney allograft pathology criteria for the diagnosis of kidney transplant rejection and other lesions seen on kidney allograft biopsies.[1]
- This classification system was first envisioned during a 1991 meeting, and every 2 years a new meeting takes place to update the criteria and incorporate new data valuable to evolution of the transplant field.
- Banff criteria define terms and assign scores to several identifiers in the renal biopsy. A combination of histologic scores and ancillary studies such as donor-specific antibodies (DSAs) testing and molecular profiling defines transplant diagnostic categories (**Table 11-1**).[2-5]
- The Banff histologic findings when present and considered significant are scored as mild (1), moderate (2), and severe (3) and are briefly summarized in **Table 11-2**.

ANTIBODY-MEDIATED REJECTION

- Antibody-mediated rejection (ABMR) is diagnosed when kidney injury or changes are present in the setting of antibody production and interaction with the tissue.
- AMBR may occur in isolation or concurrently with T-cell-mediated rejection (TCMR).
- The specific histologic features to be noted when evaluating for ABMR are glomerulitis (g), peritubular capillaritis (ptc), intimal arteritis (v), transplant glomerulopathy (cg), peritubular capillary multilayering (ptcml), and C4d positivity in ptcs (C4d).[3,4,6,7] These changes are illustrated in **Figure 11-1**.
- Antibody-mediated changes include
  - Active ABMR
  - Chronic active ABMR
  - Chronic (inactive) ABMR
  - C4d staining without evidence of rejection

TABLE 11-1 Banff Diagnostic Categories for Renal Allograft Biopsies

Category 1	Normal biopsy or nonspecific changes
Category 2	Antibody-mediated changes
Category 3	Suspicious (borderline) for acute T-cell-mediated rejection
Category 4	T-cell-mediated rejection
Category 5	Polyomavirus nephropathy

TABLE 11-2 Definitions of Banff Histologic Findings and Scoring System

Banff Finding	Mild, 1	Moderate,–2	Severe, 3
Glomerulitis (g)	Present in <25% of glomeruli	In 25%-75% of glomeruli	In >75% of glomeruli
Tubulitis (t)[a]	1-4 mononuclear cells per tubular cross section or 10 tubular epithelial cells	5-10 mononuclear cells per tubular cross section or 10 tubular epithelial cells	>10 mononuclear cells per tubular cross section or 10 tubular epithelial cells Or TBM destruction[b]
Interstitial inflammation (i)	10%-25% of cortex with inflammation	26%-50% of cortex with inflammation	>50% of cortex with inflammation
Intimal arteritis (v)	<25% luminal area lost	>25% luminal area lost	Transmural arteritis and/or fibrinoid necrosis
Glomerulopathy (cg)	Double contours by EM only or in <25% loops of most affected glomerulus	Double contours in 25%-50% loops of most affected glomerulus	Double contours in >50% loops of most affected glomerulus
Tubular atrophy (ct)	In up to 25% of proximal tubules	In 26%-50% of proximal tubules	In >50% of proximal tubules
Interstitial fibrosis (ci)	In 6%-25% of cortical area	In 26%-50% of cortical area	In >50% of cortical area
Arteriopathy (cv)	Up to 25% of vascular lumen narrowed by fibrointimal thickening	26%-50% of vascular lumen narrowed by fibrointimal thickening	>50% of vascular lumen narrowed by fibrointimal thickening
Peritubular capillaritis (ptc)	In ≥10% of cortical PTCs with 3-4 PMNs in most severe PTC	In ≥10% of cortical PTCs with 5-10 PMNs in most severe PTC	In ≥10% of cortical PTCs with >10 PMNs in most severe PTC
C4d positivity in peritubular capillaries (C4d)	Stain in <10% of PTC and medullary vasa recta	Stain in 10%-50% of PTC and medullary vasa recta	Stain in >50% of PTC and medullary vasa recta
Total inflammation (ti)	Inflammation in 10%-25% of total cortex	Inflammation in 26%-50% of total cortex	Inflammation in >50% of total cortex
Inflammation in fibrosis (i-IFTA)	Inflammation in 10%-25% of scarred cortex	Inflammation in 26%-50% of scarred cortex	Inflammation in >50% of scarred cortex

TABLE 11-2 Definitions of Banff Histologic Findings and Scoring System (Continued)

Banff Finding	Mild, 1	Moderate,–2	Severe, 3
Tubulitis in fibrosis (t-IFTA)	Mild tubulitis in tubules within scarred cortex	Moderate tubulitis in tubules within scarred cortex	Severe tubulitis in tubules within scarred cortex
Arteriolar hyalinosis (ah)	Mild to moderate hyaline thickening	Moderate to severe hyaline thickening in >1 arteriole	Severe hyaline thickening in several arterioles
Mesangial expansion (mm)	Moderate or severe mesangial matrix increase in up to 25% of nonsclerotic glomeruli	Moderate or severe mesangial matrix increase in 26%-50% of nonsclerotic glomeruli	Moderate or severe mesangial matrix increase in >50% of nonsclerotic glomeruli
Polyomavirus load (pvl)	≤1% of all tubules with viral replication	>1% to ≤10% of all tubules with viral replication	>10% of all tubules with viral replication

EM, electron microscopy; PMN, polymorphonuclear leukocytes; PTC, peritubular capillary; TBM, tubular basement membranes.
[a]Tubulitis should be scored only in tubuli that are not severely atrophic.
[b]TBM destruction has to be present in 2 areas and t2 seen elsewhere in the biopsy.

- For active ABMR, the following 3 criteria need to be met, with at least 1 criterion from each category:
  - Histologic evidence of acute (active ABMR) or chronic tissue injury (chronic active ABMR), described in **Table 11-3**.
  - Evidence of current/recent antibody interaction with vascular endothelium:
    - Linear C4d staining in peritubular capillaries or medullary vasa recta
    - Moderate or severe microvascular inflammation ([g + ptc] ≥ 2), noting that g ≥ 1 must be observed if there is concurrent borderline/TCMR or infection
    - Increased expression of validated gene transcripts/classifiers strongly associated with ABMR
  - Serologic evidence of circulating DSAs (to HLA or other antigens). This criterion may be substituted by positive C4d staining of peritubular capillaries or expression of validated transcripts/classifiers, but complete DSA investigation is strongly recommended (including non-HLA).
- Chronic (inactive) AMBR is diagnosed in patients with previous history of active/chronic active ABMR or history of positive DSA, with biopsy findings of cg or severe ptcml, and absence of current/recent antibody interaction with vascular endothelium (C4d negative, no microcirculation inflammation, no gene transcripts/classifiers).
- C4d staining without evidence of rejection implies C4d positivity in a biopsy without histologic or molecular criteria defining ABMR or TCMR.

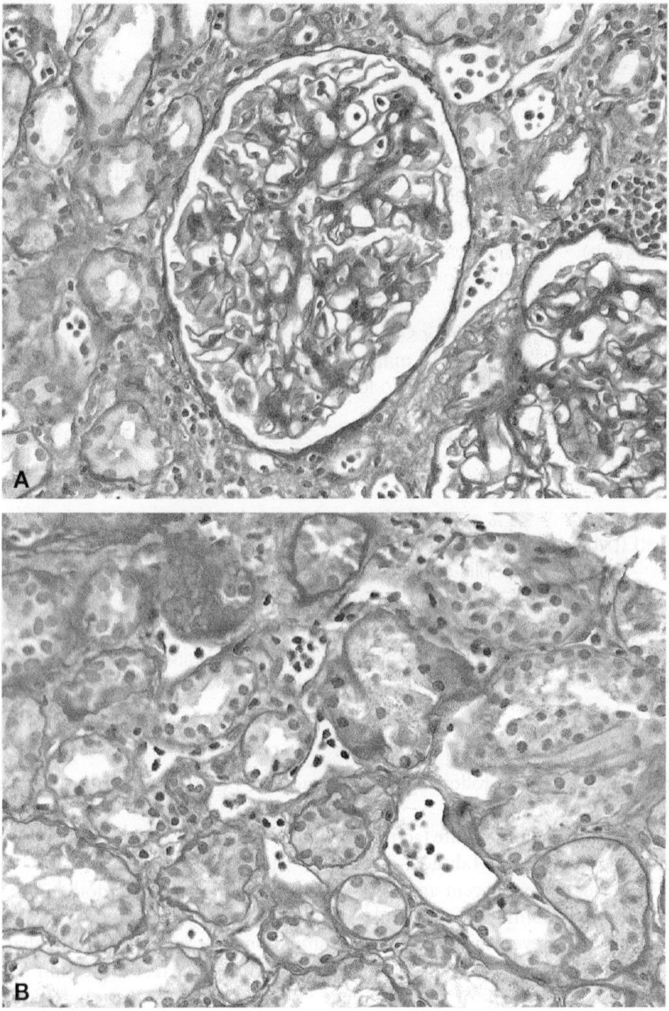

Figure 11-1. **Histologic findings in antibody-mediated changes.** Microcirculation inflammation is the hallmark of active antibody-mediated changes. Glomerulitis (g) and peritubular capillaritis (ptc) are the acute microcirculation inflammation markers and provide histologic evidence of acute tissue injury. Intimal arteritis (as seen in TCMR) and acute tubular injury and/or thrombotic microangiopathy (in the absence of other known causes) also serve as histologic evidence of tissue injury. C4d positivity on peritubular capillaries is a marker of antibody interaction with vascular endothelium and may substitute the need for positive DSA for diagnosis of active ABMR. Chronic transplant glomerulopathy and severe peritubular capillary multilayering are observed in chronic ABMR, either active or inactive. Electron microscopy examination may be required to observe these changes. Findings illustrated are A, glomerulitis (g); B, peritubular capillaritis (ptc); C, intimal arteritis with transmural fibrinoid necrosis (v3); D, C4d positivity on peritubular capillaries (duo stain—green for C4d stain, red stains the tubules in the background); E, chronic transplant glomerulopathy (cg); F, chronic transplant glomerulopathy observed on electron microscopy (cg).

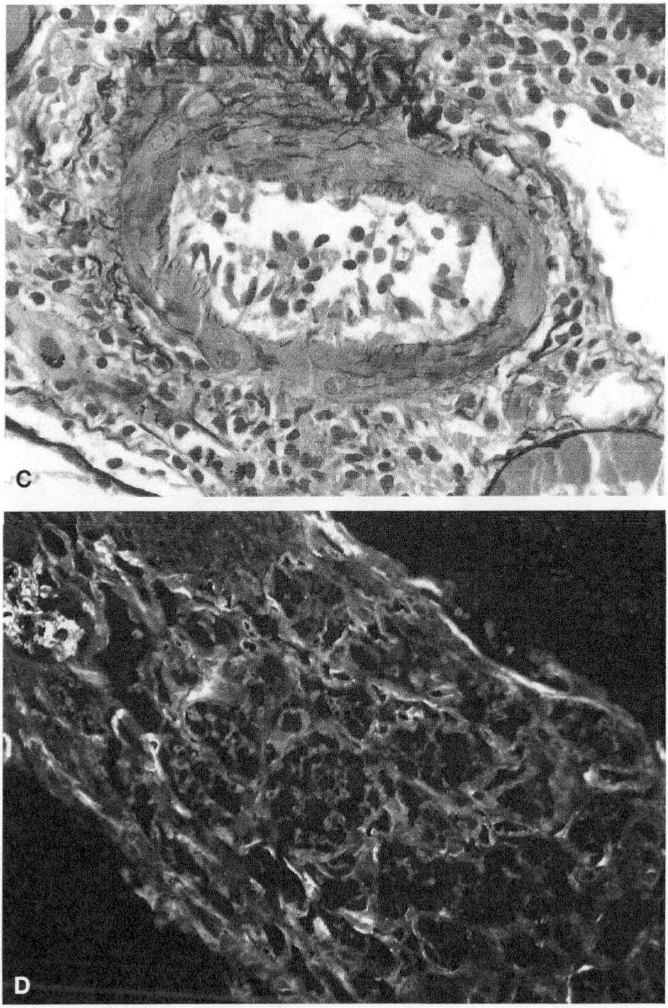

Figure 11-1. Continued

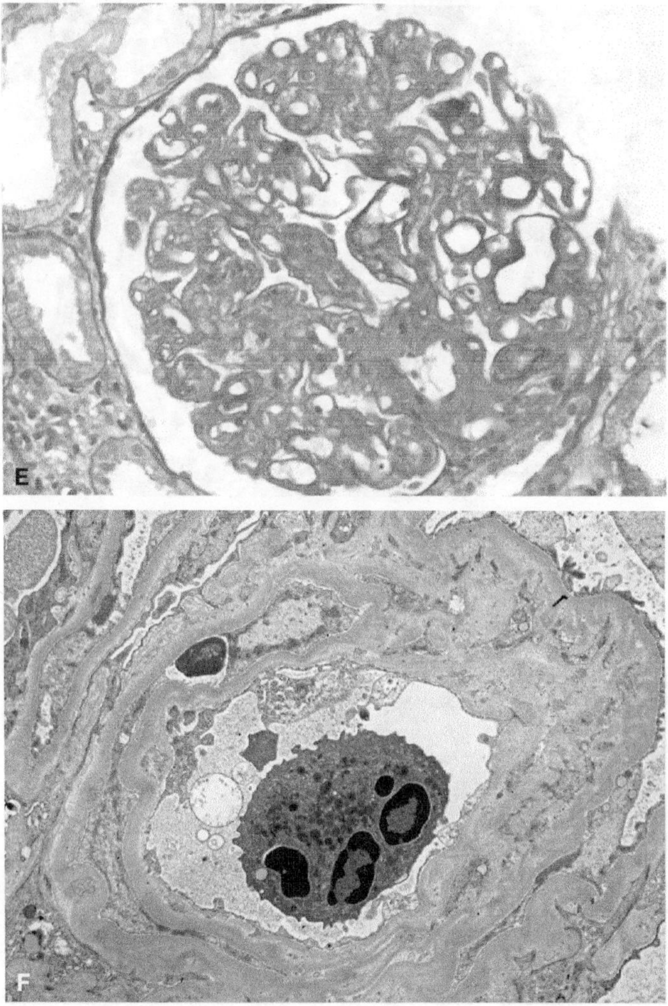

Figure 11-1. Continued

SUSPICIOUS/BORDERLINE FOR TCMR

- Histologic changes qualifying for a diagnosis of suspicious/borderline for acute TCMR are of insufficient magnitude to qualify for acute TCMR.
- Specifically, suspicious/borderline changes refer to presence of tubulitis and interstitial inflammation in minor degrees as compared with cases with acute TCMR.[3,4]
- The criteria for borderline changes have varied and evolved in different versions of the Banff classification, which may lead to confusion among pathologists and nephrologists.

TABLE 11-3 Histologic Evidence of Acute and Chronic Tissue Injury in ABMR

Acute Tissue Injury	Chronic Tissue Injury
Microvascular inflammation (g > 0 and/or ptc > 0), in the absence of recurrent or de novo glomerulonephritis, although in the presence of acute TCMR, borderline infiltrate, or infection, ptc ≥ 1 alone is not sufficient and g must be ≥1	Transplant glomerulopathy (cg > 0) if no evidence of chronic TMA or chronic recurrent/de novo glomerulonephritis; includes changes evident by EM alone (cg1a)
Intimal or transmural arteritis (v > 0)	Severe peritubular capillary basement membrane multilayering (ptcml1), defined as ≥7 basement membrane layers in the most affected PTC AND ≥5 layers in 2 additional PTCs; requires EM
Acute thrombotic microangiopathy, in the absence of any other cause and/or acute tubular injury, in the absence of any other apparent cause	Arterial intimal fibrosis of new onset, excluding other causes; leukocytes within the sclerotic intima favor chronic ABMR if there is no prior history of TCMR, but are not required

ABMR, antibody-mediated rejection; EM, electron microscopy; PTC, peritubular capillary; TCMR, T-cell-mediated rejection; TMA, thrombotic microangiopathy.

- The most recent Banff classification (2019) defines borderline changes as (1) presence of any degree of tubulitis (t1, t2, or t3) with mild interstitial inflammation (i1) or (2) mild (t1) tubulitis with moderate-severe interstitial inflammation (i2 or i3).
- While ABMR may be present in cases of suspicious/borderline acute TCMR, the presence of intimal or transmural arteritis is not allowed for borderline diagnosis.

T-CELL-MEDIATED REJECTION

- TCMR, or cellular rejection, is centered on direct presence of inflammatory cellular elements inflammatory within interstitium, tubules, and vessels.
- The specific histologic features to be noted when evaluating for TCMR are tubulitis (t), interstitial inflammation (i), intimal arteritis (v), total inflammation (ti), and inflammation in scarred cortex (i-IFTA), tubulitis in tubules within scarred cortex (t-IFTA), and chronic allograft arteriopathy (cv).[3,4,8] These changes are illustrated in **Figure 11-2**.
- While antibody-mediated changes and DSAs may be present, these do not impact the diagnostic criteria of TCMR.
- TCMR is divided into active or acute TCMR and chronic active TCMR, with different grades according to severity.
- Active TCMR refers to acute changes present in the transplant related to direct tissue injury by mononuclear inflammatory cells. Grading of acute TCMR is defined as follows and summarized in **Figure 11-3**.

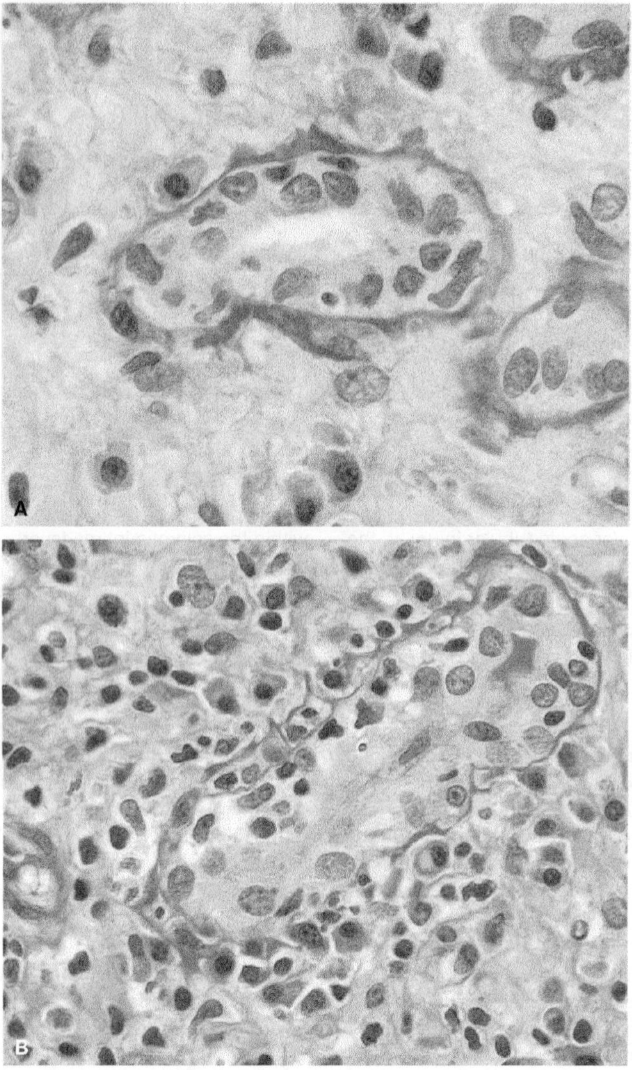

Figure 11-2. **Histologic findings in T-cell-mediated rejection (TCMR).** The diagnosis of acute TCMR relies on the presence of moderate (t2) or severe tubulitis (t3) AND moderate (i2) or severe interstitial inflammation (i3) in nonscarred cortex, OR presence of intimal arteritis (v), with (v3) or without (v1, v2) transmural changes/fibrinoid necrosis. The diagnosis of chronic active TCMR is based on total inflammation in more than 25% of the cortex AND moderate (i-IFTA2) or severe interstitial inflammation (i-IFTA3) in scarred cortex WITH moderate or severe tubulitis in nonscarred (t2/t3) or scarred cortical areas (t-IFTA2/3), OR presence of chronic allograft arteriopathy (cv). The vascular lesions described on TCMR may also be a component of ABMR. Findings illustrated are A, moderate tubulitis (t2); B, severe tubulitis (t3); C, interstitial inflammation in nonscarred cortex (i); D, intimal arteritis (v); E, total inflammation involving scarred and nonscarred cortex (ti); F, inflammation in scarred cortex (i-IFTA); G, tubulitis in scarred cortex (t-IFTA); and H, chronic allograft arteriopathy (cv).

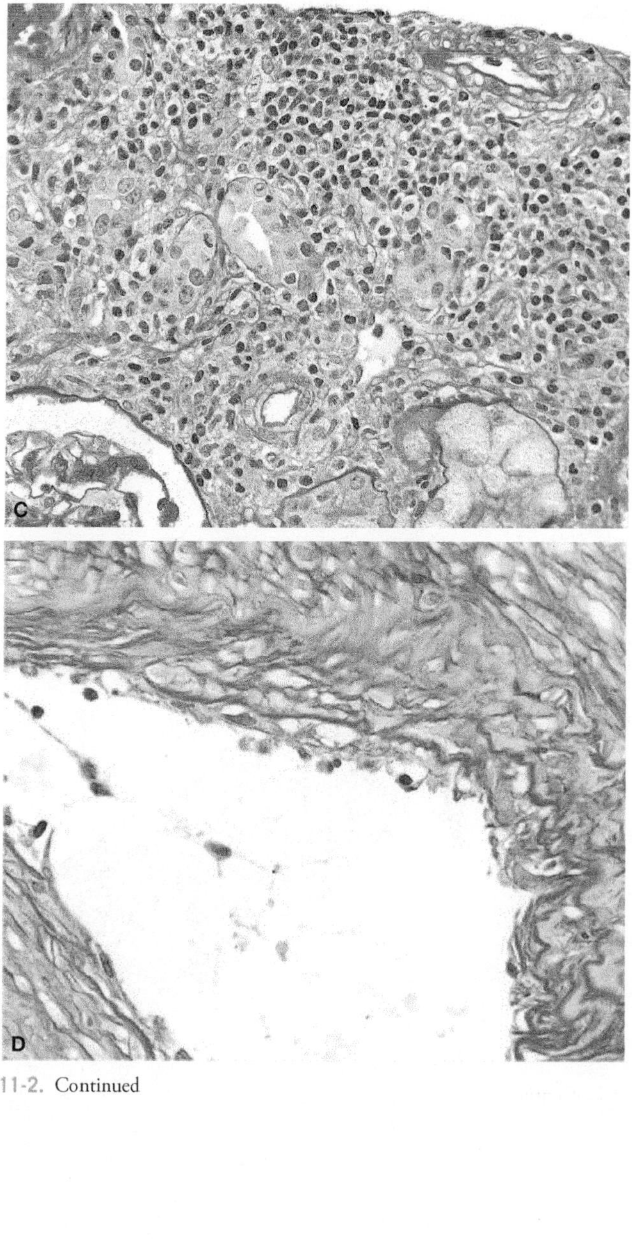

Figure 11-2. Continued

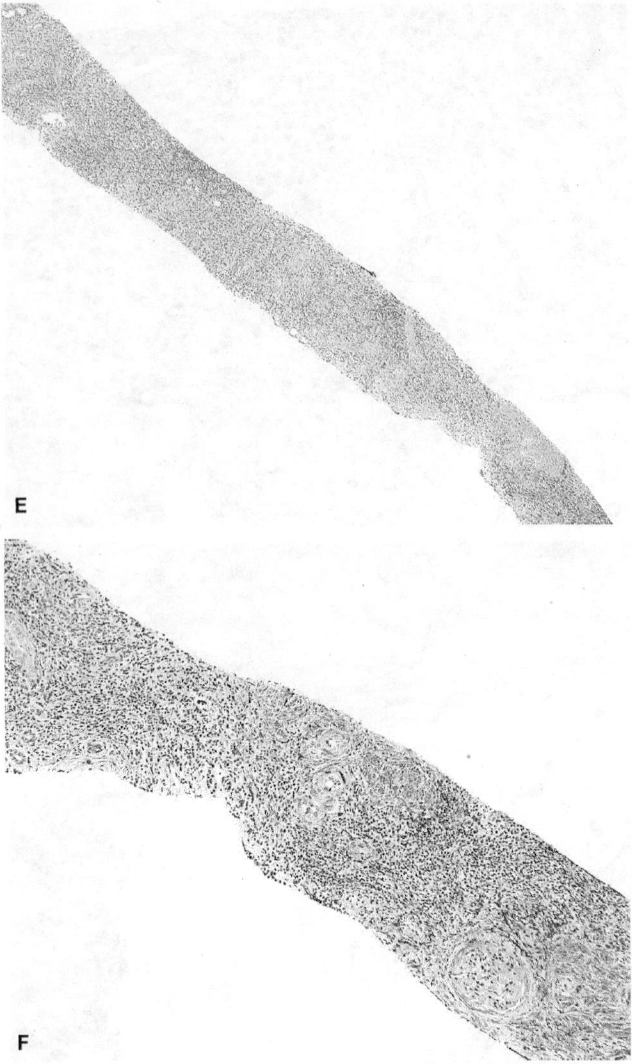

Figure 11-2. Continued

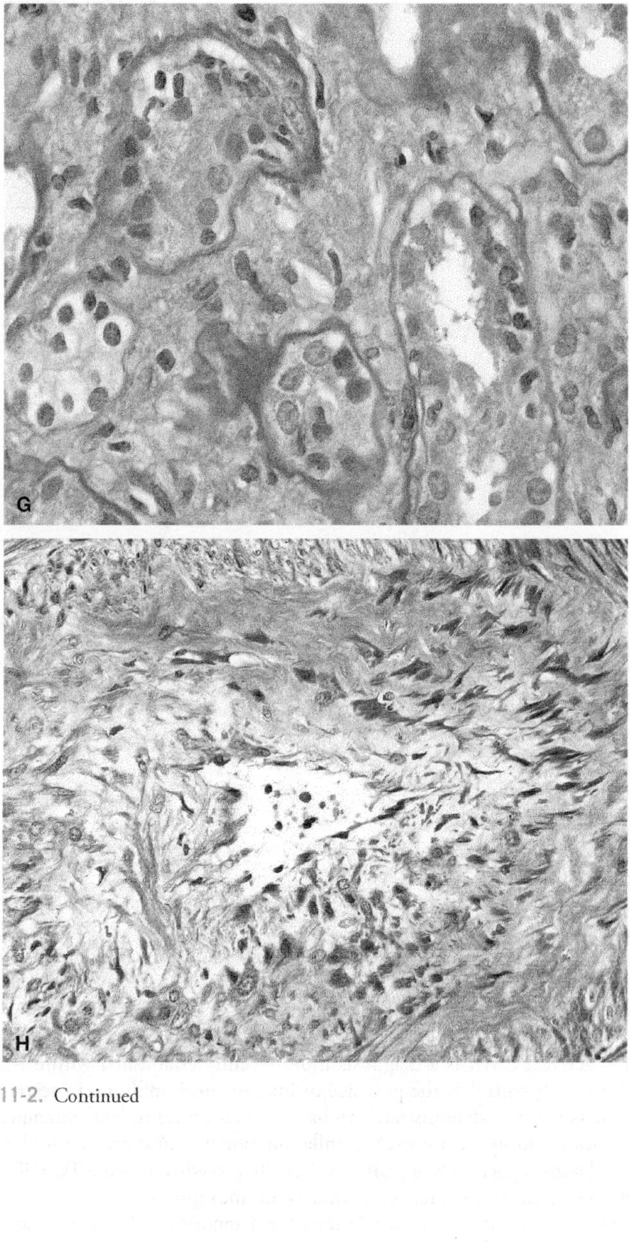

Figure 11-2. Continued

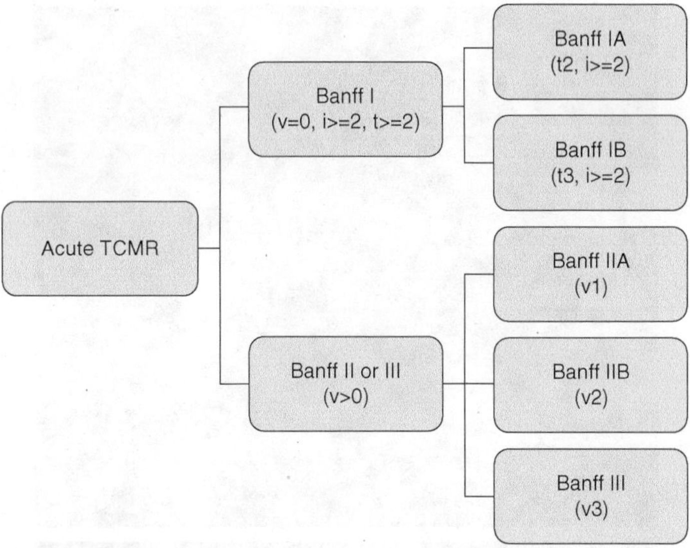

Figure 11-3. **Simplified classification of acute T-cell-mediated rejection (TCMR).** Banff I is reserved for tubulointerstitial-type rejection, when no intimal arteritis is identified. At least moderate interstitial inflammation should be present in nonscarred cortex (i2 or i3), AND moderate (t2) or severe (t3) tubulitis is seen in Banff IA and IB, respectively. Banff II and Banff III require the presence of intimal arteritis (v lesion), which may be mild or moderate (v1 and v2) for Banff IIA and IIB, respectively, or may be severe, with transmural involvement or fibrinoid necrosis (v3), defining features of Banff III.

- Grade IA: Interstitial inflammation in >25% of nonsclerotic cortex (i2 or i3) with moderate tubulitis (t2)
- Grade IB: Interstitial inflammation in >25% of nonsclerotic cortex (i2 or i3) with severe tubulitis (t3)
- Grade IIA: Mild to moderate intimal arteritis (v1), independent of interstitial inflammation and/or tubulitis
- Grade IIB: Severe intimal arteritis (v2), independent of interstitial inflammation and/or tubulitis
- Grade III: Intimal arteritis with transmural involvement and/or arterial fibrinoid necrosis in smooth muscle (v3), independent of interstitial inflammation and/or tubulitis

- Chronic active TCMR is a diagnosis more recently established within the Banff classification. It considers the presence of inflammatory infiltrate in scarred cortical areas, as this was demonstrated to have impact on transplant outcomes. Total inflammation and significant (>25%) inflammation within scarred cortex have been associated with higher rates of graft loss. Usually preceded by acute TCMR, inflammation in scarred cortex is related to underimmunosuppression.
- If features are present that fit into criteria for diagnosis of both acute and chronic active TCMR, both should be reported.
- Grading of chronic active TCMR is defined as follows:
  - Grade IA: Interstitial inflammation in >25% of sclerotic cortex (i-IFTA2 or i-IFTA3) AND >25% of total cortex (ti2 or ti3) with moderate tubulitis (t2 or t-IFTA2)

- Grade IB: Interstitial inflammation in >25% of sclerotic cortex (i-IFTA2 or i-IFTA3) AND >25% of total cortex (ti2 or ti3) with severe tubulitis (t3 or t-IFTA3)
- Grade II: Chronic allograft arteriopathy (which may also be seen with ABMR)

INFECTIONS

Polyomavirus Nephropathy

- Polyomavirus infection is common, impacting up to 90% of young adults. Although essentially asymptomatic in healthy individuals, the immunosuppression associated with kidney transplantation may lead to a clinically significant infection.
- Polyomavirus nephropathy (PVN) is one of the most common infections involving renal allografts, with an incidence of about 5% in biopsies. The polyomavirus most often present is type 1, also named BK virus, although type 2, also named JC virus, may show similar histomorphology.
- While polyomavirus infection is usually monitored and initially detected by blood polymerase chain reaction, the features on the kidney biopsy may guide therapeutics based on the prognosis.
- The histologic diagnosis relies on morphologic features and immunohistochemical staining for the SV40 large T antigen.
- This immunostain highlights nuclei positive for polyomavirus but does not distinguish BK from other types of polyomavirus.
- PVN may be identified on routine light microscopy by intranuclear viral inclusions within tubular epithelial nuclei.
- Interstitial inflammation and tubulitis may also be seen, creating a diagnostic dilemma with acute TCMR. Rapid immunohistochemical staining for SV40 large T antigen is critical to distinguish rejection from PVN.
- The inflammatory infiltrate is predominantly composed of mononuclear cells enriched with plasma cells. Plasma cell tubulitis is more typical of PVN than rejection. **Figure 11-4** illustrates some of the findings observed on PVN.
- Banff classification incorporates polyomavirus grading into their recommendations.[9] The grading and classification is based on the polyomavirus load (pvl) and interstitial fibrosis (ci).
- In summary, PVN is classified as:
  - PVN class 1—mild viral load (pvl1) and no (ci0) or mild interstitial fibrosis (ci1)
  - PVN class 2—moderate viral load (pvl2), or a combination of mild viral load (pvl1) and moderate or severe interstitial fibrosis (ci2-3) or a combination of severe viral load (pvl1) and no (ci0) or mild or severe interstitial fibrosis (ci1)
  - PVN class 3—severe viral load (pvl1) and severe interstitial fibrosis (ci3)
- Polyomavirus infects tubuli in cortex and medulla, hence distal and proximal tubuli and ducts are quantified for estimation of viral load. In fact, presence of medulla in the sample is one of the recommendations for adequate evaluation of PVN.
- PVN may occur concomitantly with rejection. A not so uncommon and challenging scenario is that in which the polyomavirus nephropathy is being addressed and a superimposed rejection takes place secondary to adjustments in the therapy.

Cytomegalovirus

- Transplanted kidneys are susceptible to cytomegalovirus (CMV).
- CMV infection shows a characteristic morphologic appearance, with large and prominent nuclear and cytoplasmic inclusions.

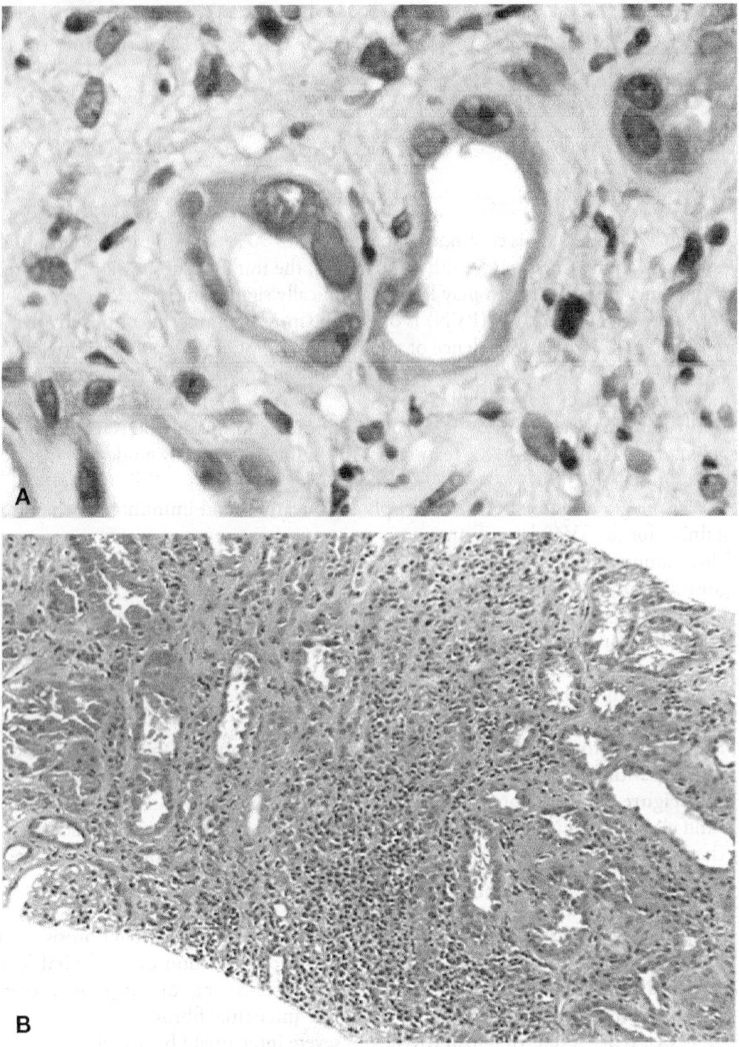

Figure 11-4. **Polyomavirus nephropathy.** Polyomavirus nephropathy is characterized by involvement of tubular cells by polyomavirus, and the viral cytopathic effects lead to nuclear inclusions (A). The viral cytopathic effects may be accompanied by interstitial inflammation (B) and tubulitis (C), which is problematic in the distinction from TCMR. Tubular injury with sloughing of tubular cells is also often observed. Plasma cell tubulitis may be noted in polyomavirus nephritis. Classification of polyomavirus nephropathy depends on the quantification of interstitial fibrosis and viral load (pvl). Polyomavirus load may be mild (D), when <1% of all tubules have viral replication; moderate (E), >1% to 10% of tubules have viral replication; or severe (F), when viral replication is seen in >10% of the tubules.

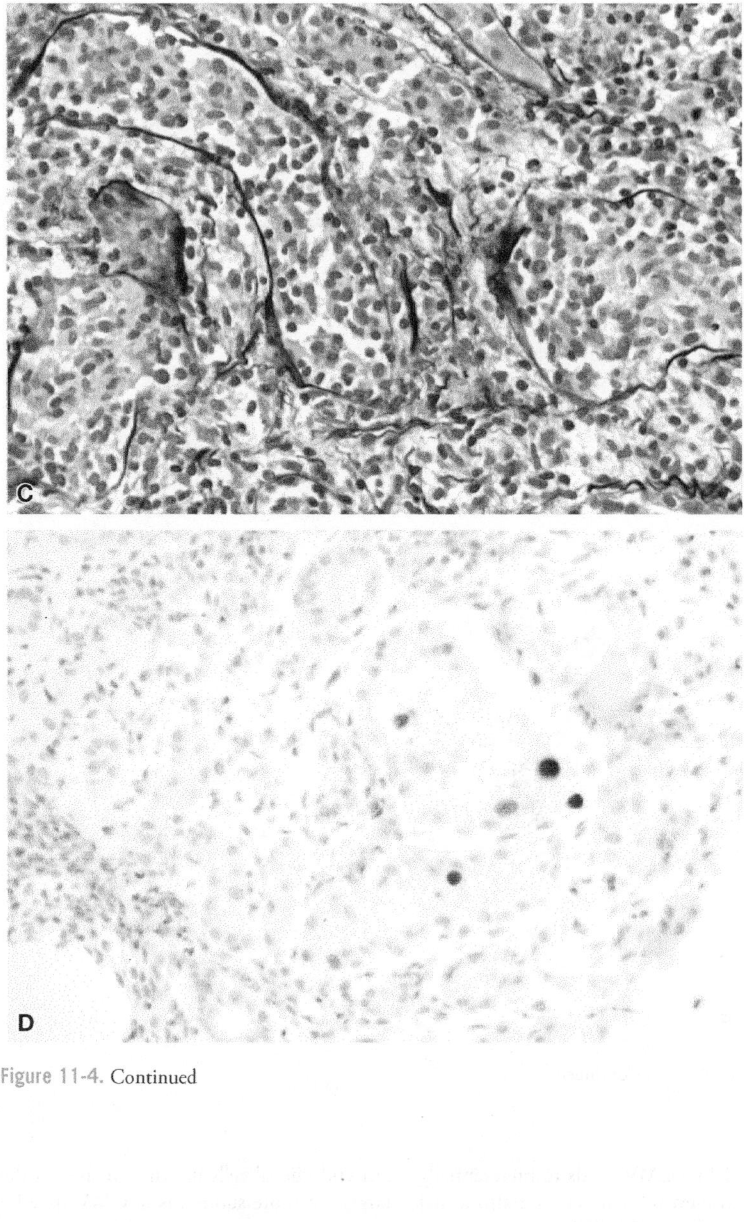

Figure 11-4. Continued

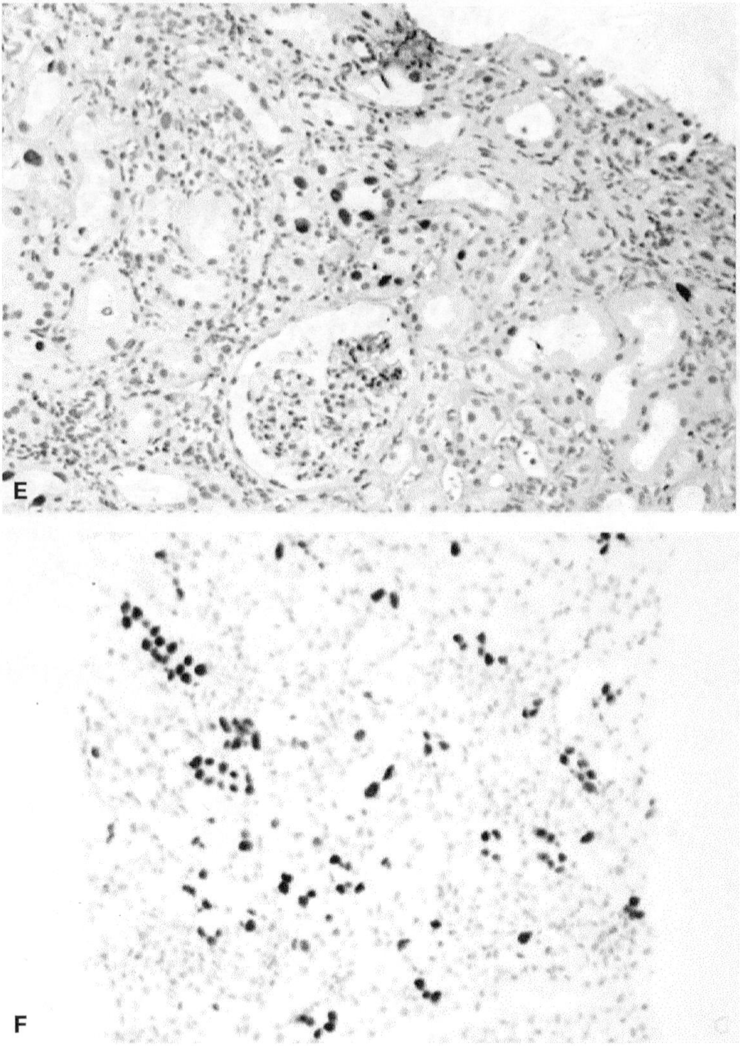

Figure 11-4. Continued

- While CMV tends to preferentially infect endothelial cells in other organs, in the kidney, tubular cells are also a major target. In more subtle cases, CMV may be confused with PVN.
- While usually not necessary, immunohistochemistry stain for CMV may be helpful to confirm cases where there is a diagnostic dilemma. **Figure 11-5** illustrates some of the findings observed on CMV nephritis.

Adenovirus

- Kidney infection with adenovirus is rare.
- It is typically associated with an intense inflammatory infiltrate including neutrophils and neutrophilic casts associated with areas of interstitial hemorrhage. Tubular injury and foci of tubular necrosis may be present.
- Viral inclusions are also present but less distinctive than with other viruses. A high degree of suspicion is needed for diagnosis. Immunohistochemistry stain for adenovirus is particularly helpful.

Other Infections

- Bacterial infections affecting the transplant kidney tend to present as pyelonephritis and are often seen in association with reflux nephropathy.
- Interstitial granulomas should raise the possibilities of fungi or acid-fast bacilli as infectious agents. Drug reactions may also cause granulomatous interstitial nephritis.
- Similar to native kidneys, the indirect effects of systemic infections may be identified in transplanted kidneys. These may manifest as glomerulonephritides like membranoproliferative glomerulonephritis in cases of hepatitis, collapsing glomerulopathy in HIV and coronavirus disease 2019 (COVID-19) infections, and proliferative glomerulonephritis in bacterial infections. Thrombotic microangiopathy may also be the defining histopathologic finding (eg, in COVID-19 infection).

EFFECTS OF TRANSPLANT MEDICATIONS

- Changes related to therapy may be observed in transplant recipients. These changes should be considered nonspecific as they may also be encountered in other pathologies.
- Most notably, calcineurin inhibitor therapy has been described in association with tubular injury, with isometric vacuolization of the tubular epithelial cytoplasm, arteriolar hyalinosis and arteriolar necrosis and vacuolization, and thrombotic microangiopathy.[10]
- Some of these findings are illustrated in **Figure 11-6**.
- Chronic changes including glomerulosclerosis, arteriolar hyaline thickening, and striped interstitial fibrosis and tubular atrophy may be seen.

RECURRING DISEASES IN TRANSPLANT

- Most diseases affecting the native kidney may recur in the kidney transplant with few exceptions. Most notably, Alport syndrome and polycystic kidney disease do not recur.
- While early recurrence plays a minor clinical role in early graft loss, it becomes more problematic in older transplants.
- Recurrent glomerulonephritis was cited as the third most frequent cause for graft loss 10 years after kidney transplantation.
- Pathologies prone to recur in transplant include IgA nephropathy, focal segmental glomerulosclerosis, membranoproliferative glomerulonephritis, C3 glomerulopathy, membranous nephropathy, and antineutrophil cytoplasmic antibodies-associated glomerulonephritis.[11]
- Lupus nephritis may recur, but less frequently. Anti-glomerular basement membrane disease is unlikely to recur in transplants.
- Since transplant patients are on an immunosuppressive therapeutic regimen, this may keep native inflammatory diseases less active than they would be otherwise. Still, proper diagnosis may lead to changes in therapy.

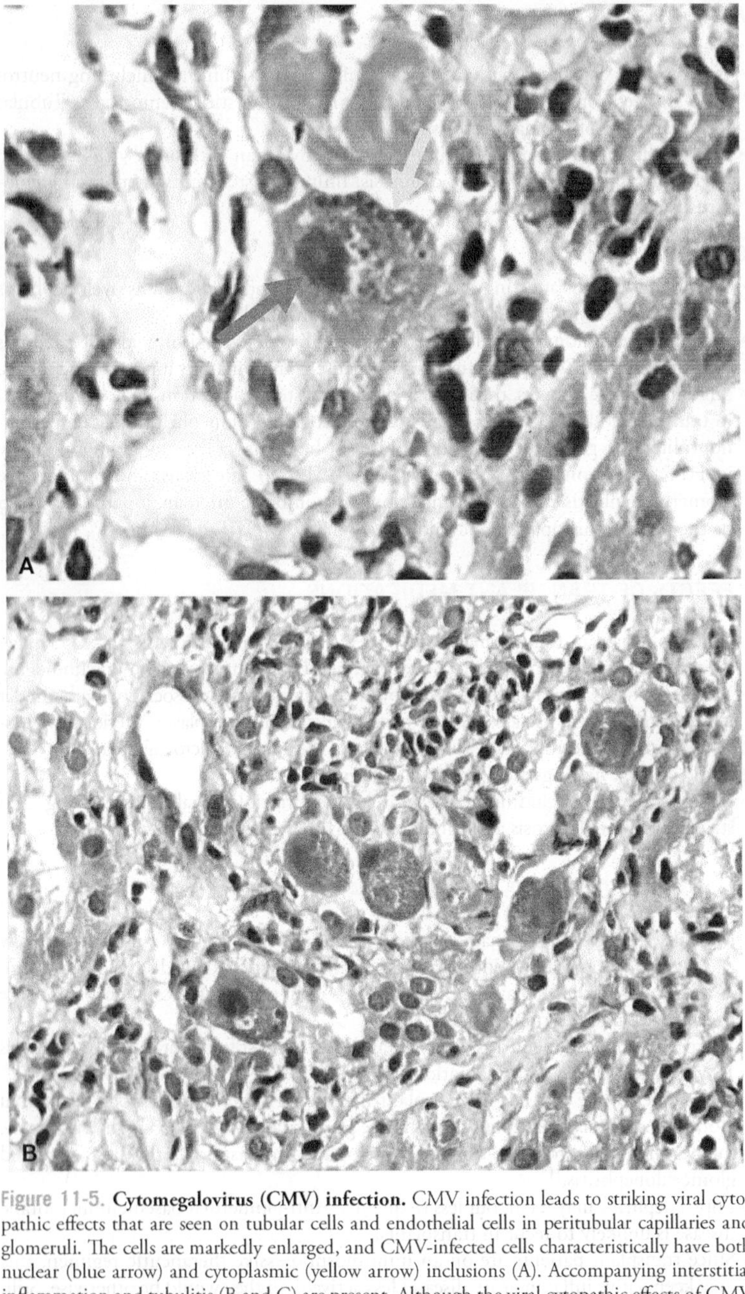

Figure 11-5. **Cytomegalovirus (CMV) infection.** CMV infection leads to striking viral cytopathic effects that are seen on tubular cells and endothelial cells in peritubular capillaries and glomeruli. The cells are markedly enlarged, and CMV-infected cells characteristically have both nuclear (blue arrow) and cytoplasmic (yellow arrow) inclusions (A). Accompanying interstitial inflammation and tubulitis (B and C) are present. Although the viral cytopathic effects of CMV are quite distinct, immunohistochemistry stain for CMV (D) may help in differentiating from other viruses, particularly polyomavirus. (Courtesy of Dr. David Campos Wanderley, Brazil.)

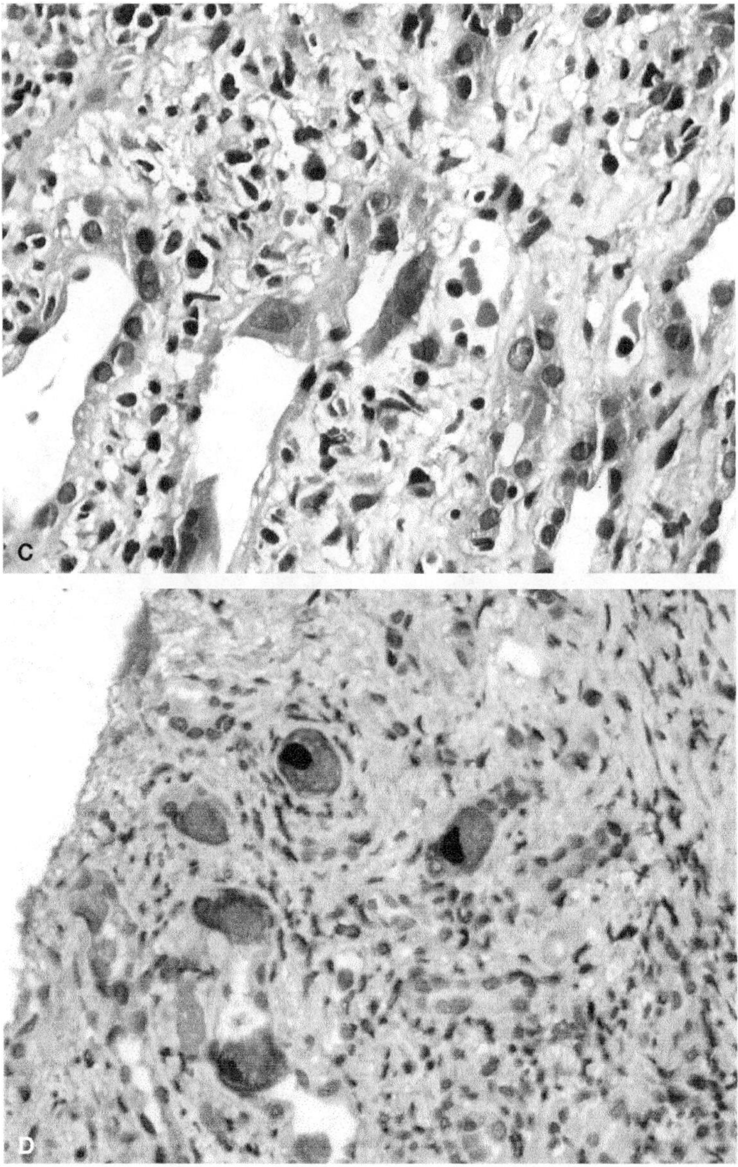

Figure 11-5. Continued

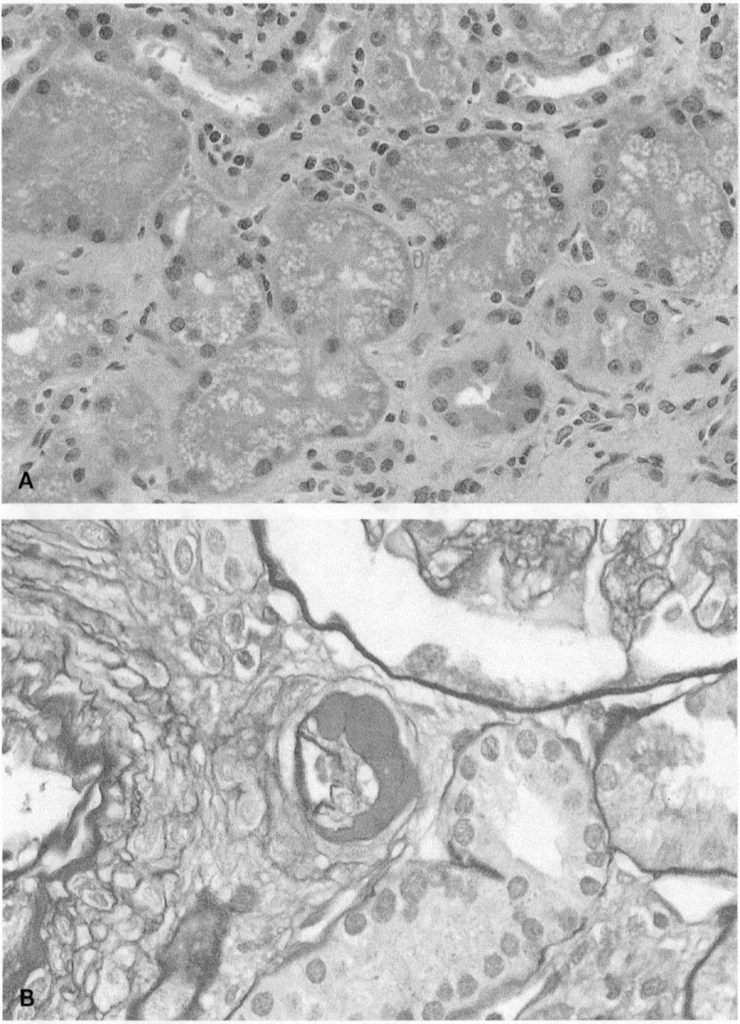

Figure 11-6. **Calcineurin inhibitor (CNI) toxicity effects.** Tubular injury with isometric cytoplasmic vacuolization has been described as a histologic feature associated with acute CNI toxicity (A). Vasculature is also involved and characterized by nodular arteriolar hyalinosis (B) and/or vacuolization of the arteriolar walls (C). Other changes associated with CNI include "stripped" interstitial fibrosis and thrombotic microangiopathy.

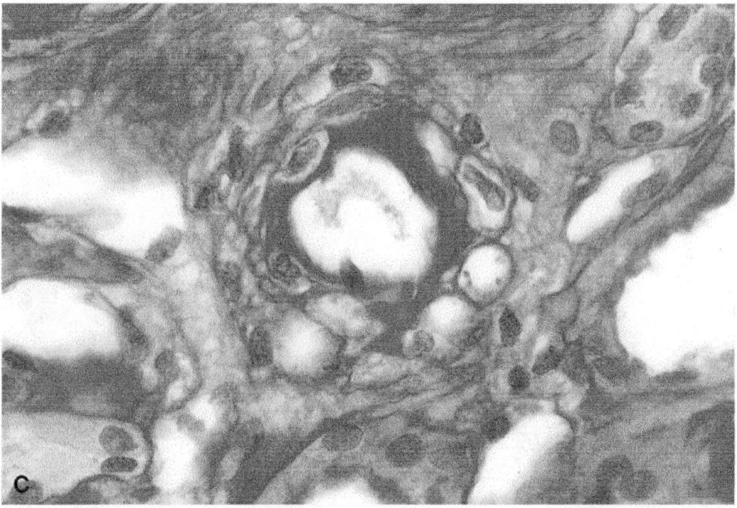

Figure 11-6. Continued

EVALUATION OF DONOR BIOPSIES

- Donor transplant biopsies are commonly performed in older, extended criteria donors or those with a kidney donor profile index >85%. In contrast to routine transplant biopsies, donor biopsies are typically frozen sections requiring immediate interpretation by nonrenal pathologists in off hours.
- Donor biopsies may be a wedge or core, depending on the transplant center and surgeon preference. A cortical sample is preferred. The United Network for Organ Sharing recommends a minimum of 25 glomeruli for adequate evaluation.
- The clinical utility of the histologic evaluation of kidney donor biopsies has been validated in several studies, and in general, signs of chronicity in the donor biopsy show correlation with graft loss and diminished kidney function.[12]
- Standard features evaluated in the donor kidney biopsy include global glomerulosclerosis, tubular atrophy, interstitial fibrosis, arterial intimal fibrosis, and arteriolar hyalinosis. Presence of fibrin thrombi and cortical necrosis are also noted. Other changes within the glomeruli, most commonly diabetic nodular glomerulosclerosis, are also reported. **Figure 11-7** shows examples of these changes.
- The evaluation of donor kidneys may reveal donor kidney disease that might have been previously unrecognized and would impact both the decision to transplant and recipient therapy.
- Digital pathology has been routinely used in our center and others for evaluation of donor transplant biopsies, as it allows for reliable and timely reading and results. With continued application of digital pathology, development of artificial intelligence methods may be applied to assist pathologists with quantitation of chronic damage, improving precision and accuracy in the challenging setting of after-hours frozen sections.[13]

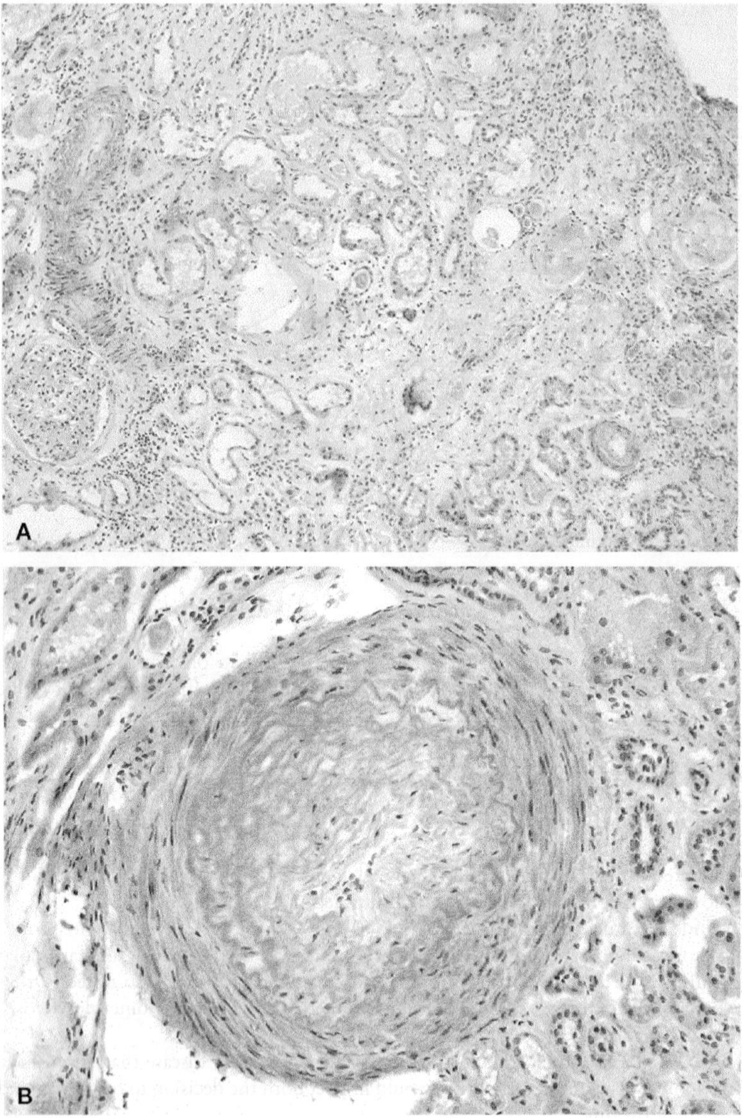

Figure 11-7. **Evaluation of donor biopsy.** Standard features evaluated on donor biopsies include global glomerulosclerosis, tubular atrophy, interstitial fibrosis (A), arterial intimal fibrosis (B), and arteriolar hyalinosis (C). In addition, other significant findings are the presence of fibrin thrombi, which may be seen in glomeruli (D, arrows) or arteries/arterioles, and cortical necrosis (E). Occasionally, pathologic findings of donor-derived disease may be diagnosed such as nodular glomerulosclerosis, characteristic of diabetic nephropathy (F). Global glomerulosclerosis is usually quantified, and all glomeruli in the sample are counted to give a percentage of global glomerulosclerosis. Interstitial fibrosis, tubular atrophy, arterial intimal fibrosis, and arteriolar hyalinosis are reported semiquantitatively as mild, moderate, or severe. The extent of cortical necrosis is usually estimated as percentage of cortical involvement, if present.

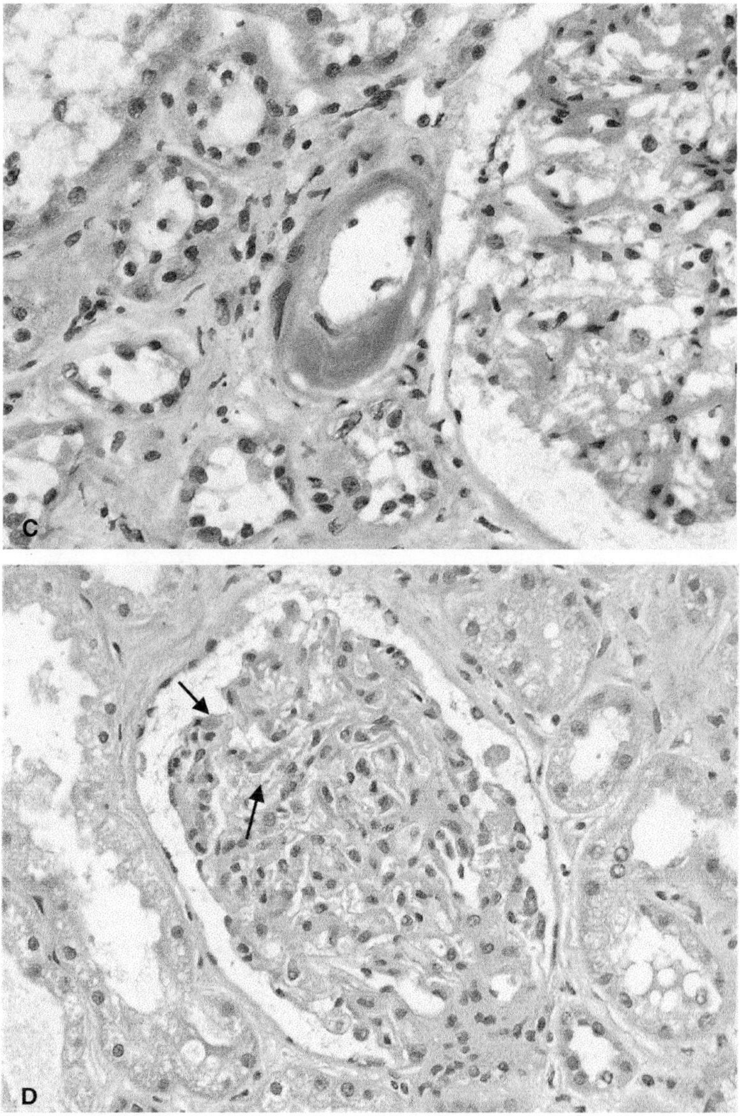

Figure 11-7. Continued

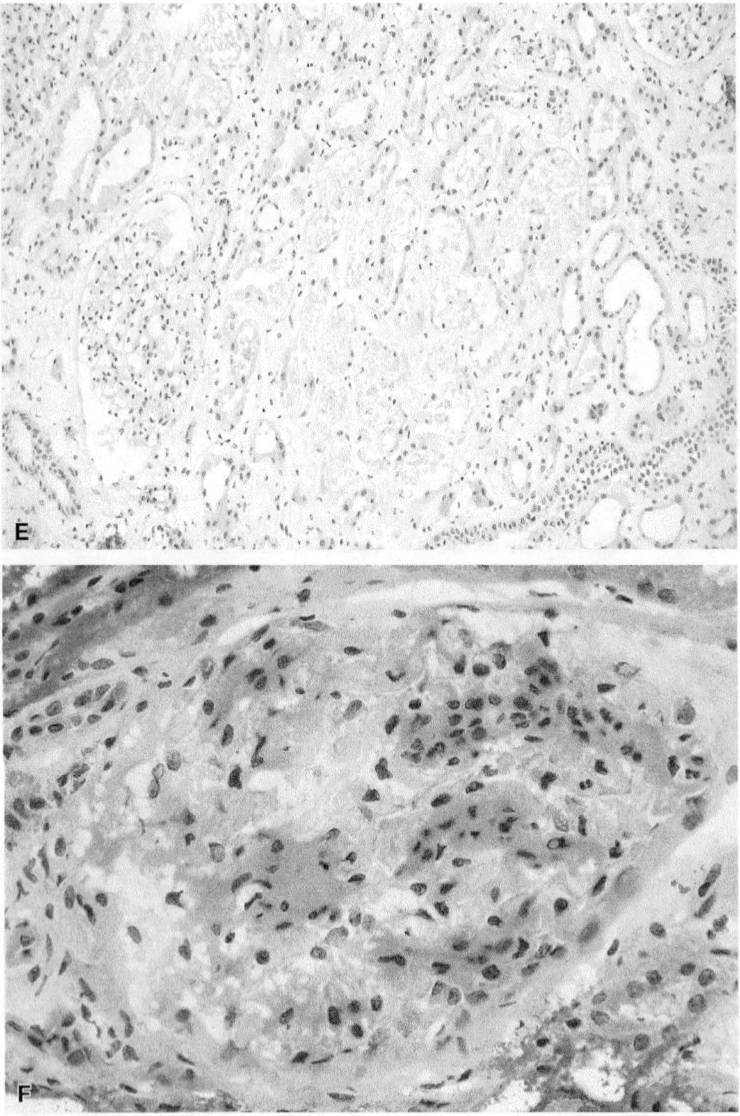

Figure 11-7. Continued

REFERENCES

1. Solez K. History of the Banff classification of allograft pathology as it approaches its 20th year. *Curr Opin Organ Transplant.* 2010;15(1):49-51.
2. Racusen LC, Solez K, Colvin RB, et al. The Banff 97 working classification of renal allograft pathology. *Kidney Int.* 1999;55(2):713-23.
3. Roufosse C, Simmonds N, Clahsen-van Groningen M, et al. A 2018 reference guide to the Banff classification of renal allograft pathology. *Transplantation.* 2018;102(11):1795-814.
4. Loupy A, Haas M, Roufosse C, et al. The Banff 2019 kidney meeting report (I): updates on and clarification of criteria for T cell- and antibody-mediated rejection. *Am J Transplant.* 2020;20(9):2318-31.
5. Loupy A, Mengel M, Haas M. Thirty years of the international Banff classification for allograft pathology: the past, present, and future of kidney transplant diagnostics. *Kidney Int.* 2022;101(4):678-91.
6. Haas M. The revised (2013) Banff classification for antibody-mediated rejection of renal allografts: update, difficulties, and future considerations. *Am J Transplant.* 2016;16(5):1352-57.
7. Haas M, Sis B, Racusen LC, et al. Banff 2013 meeting report: inclusion of c4d-negative antibody-mediated rejection and antibody-associated arterial lesions. *Am J Transplant.* 2014;14(2):272-83.
8. Haas M, Loupy A, Lefaucheur C, et al. The Banff 2017 Kidney Meeting Report: revised diagnostic criteria for chronic active T cell-mediated rejection, antibody-mediated rejection, and prospects for integrative endpoints for next-generation clinical trials. *Am J Transplant.* 2018;18(2):293-307.
9. Nickeleit V, Singh HK, Randhawa P, et al. The Banff Working Group classification of definitive polyomavirus nephropathy: morphologic definitions and clinical correlations. *JASN (J Am Soc Nephrol).* 2018;29(2):680-93.
10. Naesens M, Kuypers DR, Sarwal M. Calcineurin inhibitor nephrotoxicity. *Clin J Am Soc Nephrol.* 2009;4(2):481-508.
11. Ramos EL, Tisher CC. Recurrent diseases in the kidney transplant. *Am J Kidney Dis.* 1994;24(1):142-54.
12. Randhawa P. Role of donor kidney biopsies in renal transplantation. *Transplantation.* 2001;71:1361-5.
13. Marsh JN, Liu T-C, Wilson PC, Swamidass SJ, Gaut JP. Development and validation of a deep learning model to quantify glomerulosclerosis in kidney biopsy specimens. *JAMA Netw Open.* 2021;4(1):e2030939.

12

Cellular Rejection

April Pottebaum, Nidia Messias, and Anuja Java

GENERAL PRINCIPLES

- Kidney transplantation in non–human leukocyte antigen (HLA)-identical recipients stimulates alloimmune responses that can lead to allograft rejection.
- Rejection is characterized by an acute decline in kidney function associated with specific pathologic changes in the allograft.
- Despite a remarkable decrease in the incidence due to the availability of current immunosuppressive medications, acute rejection remains a major cause of allograft dysfunction and is a major predictor of interstitial fibrosis and tubular atrophy (IFTA) that affects long-term graft survival.[1]
- There are two main forms of acute rejection that result from distinct pathophysiological mechanisms, are associated with unique histologic findings, and require different modalities of treatment:
  - **Acute cellular (T-cell-mediated) rejection (TCMR)**, which is characterized by lymphocytic infiltration of the tubules, interstitium, and, in some cases, the arterial intima.
  - **Acute (active) antibody-mediated rejection (AMR)**, which occurs due to circulating donor-specific antibodies (DSAs) to donor alloantigens on graft endothelial cells, that results in inflammation, tissue injury, and graft dysfunction. AMR will be reviewed in Chapter 13, Antibody-mediated Rejection.
- Acute TCMR and AMR can coexist at the same time in the allograft.
- Risk factors for acute rejection commonly include level of presensitization (i.e., presence of preformed DSAs or a high panel reactive antibody), recipient age, HLA mismatches, and blood group incompatibility. In the posttransplant period, those with medication nonadherence are at increased risk for acute rejection (for example, a young patient with lower tacrolimus levels due to suspected nonadherence).[2,3]

DIAGNOSIS

Clinical Manifestations

- Patients with acute rejection are typically asymptomatic.
- Occasionally, patients may present with fever, malaise, oliguria, and allograft pain and/or tenderness, although these symptoms are rare in the setting of modern immunosuppressive regimens (unless medications have been completely discontinued).

Laboratory Features

- Acute kidney transplant rejection is suspected when patients present with a rise in the serum creatinine above their baseline (or if the creatinine stops decreasing earlier than expected in recently transplanted patients), new or worsening proteinuria, worsening hypertension, or occasionally pyuria.

- Plasma levels of donor-derived cell-free DNA (dd-cfDNA), which is released into the bloodstream by dead or injured allograft cells, may be elevated (>1%) in patients with acute rejection.[4]
- Findings on renal imaging may include increased graft size, loss of corticomedullary junction, decreased echogenicity of the renal sinus, and elevated resistance indices, but these findings are not specific. Ultrasound and Doppler studies are generally performed to exclude other causes of acute kidney injury.
- The current gold standard for diagnosis of acute cellular rejection is an allograft biopsy, which can accurately grade the severity of rejection (see Histologic Findings), differentiate between TCMR and AMR, and determine the degree of IFTA.
- Biopsy will also help to exclude other causes of elevated creatinine that should be considered in the differential diagnosis (such as BK [polyomavirus] nephropathy, cytomegalovirus [CMV]-related disease, de novo or recurrent glomerular disease, drug- or infection-related interstitial nephritis, transplant pyelonephritis, and post-transplant lymphoproliferative disease [PTLD]).

Histologic Findings[5-7]

- Histologic diagnosis of TCMR follows the Banff criteria and is classified into:
  - Acute T-cell-mediated rejection (**Figures 12-1** and **12-2**)
    - Banff IA—moderate tubulitis (t2) <u>and</u> moderate or severe interstitial inflammation (i2/3) in unscarred cortex
    - Banff IB—severe tubulitis (t3) <u>and</u> moderate or severe interstitial inflammation (i2/3) in unscarred cortex
    - Banff IIA—intimal arteritis with up to 25% arterial luminal area lost (v1)
    - Banff IIB—intimal arteritis with >25% arterial luminal area lost (v2)
    - Banff III—transmural arteritis and/or fibrinoid necrosis (v3)
  - Chronic active T-cell-mediated rejection
    - Grade IA—moderate tubulitis (t2 or t-IFTA2) <u>and</u> total inflammation >25% of the cortex (ti2/3) <u>and</u> inflammation >25% fibrotic cortex (i-IFTA 2/3)
    - Grade IB—severe tubulitis (t3 or t-IFTA3) <u>and</u> total inflammation >25% of the cortex (ti2/3) <u>and</u> inflammation >25% fibrotic cortex cortex (i-IFTA 2/3)
    - Grade II—chronic allograft arteriopathy—arterial intimal fibrosis with inflammation in fibrosis and neointima formation
  - Borderline/suspicious for rejection (**Figure 12-1**)
    - Presence of tubulitis (t1/2/3) <u>and</u> mild interstitial inflammation (i = 1) or
    - Mild tubulitis and moderate or severe inflammation (i2 or i3)
    - No intimal or transmural arteritis present
- Tubulitis, the presence of mononuclear cells within tubuli, is one of the hallmarks of TCMR. It is ranked based on the presence of mononuclear cells within tubuli (**Table 12-1**).
- Interstitial inflammation is graded based on the area of inflammation in the cortex (**Table 12-2**). Interstitial inflammation may be quantified in the total, entire cortical area (ti), in unscarred cortex only (i), and in scarred cortex only (i-IFTA), and the distribution of the inflammatory infiltrate helps to distinguish active versus chronic active TCMR.
- AMR may occur concomitant to cellular rejection.
- In cases with intimal or transmural arteritis (v) or chronic allograft nephropathy (cv), the possibility of vascular injury secondary to AMR should be considered.
- In biopsies which meet criteria for acute TCMR and chronic active TCMR, both should be reported.

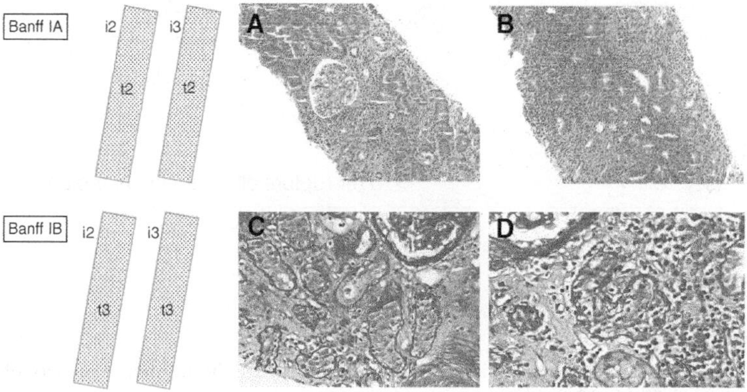

Figure 12-1. Acute T-cell-mediated rejection. Banff IA and IB are marked by moderate (A) or severe interstitial inflammation (B)—i2 and i3 scores, accompanied by moderate tubulitis (C) or severe tubulitis (D)—t2 and t3 scores—respectively.

- The Banff criteria for rejection are revised approximately every 2 years, according to new evidence available at the time.
- The use of molecular diagnostics and artificial intelligence may soon play an important role in the diagnosis of cellular rejection.
- The differential diagnosis of rejection includes other pathologies that lead to interstitial inflammation and tubulitis, and a diagnosis of rejection should be made with caution or avoided in these settings:
  - Infections: pyelonephritis, polyomavirus (BK), CMV, adenovirus
  - PTLD
  - Drug induced interstitial nephritis

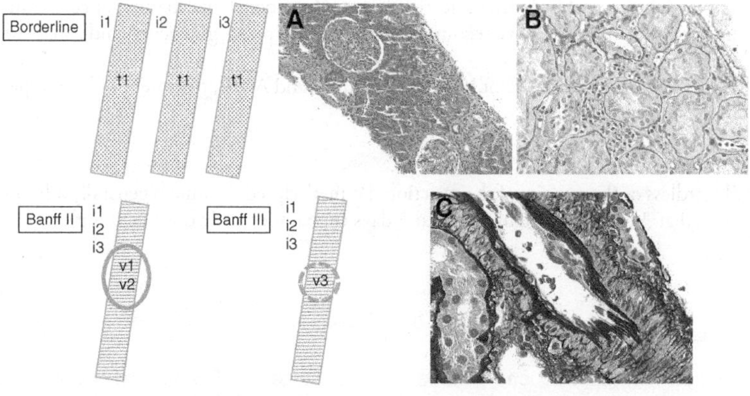

Figure 12-2. **Borderline changes and acute T-cell-mediated rejection with v-lesion.** The borderline category is for cases that show inflammation—at least i1 (A)—and mild tubulitis (B). Vascular rejection cases are graded as Banff IIA for cases with mild or moderate intimal arteritis (C), Banff IIB for severe intimal arteritis, and Banff III for transmural arteritis of fibrinoid necrosis (represented by the red circles in the illustration).

TABLE 12-1 Grading of Tubulitis

Tubulitis (t) Grade	Number of Mononuclear Cells
t1 (mild)	1-4
t2 (moderate)	5-10
t3 (severe)	>10 (or rupture of basement membrane)

TREATMENT

Selection of Therapies

- Treatment of acute TCMR is determined primarily by the histologic severity of rejection (**Table 12-3**).[8-11]
  - Glucocorticoids and/or antithymocyte globulin (ATG) should be administered.
  - Intensification of the maintenance immunosuppression regimen should be considered, as appropriate.
- For patients with Banff grade IA rejection, treatment with IV methylprednisolone is recommended.
- For patients with Banff grade IB rejection, treatment with IV methylprednisolone and/or ATG is suggested.
  - Use of IV methylprednisolone is recommended for all patients.
  - Use of ATG should be considered, especially in patients who are presenting ≤1 year after transplant and in those who do not respond to glucocorticoids.
- For patients with Banff grade II or III rejection, treatment with IV methylprednisolone and ATG is recommended.
  - Use of IV methylprednisolone is recommended for all patients.
  - Use of ATG is recommended for all patients. In **patients who cannot receive ATG**, use of alemtuzumab as a single dose of 30 mg is recommended.
- For patients with borderline rejection, intensification of the maintenance immunosuppression regimen is recommended. Use of pulse glucocorticoids may be considered.
- For patients with evidence of both acute TCMR and AMR, treatment of both types of rejection is warranted.

Dosing Recommendations

- Regardless of the severity of the rejection, IV methylprednisolone is generally administered at 3 to 5 mg/kg daily for 3 to 5 days (maximum daily dose, 500 mg).

TABLE 12-2 Grading of Interstitial Inflammation in the Cortex

Interstitial Inflammation (i) Grade	Percentage of Inflammation of Cortex
i1 (mild)	Up to 25%
i2 (moderate)	26%-50%
i3 (severe)	>50%

TABLE 12-3 Treatment Based on Histologic Severity of T-Cell-Mediated Rejection

Banff Classification	Recommended Treatment
IA	Glucocorticoids only
IB	Glucocorticoids and possibly antithymocyte globulin
II	Glucocorticoids and antithymocyte globulin
III	Glucocorticoids and antithymocyte globulin

- After completion of IV methylprednisolone, a gradual taper of oral prednisone is generally ordered before returning to the patient's maintenance dose.
  - The optimal glucocorticoid regimen remains unknown.
  - At our center, a common oral prednisone taper includes 60 mg daily for 7 days, 40 mg daily for 7 days, 20 mg daily for 7 days, 10 mg daily for 7 days, and then return to the maintenance dose.
  - The prednisone taper may be expedited for patients who are unable to tolerate this regimen (i.e., acute hyperglycemia, psychiatric disturbances).
- The dosing of ATG is dependent on the histologic severity of rejection.
  - For Banff grade IB rejection, ATG is generally administered daily at 1.5 to 3 mg/kg per dose for a total dose of 3 to 6 mg/kg.
  - For Banff grade II or III rejection, ATG is generally administered daily at 1.5 to 3 mg/kg per dose for a total dose of 5 to 10 mg/kg. The total number of doses is dependent on the severity of rejection and the patient's clinical response.

Additional Considerations

For patients who are treated with high-dose glucocorticoids and ATG (or alemtuzumab), antimicrobial and antiviral prophylaxis should be resumed for at least 3 months.

RESPONSE AND MONITORING AFTER TREATMENT

- In most patients with TCMR who do not have significant IFTA, a favorable response to treatment is expected within three to 5 days of treatment initiation.
- Patients with evidence of chronic injury and fibrosis are less likely to demonstrate reversal of allograft dysfunction with treatment.
- A decrease in serum creatinine to within 10% of the baseline level is considered to be successful treatment of rejection, although some patients may have persistent rejection even after treatment, suggesting that histology is equally important in determining remission (which is why some centers utilize follow-up biopsies).
- While admitted for treatment, we monitor serum creatinine daily to assess response to therapy. After discharge, we monitor serum creatinine on a weekly basis until it has returned to the patient's baseline level or until it achieves and plateaus at a new baseline, after which routine monitoring of kidney function can be resumed (which is done monthly at our center).
- Measurement of dd-cfDNA can also be used to assist monitoring for response to therapy. At our center, we obtain a repeat dd-cfDNA level one to 2 months after treatment. In patients who respond to treatment, the dd-cfDNA fraction should decrease back to the normal range (<1%) within 2 months of therapy.[12]

REFERENCES

1. Bouatou Y, Viglietti D, Pievani D, et al. Response to treatment and long-term outcomes in kidney transplant recipients with acute T cell-mediated rejection. *Am J Transplant.* 2019;19(7):1972-88.
2. Lebranchu Y, Baan C, Biancone L, et al. Pretransplant identification of acute rejection risk following kidney transplantation. *Transpl Int* 2014;27(2):129-38.
3. Cippà PE, Schiesser M, Ekberg H, et al. Risk stratification for rejection and infection after kidney transplantation. *Clin J Am Soc Nephrol* 2015;10(12):2213-20.
4. Bloom RD, Bromberg JS, Poggio ED, et al. Cell-free DNA and active rejection in kidney allografts. *J Am Soc Nephrol* 2017;28(7):2221-32.
5. Roufosse C, Simmonds N, Clahsen-van Groningen M, et al. A 2018 reference guide to the Banff classification of renal allograft pathology. *Transplantation* 2018;102(11):1795-814.
6. Loupy A, Haas M, Roufosse C, et al. The Banff 2019 kidney meeting report (I): updates on and clarification of criteria for T cell- and antibody-mediated rejection. *Am J Transplant* 2020;20(9):2318-31.
7. Loupy A, Mengel M, Haas M. Thirty years of the international Banff classification for allograft pathology: the past, present, and future of kidney transplant diagnostics. *Kidney Int* 2022;101(4):678-91.
8. Kidney disease: improving global outcomes (KDIGO) transplant work group. KDIGO clinical practice guidelines for the care of kidney transplant recipients. *Am J Transplant.* 2009;9(suppl 3):S1-155.
9. Hoitsma AJ, van Lier HJ, Reekers P, Koene RA. Improved patient and graft survival after treatment of acute rejections of cadaveric renal allografts with rabbit antithymocyte globulin. *Transplantation.* 1985;39(3):274-9.
10. Theodorakis J, Schneeberger H, Illner WD, Stangl M, Zanker B, Land W. Aggressive treatment of the first acute rejection episode using first-line anti-lymphocytic preparation reduces further acute rejection episodes after human kidney transplantation. *Transpl Int.* 1998;11(suppl 1):S86-9.
11. Gaber AO, First MR, Tesi RJ, et al. Results of the double-blind, randomized, multicenter, phase III clinical trial of Thymoglobulin versus Atgam in the treatment of acute graft rejection episodes after renal transplantation. *Transplantation.* 1998;66(1):29-37.
12. Wolf-Doty TK, Mannon RB, Poggio ED, et al. Dynamic response of donor-derived cell-free DNA following treatment of acute rejection in kidney allografts. *Kidney360.* 2021;2(4):729-36.

13 Antibody-Mediated Rejection

Haris F. Murad, Parker C. Wilson, and
Casey A. Dubrawka

GENERAL PRINCIPLES

- Antibody-mediated rejection (AMR), also known as humoral rejection, is defined as specific histologic signs of allograft injury associated with evidence of current or recent antibody interaction with vascular endothelium as well as serologic evidence of circulating donor-specific antibodies.[1,2]
- Subclinical AMR is an ongoing AMR that has not resulted in a change in allograft function. So it is an AMR without an elevation of creatinine, proteinuria, or azotemia.
- The definitions and criteria for AMR have undergone substantial changes over the decades. The biggest recent change in the Banff guidelines is the division of AMR into active and chronic active AMR. The histological differences of which are detailed here.[3]

EPIDEMIOLOGY

- Due to the evolving definition of AMR, the data vary considerably, but most studies report an incidence of AMR between 3% and 12% among renal transplants.[1,2,4,5]
- The incidence is higher in the first posttransplant year and decreases with time.[4,5]
- AMR is often associated with concomitant cellular rejection.

RISK FACTORS

Risk factors for AMR are shown in **Table 13-1**.[4,5]

PATHOPHYSIOLOGY

- As the name suggests, circulating antibodies against the renal allograft have a central role in development of AMR.[3-6]
- Antibodies can be preformed or de novo (formed after transplant).
- These antibodies are most often against major histocompatibility complex antigens also known as human leukocyte antigens (HLAs). However non-HLA-mediated antibodies are increasingly being found as a cause of AMR as well.[6,7] Some of the common non-HLA causes of AMR in renal allografts are antibodies against angiotensin 1 receptor, MICA, and vimentin.
- Very early AMR (within hours after transplant) can occur secondary to preformed circulating antibodies. This was the basis of the dreaded hyperacute rejection from ABO-incompatible transplants.
- Antigens are presented to T helper cells (CD4) by donor and recipient antigen-presenting cells. These then activate B cells via cytokines and mediators to differentiate into plasma cells or memory B cells (**Figure 13-1**). Plasma cells produce antibodies against a specified antigen.[2,4]

TABLE 13-1 Risk Factors for Antibody-Mediated Rejection

Pre-Transplant Factors	Factors at Time of Transplant	Post-Transplant Factors
• Sensitization (e.g., prior transplant, transfusion) • Higher number of HLA mismatches in donor-recipient pair • Pre-existing donor-specific antibodies • Higher levels of panel reactive antibodies	• ABO blood type-incompatible transplant • Non (lymphocyte) depleting induction therapy • Tissue injury, e.g., ATN from delayed graft function	• Prior rejection episodes • Nonadherence with immunosuppression medications • Lower maintenance immunosuppression doses/target levels • Certain viral infections: e.g., CMV

ATN, acute tubular necrosis; CMV, cytomegalovirus; HLA, human leukocyte antigen.

- Antibodies themselves do not cause injury to cells directly, but rather rely on activation of complement and CD8 cytotoxic T cells (**Figure 13-2**).[2,7,8]
  - Complement-mediated damage entails the binding of complement factor 1 to the antigen-antibody complex. This sets forth a cascade along the target cell membrane, ultimately forming the membrane attack complex (MAC).
    - Complement factors within this cascade also work as mediators and inflammatory markers to attract and recruit further immune cells like neutrophils and macrophages, which further implicate the immune system and injury.
    - One of the complement split proteins (C4d) binds to collagen in the basement membrane and endothelium, serving as evidence of complement activation and AMR (see diagnosis).
  - Complement independent injury is via antibody-mediated cell mediated cytotoxicity, which involves macrophages and natural killer cells (**Figure 13-2**).

PROGNOSIS AND LONG-TERM EFFECTS

- AMR is associated with deleterious long-term effects including subsequent rejection, chronic AMR, and graft failure. Some biopsy-based studies have shown that AMR is the leading cause of renal allograft failure.[1,7,8]

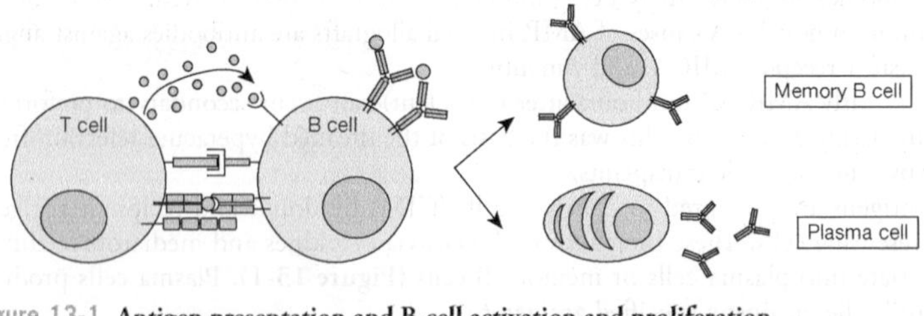

Figure 13-1. **Antigen presentation and B-cell activation and proliferation.**

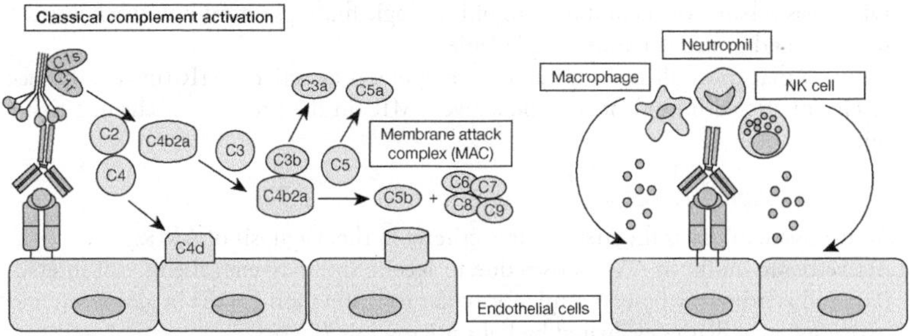

Figure 13-2. **Mechanisms of antibody-mediated graft injury via complement pathway activation, recruitment of innate immune cells, and direct endothelial cell activation.**

- A multicenter cohort showed late allograft dysfunction in nearly 60% of renal transplant recipients with AMR.[1,5]
- If AMR treatment is not successful, there is a 20% to 30% rate of allograft loss at 1 year.[9]
- Predictors for worse outcomes of AMR include the following:
  - Severity of histological grade
  - Type and strength of donor-specific antibodies
  - Presence of concomitant cellular rejection
  - Pre-existing graft function
  - Positive/high molecular markers of injury (see below)

DIAGNOSIS OF ANTIBODY-MEDIATED CHANGES

- The Banff kidney allograft criteria are used to evaluate biopsies for AMR.[3]
- Diagnosis of AMR requires the presence of all three criteria (**Table 13-2**)[5]:
  - Histologic evidence of active tissue injury ± chronic tissue injury
  - Evidence of antibody-endothelial cell interaction
  - Donor-specific antibodies

TABLE 13-2 Major Diagnostic Criteria for AMR

Histologic evidence of active tissue injury
MVI (g + ptc > 0), TMA, or AKI. In the presence of glomerulonephritis, borderline, or TCMR g ≥ 1
Evidence of antibody-endothelial cell interaction.
Linear C4d staining in ptc OR moderate MVI (g + ptc ≥ 2) OR molecular classifier. In the presence of glomerulonephritis, borderline, or TCMR g ≥ 1
Donor-specific antibodies
Anti-HLA or non-HLA antibody serology OR linear C4d staining OR molecular classifier

AKI, acute kidney injury; HLA, human leukocyte antigen; MVI, microvascular inflammation; TCMR, T-cell-mediated rejection; TMA, thrombotic microangiopathy.

- Diagnosis is based on a combination of histologic findings, immunohistochemistry, serology, and molecular assays as available.
- Biopsies that meet all three criteria are diagnosed as active AMR (in the absence of chronic tissue injury) or chronic active AMR (in the presence of chronic tissue injury).

Histologic Evaluation of Tissue Injury

- Active tissue injury is the first of three criteria in the diagnosis of AMR.
- Active tissue injury in AMR arises due to recent antibody-endothelial cell interaction and is primarily based on microvascular inflammation (MVI) in glomeruli and peritubular capillaries evaluated by light microscopy (LM):
  - Glomerulitis (g) is scored on the proportion of glomeruli with complete or partial occlusion of a capillary loop by leukocyte infiltration and endothelial cell enlargement.
    - g0—No glomerulitis
    - g1—Segmental or global glomerulitis in <25% of glomeruli
    - g2—Segmental or global glomerulitis in 25% to 75% of glomeruli
    - g3—Segmental or global glomerulitis in more than 75% of glomeruli
  - Peritubular capillaritis (ptc) is a measure of the amount of inflammation within the most severely affected peritubular capillary.
    - ptc0—Fewer than 3 leukocytes
    - ptc1—At least 1 leukocyte in at least 10% of cortical peritubular capillaries with 3 to 4 leukocytes in the most severely involved capillary
    - ptc2—At least 1 leukocyte in at least 10% of cortical peritubular capillaries with 5 to 10 leukocytes in the most severely involved capillary
    - ptc3—At least 1 leukocyte in at least 10% of cortical peritubular capillaries with >10 leukocytes in most severely involved capillary
  - MVI is the sum of the ptc and g scores. The presence of MVI (ptc > 0 and/or g > 0) in the absence of glomerulonephritis meets criteria 1 for acute tissue injury due to AMR with a few exceptions. Biopsies with T-cell-mediated rejection (TCMR), borderline infiltrate, or infection must have g ≥ 1. MVI is a precursor to chronic lesions like cg and peritubular capillary basement membrane multilayering (ptcml) and has been associated with worse allograft outcomes independent of C4d positivity.
  - Acute thrombotic microangiopathy or acute tubular injury may also serve as histologic evidence of acute tissue injury in the absence of another cause. These findings may be especially useful in patients with a high suspicion for AMR that already meet other criteria.
- Chronic tissue injury in AMR arises due to prolonged tissue injury from antibody-endothelial cell interaction in glomeruli, peritubular capillaries, and arteries. Histologic evidence of chronic tissue injury requires at least 1 of the following:
  - Transplant glomerulopathy (cg) is based on the presence of glomerular basement membrane double contours in the most severely affected glomerulus. The earliest stages are only detectable by electron microscopy (EM). Later stages are visible by LM and EM.
    - cg1a—GBM double contours in at least 3 capillaries by EM only
    - cg1b—GBM double contours in 1% to 25% of capillary loops by LM
    - cg2—GBM double contours in 26% to 50% of capillary by LM
    - cg3—GBM double contours in >50% of capillary loops by LM
  - ptcml is visible by EM in patients with chronic AMR. ptcml—7 or more layers of basement membrane in at least 1 cortical ptc and 5 or more in at least 2 additional capillaries.

- Arterial intimal fibrosis of new onset is visible by LM in patients with chronic AMR.
    - cv1—Vascular narrowing up to 25% of lumen
    - cv2—Vascular narrowing of 26% to 50% of lumen
    - cv3—Vascular narrowing of >50% of lumen

Histologic Evaluation of Antibody-Endothelial Cell Interaction

- Antibody-endothelial cell interaction is the second of three criteria in the diagnosis of AMR.
- Antibody-endothelial cell interaction is primarily evaluated on the presence of MVI and/or deposition of complement C4d in peritubular capillaries. Molecular assays may be useful in cases that are equivocal for an AMR diagnosis.
- Active antibody-endothelial cell interaction requires at least one of the following:
    - MVI (g + ptc ≥ 2) in the absence of glomerulonephritis. Biopsies with TCMR, borderline infiltrate, or infection must have g ≥ 1.
    - Linear C4d **staining** in peritubular capillaries (C4d2 or C4d3 by immunofixation on frozen sections or C4d > 0 by immunohistochemistry on paraffin sections).
        - C4d0—No staining of capillaries
        - C4d1—Staining in 0% to 10% of capillaries
        - C4d2—Staining in 10% to 50% of capillaries
        - C4d3—Staining in >50% of capillaries
    - Increased expression of gene transcripts/classifiers in biopsy tissue strongly associated with AMR.
    - Biopsies with isolated linear C4d staining that do not have evidence of active tissue injury or increased expression of gene transcripts/classifiers may be diagnosed as C4d staining without evidence of rejection.
- An estimated 25% to 50% of AMR cases are C4d negative, which may be due to differences in detection methods (immunofluorescence vs. immunoperoxidase), interobserver variability of what constitutes a positive C4d, and the patient population at the treatment facility.
- Molecular diagnostics for AMR may be useful when histologic, immunohistochemical, and serologic data are equivocal for diagnosis of AMR. These may include the following scenarios where one or more of the criteria are satisfied, but the biopsy does not yet meet criteria for AMR:
    - Mild MVI with a positive donor-specific antibody (DSA) (g + ptc = 1), C4d0, DSA+ve
    - Moderate-to-severe ptc with a DSA (ptc ≥ 2, g0), C4d0, DSA+ve
    - Moderate-to-severe MVI without a DSA (g + ptc ≥ 2), C4d0, DSA-ve
    - No MVI with a positive C4d (g + ptc = 0), C4d+ve, DSA±
    - Transplant glomerulopathy (cg > 0) with or without mild MVI (g + ptc ≤ 1), C4d0, DSA+ve
    - Isolated arteritis with a DSA

Serologic Evidence of Donor-Specific Antibodies

- Serologic evidence of DSAs is the third of three criteria in the diagnosis of AMR.
- Anti-HLA DSAs are routinely evaluated by ELISA.
- Non-HLA DSA can form independently of anti-HLA DSA and are not routinely evaluated. There are a wide variety of non-HLA DSAs, including anti-AT1R.
- Patients with a high suspicion for AMR with a negative anti-HLA should be considered for evaluation of non-HLA DSA.

- Linear C4d staining of ptc (as defined in the section above) or expression of validated transcripts/classifiers may substitute for a positive DSA. Linear C4d staining in ptc is ≥90% specific for humoral immunity.

Biomarkers

- While biomarkers of renal injury and rejection are not yet formally a part of the diagnostic criteria for AMR, they are increasingly being used to aid in the diagnosis of rejection.[10,11]
- Benefits include the following:
  - Being able to detect rejection early (e.g., subclinical AMR).
  - Patients in whom a biopsy is very high risk (e.g., bleeding dyscrasias).
  - Aiding in the diagnosis when histological evidence is unclear or equivocal.
- Donor-derived cell-free DNA is one such biomarker that has been shown to predict biopsy proven AMR.[10]
  - The negative predictive value for AMR in donor-derived cell-free DNA levels of >1% is up to 96%.
  - Values of >0.5% were associated with nearly a threefold rise in risk of development of de novo DSAs.
- Other biomarkers include mRNA transcripts in the urine of CXCR3, perforin, CD3ε, proteinase-inhibitor-9, and others. Protein biomarkers in the urine of CXCL9 and CXCL10 have also been studied.[11]

TREATMENT

Treatment Challenges

- AMR in kidney transplant recipients remains a significant barrier to long-term graft survival, making both prevention and treatment essential foci of posttransplant management.[1,12,13]
- Despite this, a multitude of challenges remain regarding optimal management, available treatment agents, and response to therapy.
- Presently, there are no U.S. Food and Drug Administration (FDA)–approved therapies for AMR prevention or treatment in solid organ transplant recipients and development of successful treatments remains an unmet need.
- Established conventional therapies for AMR are supported by limited, lower-quality evidence and are associated with variable success rates.[1]
- As the understanding and diagnosis of AMR evolve, novel and experimental treatments continue to be investigated, especially in the setting of resistant and/or refractory episodes of AMR.

Treatment Approach

- Prioritization is given to minimize risk factors for AMR and DSA development.
- Strategies include donor/recipient HLA-matching, desensitization, optimization of maintenance immunosuppression, infection prevention, and promotion of medication adherence (see risk factors for AMR in **Table 13-1**).[2]
- The treatment approach to AMR is complex and can be highly variable across transplant centers, though generally consists of a combination of modalities directed against AMR pathogenesis and its deleterious effects on the allograft.[12-15]
- Overarching targets include direct antibody removal, interference with various stages of antibody production, and inhibition of ongoing antibody-mediated graft injury (**Table 13-3**).[2,4,8]

TABLE 13-3 Treatment Agents for Antibody-Mediated Rejection

Removal of Circulating Antibodies	Reduction and/or Prevention of Further Antibody Production	Minimization of Antibody-Mediated Allograft Injury
• Therapeutic plasmapheresis • IVIg	• IVIg • Antithymocyte globulin • Corticosteroids • Rituximab • Bortezomib • Carfilzomib • Tocilizumab	• Corticosteroids • Eculizumab

IVIg, intravenous immunoglobulin.

- Based on these targets, treatment is focused on recipient T cell, B cell, and/or plasma cell populations, the complement cascade, and inflammatory pathways.[2,4]
- These components of the immune system are key mediators of both antibody production and propagation of antibody-mediated graft injury.[2,4]
  - Following donor antigen presentation, T-cell signaling facilitates B-cell differentiation and proliferation of antibody-secreting plasma cells (**Figure 13-1**).
  - Circulating antibodies can mediate graft injury via complement-dependent cytotoxicity (CDC), antibody-dependent cellular toxicity (ADCC), and direct vascular endothelial cell activation and injury (**Figure 13-2**).
- Due to the complexity and multitude of contributing pathways of AMR, a single intervention cannot effectively address all facets and a multimodal treatment approach is often necessary.
- Conventional treatment in kidney transplant recipients consists of therapeutic plasma exchange (TPE), intravenous immunoglobulin (IVIg), and corticosteroids, with or without the incorporation of rituximab (**Table 13-3**).[4,5,8,12-18]
- In addition to the definitive AMR treatment options that are being discussed here, it is important to also strengthen and/or augment the maintenance immunosuppression regimen:
  - Assess medication adherence.
  - Target higher calcineurin inhibitor trough levels.
  - Consider addition or increase in dose of antimetabolite (e.g., mycophenolate or azathioprine).

Treatment Agents

Therapeutic Plasma Exchange

- TPE is a mechanical, nonselective intervention for removal of DSA.[4]
- TPE does not directly suppress antibody production.[4]
- Human plasma, containing circulating IgG antibodies, is fractionated from whole blood, and removed via extracorporeal circuit employing either continuous flow centrifugation or membrane-based filtration.[16]
- This is followed by replacement with either plasma and/or 5% albumin as TPE facilitates nonspecific removal of plasma, thereby also removing beneficial plasma proteins including immune-protective antibodies, albumin, clotting factors, and fibrinogen.[16]

- Fresh frozen plasma (FFP) repletion attenuates depletion coagulopathy and relative immunoglobulin deficiency.
- Low-dose IVIg (0.1 g/kg) may also be given between sessions.
- Only antibodies in the intravascular space can be removed by TPE.
- Effectiveness of antibody removal is influenced by plasma volume and the rate of antibody redistribution, synthesis, and half-life. TPE may not be as effective for high-level DSA burden.[16,17]
- Dosing[4,16,17]
  - Plasma volume to be exchanged is determined by the patient's estimated plasma volume. A typical exchange is 1 to 1.5 plasma volume per session.
  - A treatment course generally consists of 3 to 5 sessions separated by 24 to 48 hours each to allow for redistribution of antibodies into the vascular space.
- Possible adverse effects include hypocalcemia secondary to citrate anticoagulation within the circuit, muscle cramping, urticaria, coagulopathies, hypotension, dyspnea, and chest pain.[4,17]

Intravenous Immunoglobulin

- IVIg is a purified, fractionated blood product preparation containing IgG extracted from pooled plasma of thousands of human donors.[4,17-19]
- Preformed IgG antibodies provide passive immunity, immunomodulation, and anti-inflammatory effects.
- Administration of IVIg for AMR has been proposed to offer several potential pleiotropic effects, some of which remain to be completely understood (**Table 13-4**).[18,19]
- There are low-dose (0.1 g/kg) or high-dose (0.5-2.0 g/kg) regimens[2,7]
  - Dosing is highly variable and a standard dosing approach for AMR has not been universally defined.

TABLE 13-4 Proposed Mechanisms of IVIg for the Treatment of Antibody-Mediated Rejection

Proposed mechanisms of IVIg for the treatment of AMR	Neutralization of circulating DSA Immunomodulatory effects on T and B cells • Inhibition of T-cell activation, interference with B-cell signaling, and induction of B-cell apoptosis F_{ab} and F_c-mediated inhibition of complement activation and/or activated complement component Saturation of endothelial F_c receptors responsible for endogenous IgG recycling, thus reducing antibody half-life F_c receptor-mediated inhibition of immune activation and anti-inflammatory effects Suppression of endogenous antibody rebound following depletion with plasmapheresis Restoration of immune-protective antibodies removed during plasmapheresis

AMR, antibody-mediated rejection; DSA, donor-specific antibody; IVIg, intravenous immunoglobulin.

- Low-dose regimen may be used between sessions of TPE to dampen endogenous antibody rebound.
- Adverse effects[19]
  - Many IVIg products exist. Individual products should be reviewed and chosen based on patient-specific factors.
  - When selecting a product, consider sodium, sugar, and IgA content, osmolality, and concentration.
  - Side effects include flu-like symptoms, hypotension, headache, and arthralgia. Rarer, but severe manifestations may include bronchospasm, anaphylaxis, thrombotic events, and renal dysfunction.
- Drug-drug interactions: IVIg may contain neutralizing antibodies that may diminish the therapeutic effects of monoclonal and polyclonal antibody therapies when given concomitantly.

Corticosteroids

- Corticosteroids lead to upregulation of anti-inflammatory gene expression and inhibition of nuclear factor KB-mediated production of cytokines.[4]
- The role of corticosteroids in AMR is multifactorial and includes reduction in inflammation and ongoing graft injury and suppression of T-cell and B-cell responses.[4]
- Dosing
  - Methylprednisolone 250 to 1,000 mg/d intravenous × 3 to 5 days
  - Prednisone 1 to 3 mg/kg oral daily × 3 to 5 days
- Adverse effects are often dose related and include hyperglycemia, mental status changes, leukocytosis, hypertension, peptic ulcer disease, infection, and impaired wound healing.

Rituximab

- Rituximab is a chimeric monoclonal IgG antibody targeting the CD20 surface antigen on B cells.
- CD20 is a transmembrane protein receptor located on pre- and mature B cells responsible for regulating cell cycle initiation. Plasma cells do not display CD20.[2,4]
- Rituximab binds CD20 and induces apoptosis and prolonged depletion of pre-B and mature B cells via CDC, antibody-dependent cell-mediated cytotoxicity (ADCC), and cell-mediated apoptosis (**Figure 13-3**).[2,4]
- Rituximab induces rapid peripheral B-cell depletion within 24 to 72 hours of administration and can suppress B-cell populations for up to 1 to 2 years.[4]
- Rituximab will have no effect on depleting existing antibodies and will only aid in suppression of further production via prevention of B-cell proliferation.
- Despite inconsistent results of rituximab, consensus guidance suggests the consideration of rituximab as adjunctive therapy for AMR (**Figure 13-4**).[7]
  - RITUX-ERAH: Multicenter, prospective, randomized, double-blind trial of 38 adult kidney transplant recipients with acute AMR within 1 year of transplant. Patients were randomized to receive rituximab 375 mg/m^2 or placebo in addition to usual care of corticosteroids, TPE, and IVIg. No difference was found in the primary composite outcome of treatment failure (52.6% vs. 57.9%), though the study was underpowered, and timing of concomitant interventions may have limited rituximab effectiveness.[14]
  - Several retrospective investigations of rituximab added to standard of care with IVIg and/or TPE for AMR have suggested improved graft survival.[12,13]
- Dosing: The FDA-approved dose is rituximab 375 mg/m^2 (intravenous).[4]

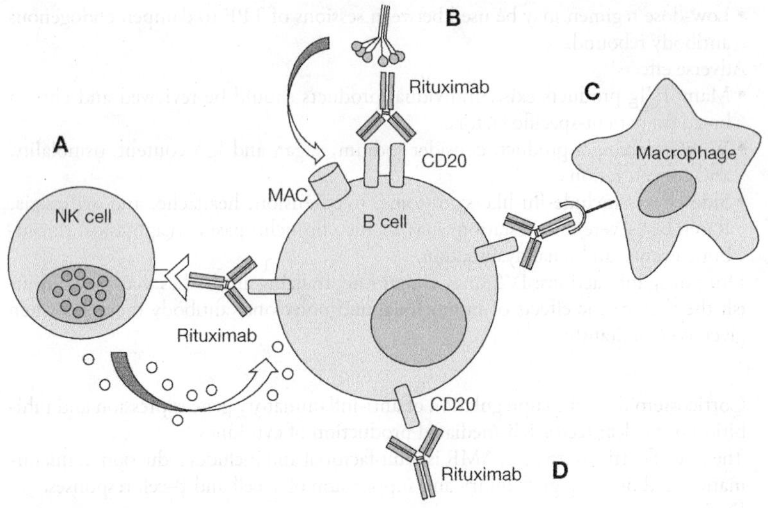

Figure 13-3. Mechanism of rituximab-induced B-cell depletion. A, Antibody-dependent cell-mediated cytotoxicity (ADCC); B, complement-dependent cytotoxicity (CDC); C, Fc-receptor-mediated phagocytosis or ADCC; D, direct cell-mediated apoptosis.

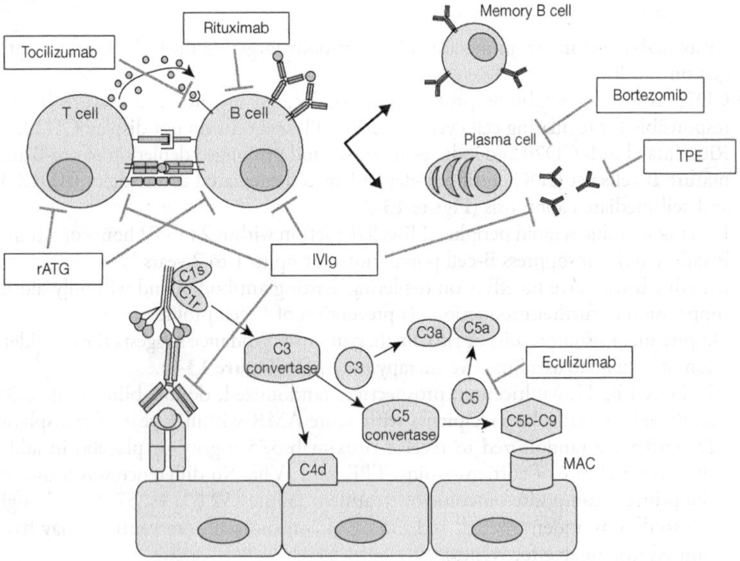

Figure 13-4. Site of action of available therapeutic agents for the treatment of antibody-mediated rejection. IVIg, intravenous immunoglobulin; MAC, membrane attack complex; rATG, rabbit antithymocyte globulin; TPE, therapeutic plasma exchange.

- Adverse effects/monitoring[2,4]
  - Infusion reactions may occur and typically present as a first-dose effect.
    - Can manifest as transient hypotension, low-grade fever, tachycardia, arthralgias, urticaria, angioedema, hypoxia, bronchospasm, or shock.
    - Premedication is recommended with an antihistamine, acetaminophen, and/or corticosteroid.
    - If reaction occurs, stop infusion and manage symptoms. Depending on severity, infusion may be resumed once symptoms have resolved at 50% of previous infusion rate with close monitoring.
  - Hepatitis B reactivation may occur. Screen patients for Hepatitis B infection prior to initiation.
  - Increased risk of bacterial, fungal, and new or reactivated viral infection is possible.
  - Avoid immunization with live virus vaccines. Administer nonlive virus vaccines at least 4 weeks prior to rituximab administration.

Rabbit Antithymocyte Globulin

- Rabbit antithymocyte globulin (rATG) is a rabbit-derived polyclonal lymphocyte-depleting antibody therapy with a well-defined role in for use as induction immunosuppression and treatment of acute cellular rejection.
- However, due to its ability to induce depletion of a variety of immune cells, rATG may offer benefit in AMR.[4]
- rATG leads to B-cell depletion through CDC, ADCC, direct B-cell apoptosis, blockage of costimulatory signals, and inhibition of $CD4^+$ helper T-cell activity required for B-cell activation.[4]
- Though not routinely employed in all presentations of AMR, rATG may be considered in select cases or mixed rejection episodes, where both B- and T-cell features are present.[4,8]
- The risks and benefits should be weighed carefully when considering addition of rATG due to the substantial increased risk of infection and malignancy.

Tocilizumab

- Tocilizumab is a humanized monoclonal antibody directed against the interleukin-6 (IL-6) receptor.[20]
- IL-6 is a cytokine that mediates multiple inflammatory and immunomodulatory pathways, including expansion and activation of B and T cells.[20]
  - In B cells, IL-6 promotes maturation into plasma cells and facilitates antibody production via T cells aid.
  - In T cells, IL-6 promotes proliferation and survival. IL-6 regulates differentiation of $CD4^+$ T cells and conversion to regulatory T cells (T_{reg}).
- Tocilizumab binds both soluble and membrane-bound IL-6 receptors to prevent interaction of IL-6 with its receptor and inhibit IL-6-mediated signaling pathways.
- In AMR, tocilizumab may aid in reducing antibody production by inhibiting B-cell development into antibody-secreting plasma cells, decrease inflammation, and lead to an increase in T_{reg} cells.[8,20]
- Tocilizumab has shown some promise in treatment of both acute and chronic AMR and is an agent that continues to be investigated (**Figure 13-5**).[8,20]
- Dosing
  - Dosing is based on other FDA-approved indications of tocilizumab of 8 mg/kg intravenous (maximum dose: 800 mg).
  - For FDA-approved indications, dosing adjustments are recommended for hepatic impairment.

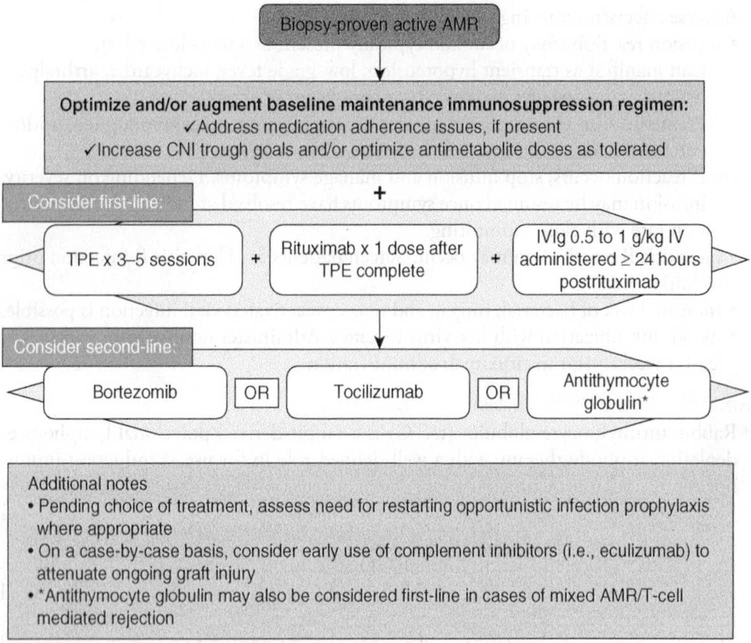

Figure 13-5. **Treatment algorithm for management of active antibody-mediated rejection in kidney transplant recipients.** CNI, calcineurin inhibitor; IVIg, intravenous immunoglobulin; TPE, therapeutic plasma exchange.

- Adverse effects
  - Infusion-related reactions are possible. Premedication with an antihistamine, acetaminophen, and a corticosteroid is recommended.
  - May cause elevations in liver enzymes, hypercholesterolemia, hyperlipidemia, and neutropenia.
  - A black box warning exists for increased risk of serious and potentially fatal infections, including active TB. Screen for latent TB prior to initiation and during therapy.

Bortezomib

- Bortezomib is a synthetic selective and reversible inhibitor of the 26S proteosome.[4]
- The 26S proteosome is expressed in the nucleus and cytoplasm of eukaryotic cells with a primary role in degradation of ubiquitinated proteins and regulation of intracellular signaling, including activation of nuclear factor-kB activity involved in cytokine production.[4]
- Inhibition of the 26S proteosome results in accumulation of misfolded proteins and intracellular endoplasmic reticulum stress, ultimately leading to apoptotic cell death.[4]
- In the treatment of AMR, bortezomib induces apoptosis of antibody-secreting plasma cells to inhibit ongoing antibody production.[2]

- Due to high antibody synthesis rates, plasma cells may be particularly sensitive to bortezomib-induced apoptosis.[2]
- Overall, bortezomib and other proteosome inhibitors, such as carfilzomib, are not universally employed in the treatment of AMR due to mixed benefit coupled with well-established risk of treatment-limiting side effects.[2]
- Dosing[2,4]
  - Dosing strategies in AMR can be variable and are largely based on dosing for other FDA-approved indications, including mantel cell lymphoma and multiple myeloma.
  - Dose: bortezomib 1.3 to 1.5 mg/m^2 intravenous on days 1, 4, 8, and 11
  - Doses should be separated by ≥72 hours to allow time for restoration of proteasome function.
  - Bortezomib is metabolized primarily by cytochrome P-450 (CYP) enzymes CYP-2C19 and CYP-3A4 and to a lesser extent by CYP-1A2. Dose adjustments are recommended for moderate-to-severe hepatic impairment.
- Adverse effects[2,4]
  - Adverse effects commonly limit tolerability of therapy and generally resolve with dose reduction or treatment discontinuation.
  - These may include peripheral neuropathy, gastrointestinal toxicities (nausea, vomiting, and diarrhea), hypotension, bone marrow suppression, fatigue, and malaise.
  - Dose modifications or cessation of therapy based on degree of toxicities are provided in the package labeling for FDA-approved indications of bortezomib.

Eculizumab

- Eculizumab is a humanized monoclonal IgG antibody that binds to complement protein C5 to prevent cleavage into C5a and C5b by C5 convertase.[2,4,20]
- Inhibition of C5 subsequently inhibits the formation of terminal complex C5b-9, otherwise known as the MAC.[4]
- In AMR, eculizumab may be utilized in select cases to inhibit ongoing complement-mediated graft injury but does aid in suppressing antibody production or interfering with the circulating antibody burden.
- Eculizumab has demonstrated benefit in desensitization and management of early AMR, but long-term impact remains unknown.[8,20]
- Dosing
  - Dosing for AMR is based on dosing for other FDA-approved indications of eculizumab, including atypical hemolytic uremic syndrome and paroxysmal nocturnal hemoglobinuria.
  - Eculizumab 900 to 1,200 mg intravenous, followed by 900 mg weekly if continuing therapy.
  - In patient receiving plasma exchange or FFP, supplemental dosing of eculizumab is recommended.
- Adverse effects
  - Eculizumab increases the risk of serious infections, including meningococcal infections (*Neisseria meningitidis*) and infections caused by other encapsulated bacteria (*Streptococcus pneumoniae* and *Haemophilus influenzae*).
  - Immunize with meningococcal vaccines (MenACWY and MenB) at least 2 weeks prior to the first dose of eculizumab unless the risk of delaying treatment outweighs the risk of serious infection.
  - If treatment cannot be delayed in an unvaccinated patient, at least 2 weeks of antimicrobial prophylaxis with either a penicillin or ciprofloxacin is recommended.

- Revaccinate according to Advisory Committee on Immunization Practices guidelines when appropriate and pending duration of eculizumab therapy.
- Prescribers must enroll in the REMS program aimed at mitigating the risk of meningococcal infections.
- Drug-drug interactions: Due to inhibition of complement component, C5, caution should be given to coadministration and timing of eculizumab with other antibodies therapies that rely on complement-dependent pathways, such as rituximab.

Novel Agents for Treatment of AMR

- Due to lack of consistent benefit of currently available agents for treatment of AMR, novel agents and treatment approaches continue to emerge.
- Investigated agents have explored the role of costimulatory blockade, complement inhibition via C1 esterase, direct cleavage of IgG antibodies via recombinant proteases, anti-B-cell therapies targeting B-cell activation and enhanced anti-CD20 activity, and plasma cell targeting via anti-CD38 antibodies.[20]

REFERENCES

1. Hart A, Singh D, Brown SJ, Wang JH, Kasiske BL. Incidence, risk factors, treatment, and consequences of antibody-mediated kidney transplant rejection: a systematic review. *Clin Transplant.* 2021;35(7):e14320.
2. Kim M, Martin ST, Townsend KR, Gabardi S. Antibody-mediated rejection in kidney transplantation: a review of pathophysiology, diagnosis, and treatment options. *Pharmacotherapy.* 2014;34(7):733-44.
3. Haas M, Loupy A, Lefaucheur C, et al. The Banff 2017 Kidney Meeting Report: revised diagnostic criteria for chronic active T cell-mediated rejection, antibody-mediated rejection, and prospects for integrative endpoints for next-generation clinical trials. *Am J Transplant.* 2018;18(2):293-307.
4. Lucas JG, Co JP, Nwaogwugwu UT, Dosani I, Sureshkumar KK. Antibody-mediated rejection in kidney transplantation: an update. *Expert Opin Pharmacother.* 2011;12(4):579-92.
5. Cooper JE. Evaluation and treatment of acute rejection in kidney allografts. *Clin J Am Soc Nephrol.* 2020;15(3):430-8.
6. Chong AS, Rothstein DM, Safa K, Riella LV. Outstanding questions in transplantation: B cells, alloantibodies, and humoral rejection. *Am J Transplant.* 2019;19(8):2155-63.
7. Sellarés J, De Freitas D, Mengel M, et al. Understanding the causes of kidney transplant failure: the dominant role of antibody-mediated rejection and nonadherence. *Am J Transplant.* 2012;12(2):388-99.
8. Schinstock CA, Mannon RB, Budde K, et al. Recommended treatment for antibody-mediated rejection after kidney transplantation: the 2019 expert consensus from the transplantion society working group. *Transplantation.* 2020;104(5):911-22.
9. de Sousa MV, Gonçalez AC, de Lima Zollner R, Mazzali M. Treatment of antibody-mediated rejection after kidney transplantation: immunological effects, clinical response, and histological findings. *Ann Transplant.* 2020;25:e9254888.
10. Bu L, Gupta G, Pai A, et al. Clinical outcomes from the assessing donor-derived cell-free DNA monitoring insights of kidney allografts with longitudinal surveillance (ADMIRAL) study. *Kidney Int.* 2022;101(4):793-803.
11. Eikmans M, Gielis EM, Ledeganck KJ, Yang J, Abramowicz D, Claas FFJ. Non-invasive biomarkers of acute rejection in kidney transplantation: novel targets and strategies. *Front Med.* 2018;5:358.
12. Wan SS, Ying TD, Wyburn K, Roberts DM, Wyld M, Chadban SJ. The treatment of antibody-mediated rejection in kidney transplantation: an updated systematic review and meta-analysis. *Transplantation.* 2018;102(4):557-68.

13. Kaposztas Z, Podder H, Mauiyyedi S, et al. Impact of rituximab therapy for treatment of acute humoral rejection. *Clin Transplant.* 2009;23(1):63-73.
14. Sautenet B, Blancho G, Büchler M, et al. One-year results of the effects of rituximab on acute antibody-mediated rejection in renal transplantation: RITUX ERAH, a multicenter double-blind randomized placebo-controlled trial. *Transplantation.* 2016;100(2):391-9.
15. Lefaucheur C, Loupy A, Vernerey D, et al. Antibody-mediated vascular rejection of kidney allografts: a population-based study. *Lancet.* 2013;381(9863):313-9.
16. Williams ME, Balogun RA. Principles of separation: indications and therapeutic targets for plasma exchange. *Clin J Am Soc Nephrol.* 2014;9(1):181-90.
17. Kaplan AA. Therapeutic plasma exchange: core curriculum 2008. *Am J Kidney Dis.* 2008;52(6):1180-96.
18. Jordan SC, Toyoda M, Vo AA. Intravenous immunoglobulin a natural regulator of immunity and inflammation. *Transplantation.* 2009;88:1-6.
19. Jordan S, Toyoda M, Kahwaji J, Vo A. Clinical aspects of intravenous immunoglobulin use in solid organ transplant recipients. *Am J Transplant.* 2011;11(2):196-202.
20. Jordan SC, Ammerman N, Choi J, et al. The role of novel therapeutic approaches for prevention of allosensitization and antibody-mediated rejection. *Am J Transplant.* 2020;20(suppl 4):42-56.

14 Posttransplant Glomerular Disease

Andrew Malone

GENERAL PRINCIPLES

- Most primary glomerulonephritis (GN) can recur in the transplanted kidney.
- Glomerulonephritis as a cause of end-stage kidney disease (ESKD) varies between regions around the world (**Table 14-1**).[1-3]
- The incidence of primary glomerulonephritis may be underestimated due to variable biopsy frequency.
- Glomerulonephritis is a heterogenous group of disorders. Each subtype has risks factors that affect recurrence risk and allograft survival.
- The incidence and prognosis of the recurrence of glomerular disease post transplantation is dependent on the type of native glomerular disease.
- The incidence of allograft GN varies between reports (**Table 14-2**).[4-7] This variation is likely due to variable biopsy practice post transplantation (ie, protocol biopsies vs. indication biopsies).
- Typically, time post transplantation is proportional to the risk of recurrence of GN. In one report, this ranges from 4% in the first year to 13% of clinically indicated biopsies.[8] However, some forms of GN such as focal segmental glomerulosclerosis (FSGS), atypical hemolytic uremic syndrome, or C3 GN can recur early post transplantation.
- Recurrent GN can remain subclinical for months to years. Therefore, recurrent GN may be advanced and severe at the time of clinical diagnosis and indication biopsy. A protocol biopsy approach can mitigate this issue.
- The histology of early recurrent GN may be subtle when compared with histology found in native disease. For example, early recurrent FSGS may only have foot process effacement on electron microscopy with normal light microscopy.
- Please see Chapter 15 for recurrence of complement-related glomerular diseases, such as atypical hemolytic uremic syndrome, C3 glomerulonephritis, and thrombotic microangiopathies.

TABLE 14-1 The Incidence of Glomerulonephritis as an Etiology of End-Stage Renal Disease Among Different Databases

Database	USRDS	UKRR	China	ANZDATA
GN as etiology for ESKD	7%	14%	46.5%	17%

ANZDATA, Australia and New Zealand Dialysis and Transplant Registry; ESKD, end-stage kidney disease; GN, glomerulonephritis; UKRR, The UK Research Reserve; USRDS, United States Renal Data System.
Data from Liu ZH. Nephrology in China. *Nat Rev Nephrol.* 2013;9:523-8; ANZDATA Registry. *40th Report, Chapter 1: Incidence of End Stage Kidney Disease.* Australia and New Zealand Dialysis and Transplant Registry; 2018. Accessed April 13, 2023. http://www.anzdata.org.au; and Evans K, Pyart R, Steenkamp R, et al. UK renal registry 20th annual report: introduction. *Nephron.* 2018;139:1-12.

TABLE 14-2 The Prevalence of Recurrent Glomerulonephritis Among Different Databases

Database	Mayo	Korea	ANZDATA
Recurrent GN prevalence	39.5% @ 5 y	9.7% @ 5 y 17% @ 10 y	10.3% @~7 y

ANZDATA, Australia and New Zealand Dialysis and Transplant Registry; GN, glomerulonephritis.
Data from Hariharan S, Adams MB, Brennan DC, et al. Recurrent and de novo glomerular disease after renal transplantation: a Report from Renal Allograft Disease Registry (RADR). *Transplantation.* 1999;68:635-41; Halloran PF, Pereira AB, Chang J, et al. Microarray diagnosis of antibody-mediated rejection in kidney transplant biopsies: an International Prospective Study (INTERCOM). *Am J Transplant.* 2013;13:2865-74; Sellarés J, De Freitas DG, Mengel M, et al. Understanding the causes of kidney transplant failure: the dominant role of antibody-mediated rejection and nonadherence. *Am J Transplant.* 2012;12:388-99; and An JN, Lee JP, Oh YJ, et al. Incidence of post-transplant glomerulonephritis and its impact on graft outcome. *Kidney Res Clin Pract.* 2012;31:219-26.

RECURRENCE VERSUS DE NOVO GLOMERULONEPHRITIS

- In the posttransplant setting, de novo GN refers to the occurrence of GN in a patient with a non-GN primary diagnosis. However, the primary kidney disease is often not known, making the distinction between recurrent GN and de novo GN less clear.
- In general, recurrent GN occurs earlier post transplantation than de novo GN.
- There is a greater incidence of recurrent GN than of de novo GN, 39.5% for recurrent GN and 14.6% for de novo GN at 5 years post transplantation.[9]

RECURRENT FOCAL SEGMENTAL GLOMERULOSCLEROSIS

Epidemiology and Risk Factors

- FSGS will recur post transplantation in about 30% of patients with primary FSGS.[10]
- The proportion of patients with recurrence varies according to time post transplantation, from 10.5% at 1 year to 35.1% at 5 years, according to one study.[9]

Risk Factors

- Factors that increase the risk of recurrence of FSGS include recurrence in a previous transplant, younger patients at diagnosis of FSGS, progression to ESRD within 3 years, high proteinuria before transplant, white recipient, and pretransplant bilateral nephrectomy.[9]
- The most reliable risk factor for recurrence of FSGS is recurrence in a previous kidney transplant. The likelihood of recurrence in a second transplant is approximately 80%.
- The Columbia classification histological subtype, nonnephrotic range proteinuria before transplant, and familial forms of FSGS are thought not to increase risk of recurrence. However, one study reported recurrence of FSGS in children with NPHS2 mutations as a cause for their primary disease. The recurrence rate in this study, 38%, was comparable with the recurrence rate of primary FSGS.[11]

Etiology

- The cause of FSGS recurrence post transplant has not been fully elucidated. Evidence to date points toward the presence of a circulating factor as a cause for recurrent FSGS.[12]
- Early recurrent FSGS targets the podocyte, and glomerular damage is only evident on electron microscopy.[13] Light microscopy changes of FSGS occur in biopsies performed later in the disease process.
- Early in the disease process podocyte injury is reversible.[14]
- An important care report confirmed that a circulating factor is likely the cause of recurrent FSGS. A kidney transplant that developed recurrence of FSGS early post transplant was retransplanted into a second recipient. On retransplantation proteinuria resolved.[14]
- One group has suggested soluble urokinase plasminogen activator receptors (suPARs) are a cause of FSGS.[15] suPAR is thought to mediate podocyte injury by activating integrin β(3) resulting in podocyte foot process effacement and proteinuria. Other studies have shown that higher serum suPAR levels associate with primary FSGS and that reduction of suPAR levels with immunosuppression is associated with greater likelihood of clinical remission.[16] These data have not been reproduced.
- B cells are thought to play an important role in the pathogenesis of recurrent FSGS as rituximab has been successfully used to treat recurrent FSGS.[17]
- Sphingomyelin phosphodiesterase acid-like 3b (SMPDL-3b) may also play a role in recurrent FSGS. Rituximab treatment was associated with SMPDL-3b expression in podocytes and prevention of FSGS recurrence.[18]
- High-risk variants in the APOL1 gene have been associated with native kidney FSGS and chronic kidney disease.[19] The relationship between APOL1 variants and recurrent FSGS will be discussed in more detail below.

Graft Survival

- The recurrence of FSGS post transplantation increased the risk of graft loss in patients with native kidney primary FSGS. One study estimates a 5-year graft survival of 57% in patients who have recurrence of FSGS.[20]
- Another study of nearly 5,000 patients reported a relative risk of 2.25 for graft failure among those with recurrent FSGS.[4]
- The Mayo Clinic group reported a hazards ratio for graft failure post FSGS recurrence of 4.97.[9]
- Data from the Australia and New Zealand Dialysis and Transplant Registry (ANZDATA) showed all-cause 10-year incidence of graft loss was 51% for those with biopsy-proven native kidney FSGS.[21]

Prevention

- Rituximab has been successfully used to prevent the recurrence of FSGS post transplantation. However, data are limited to small case series and case reports.
- The choice of induction agent used at the time of transplant surgery is associated with risk of glomerular disease recurrence. Use of thymoglobulin had a lower rate of recurrent FSGS post transplantation when compared with alemtuzumab and anti-IL2RA induction.[22]

Treatment

- It is important to rule out secondary causes of FSGS post transplantation, particularly in disease occurring late post transplant. Secondary causes include viruses such as hepatitis C, cytomegalovirus (CMV), parvovirus B19, Epstein-Barr virus, BK virus, and HIV and toxins such as sirolimus and bisphosphonates. However, secondary causes are less likely in early recurrence.

- There is no widely accepted treatment of recurrent FSGS.
- Response to treatment is usually measured by monitoring serial urinary protein level. This can be done by collecting a 24-hour urine specimen; however, this is not practical for serial measurements. Thus, a single sample urine protein to creatinine ratio can be used to estimate total urine protein.
- Plasmapheresis is usually used for treatment of FSGS recurring in the first year post transplant. Plasmapheresis is only effective in some patients, and it is not possible to predict who will respond to this treatment. Furthermore, some patients are responsive to, but dependent on, plasmapheresis. The presumed mechanism of action is the removal of a circulating factor.
- One study reported a response rate to plasmapheresis of 63% and 70% in adults and children, respectively.[23]
- Rituximab has also been used to successfully treat recurrent FSGS, with some authors noting the therapeutic effects of plasmapheresis and rituximab may be synergistic.[24] However, the efficacy of rituximab for the treatment of recurrent FSGS has not been widely studied.
- One study of 39 patients with recurrent FSGS reported that 64.1% of these patients has some response to rituximab.[25]
- Adrenocorticotropic hormone (ACTH) gel has also been used with some success for the treatment of recurrent FSGS. A study of 20 patients with recurrent FSGS demonstrated a 50% complete or partial remission. The majority of these patients had also received plasmapheresis and/or rituximab prior to receiving ACTH gel.[26]

RECURRENT MEMBRANOUS NEPHROPATHY

Epidemiology

- Primary membranous nephropathy will recur in 40% to 50% kidneys transplanted into patients with native membranous nephropathy.[9,27]
- Incidence rates are influenced by biopsy indication. Studies that included centers performing protocol biopsies report a higher incidence of recurrent membranous nephropathy.
- Histologic recurrence of primary membranous nephropathy usually occurs in the first year post transplant, but a second incidence peak occurs at about 5 years.[27]
- Histologic findings can be subtle in posttransplant membranous nephropathy with few or no light microscopy changes and IgG with few C3 deposits seen on immunofluorescence.

Etiology

- Most patients (70%) with primary membranous nephropathy have autoantibodies to podocyte phospholipase A2 receptor (PLA2R).[28] The number of patients transplanted with anti-PLA2R autoantibodies is similar.[27]
- It is assumed that antibody binding to the PLA2R antigen triggers a pathologic response resulting in the clinical and histologic findings.
- Other antigens have been described as targets for autoantibodies causing primary membranous nephropathy in the native kidney but less is known about these antibodies in the posttransplant setting. These include Thrombospondin type-1

domain-containing 7A (THSD7A), Neural epidermal growth factor-like 1 (NELL1), and Semaphorin 3B (Sema3B).

Anti-PLA2R and Recurrent Membranous Nephropathy

- Anti-PLA2R antibodies in the serum of patients before transplantation can predict the risk of recurrence of membranous nephropathy post transplantation (**Figure 14-1**).
- Risk of histologic recurrence is 60% to 76% in those with pretransplant anti-PLA2R antibodies and 28% to 30% in those without.[29,30]
- Anti-PLA2R antibody titers usually drop by about 50% post transplantation.
- Monitoring for persistent or rising anti-PLA2R antibody titers post transplantation can be used to predict recurrence.
- Positive PLA2R antigen staining in a biopsy is associated with recurrent membranous nephropathy and not with de novo membranous nephropathy with a sensitivity of 83% and specificity of 92% for recurrent membranous nephropathy.[31]

Graft Survival

- Compared with patients with a primary membranous nephropathy diagnosis before transplantation but without recurrence, recurrent membranous is not associated with increased graft failure, HR 1.36 (0.27-6.76, $P < .0001$).[9]
- Actual graft survival for patients with a diagnosis of primary membranous nephropathy as a cause for their ESKD is 79.6% with 99.7 ± 51 months of follow-up.[9]

Treatment

- There is some consensus to treat recurrent membranous nephropathy early and when proteinuria levels are still in the subnephrotic range (contrary to the approach commonly used in native membranous nephropathy).
- For mild disease (proteinuria below 1 g/d) it is reasonable to treat conservatively with strict blood pressure control, renin-angiotensin inhibition, and dyslipidemia treatment. There is no good evidence for the efficacy of this approach.
- The mainstay of treatment of membranous nephropathy post transplantation (proteinuria above 1 g/d) is rituximab.
- High clinical response rates have been noted with rituximab treatment.[27,32]
- The optimal dosing schedule of rituximab is not known. Some example dosing regimens include 200 g once and 1 to 4 doses of 375 mg/m^2 body surface area.
- Some centers monitor CD20 or CD19 B cell levels to measure the response to rituximab. If the patient had anti-PLA2R-positive membranous disease some centers

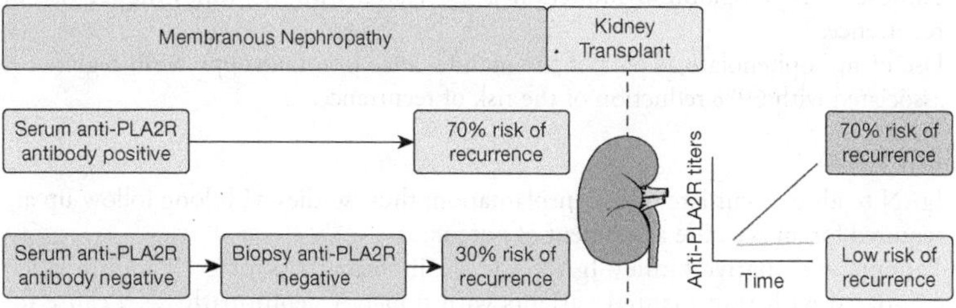

Figure 14-1. **Risk for posttransplant recurrence of membranous nephropathy according to anti-PLA2R antibody levels.**

measure this antibody after treatment to monitor response to treatment. An ideal response is an antibody titer that declines to undetectable.

- Monitoring response to treatment is probably best done by measurement of proteinuria.

RECURRENT IGA NEPHROPATHY

Epidemiology

- The incidence of recurrent or posttransplant IgA nephropathy (IgAN) varies depending on definition (clinical or histologic), criteria for biopsy, ethnicity, and time post transplant.
- The reported incidence is 33%.[33]
- The incidence increases to 50% in protocol biopsy studies.
- In biopsy studies approximately half of patients had no abnormalities in urinalysis.[34]

Etiology

- IgAN is caused by the deposition of IgA1 immune complexes.
- For IgA1 antibodies to become pathologic in the kidney they need to have certain chemical and biological features.
- Pathologic IgA1 antibodies are poorly O-galactosylated and have abnormal sialylation.
- Certain infections, including CMV, *Haemophilus parainfluenzae*, *Staphylococcus aureus*, and toxoplasmosis, have been implicated as triggers for abnormal IgA1 immune complex formation and IgAN.
- There is also a genetic predisposition to IgAN.[35]

Risk Factors

- Younger recipients, rapid progression of disease before transplant, degree of HLA matching, living increased versus deceased donors, IL-10 polymorphisms (G1082A), HLA-B8-DR3 haplotype.[9] It must be noted that not all of these findings have been reproduced in other studies.
- No commonly used clinical biomarkers can predict recurrence of IgAN.
- High pretransplant levels of circulating galactose-deficient IgA1 and IgA-IgG complexes and lower levels of circulating complexes of IgA-soluble CD89 are associated with an increased risk of recurrence of IgAN.[36]
- Corticosteroid-free or early withdrawal of corticosteroid from the maintenance immunosuppression regimen infer a hazard risk for recurrence of 8.59.[37]
- Nonuse of thymoglobulin induction is associated with 4.5 times higher risk of recurrence.[37]
- Use of mycophenolate as part of the maintenance immunosuppression regimen is associated with 60% reduction of the risk of recurrence.[37]

Graft Survival

- IgAN tends to recur late post transplantation; thus, studies with long follow-up are required for an accurate assessment of outcomes.
- Patients with native kidney IgAN had no increased risk of graft failure when compared with transplanted patients with non-IgA nephropathy as a cause for ESKD.[9]

- Patients with recurrent IgAN post transplantation have 3.4 times higher risk of graft loss compared with transplantation patients with IgAN who do not have recurrence of disease post transplant.[9]
- Australasian data reported a 10-year graft loss of 4.3% overall cumulative incidence.[38]

Prevention

The approach to the prevention of recurrent IgAN is the use of thymoglobulin induction and mycophenolate-based maintenance therapy.

Treatment

- There are no good studies to support the use of any particular therapy.
- There is some suggestion for potential benefit with the use of angiotensin-converting-enzyme inhibitors and angiotensin receptor blockers.[39]
- If patients were not on corticosteroid maintenance, a switch to corticosteroid maintenance is a reasonable approach.
- Other treatments used by some centers include high-dose glucocorticoids, rituximab, and tonsillectomy.

APOL1 AND KIDNEY TRANSPLANTATION

- Overexpression of APOL1 risk alleles in mouse podocytes induces kidney disease.[40]
- APOL1 risk variants are common only in people of African descent.
- APOL1 risk alleles are known to increase the risk of chronic kidney disease and certain nondiabetic causes of kidney disease.[19,41]

Donor APOL1 and Graft Survival

Donor kidneys with 2 APOL1 risk alleles reduce graft survival time with a hazard ratio of between 2 and 4 (**Figure 14-2**).[42,43]

Recipient APOL1 and Graft Survival

One study, using 2 independent datasets, showed that recipient APOL1 risk variants increased risk of death-censored allograft loss, independent of the recipient's ancestry and the donor's APOL1 genotype (**Figure 14-2**).[44]

RECURRENCE OF OTHER GLOMERULAR DISEASES POST TRANSPLANTATION

- Complement-related glomerular diseases and their recurrence post transplant will be discussed in Chapter 15.
- The recurrence of other glomerular diseases post transplantation is rarer than those discussed above.
- A positive antineutrophil cytoplasmic antibodies (ANCA) test does not increase risk of recurrence of ANCA-associated vasculitis post transplant and therefore should not be considered on its own a contraindication to transplantation.[45,46]
- It is usual practice to ensure patients with ANCA-associated vasculitis causing ESKD are in clinical remission before transplantation.
- One pooled analysis estimates the rate of ANCA-associated vasculitis recurrence post transplant to be between 20% and 25%.[46]

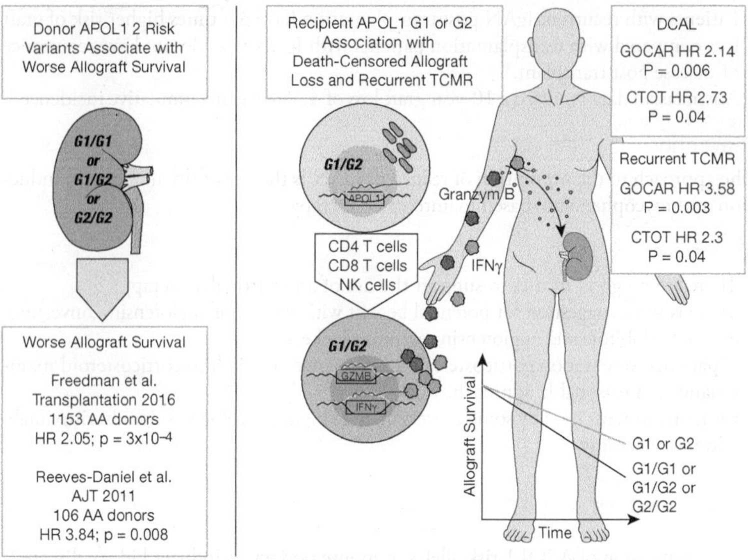

Figure 14-2. **APOL1 variants and the influence on kidney transplantation outcomes.** AA, African American; CTOT, Clinical Trials in Organ Transplantation; DCAL, death-censored allograft loss; GOCAR, Genomics of Chronic Allograft Rejection; HR, hazard ratio; TCMR, T-cell-mediated rejection. (Data from Freedman BI, Pastan SO, Israni AK, et al. APOL1 genotype and kidney transplantation outcomes from deceased african american donors. *Transplantation*. 2016;100:194-202; Reeves-Daniel AM, DePalma JA, Bleyer AJ, et al. The APOL1 gene and allograft survival after kidney transplantation. *Am J Transplant*. 2011;11:1025-30; and Zhang Z, Sun Z, Fu J, et al. Recipient APOL1 risk alleles associate with death-censored renal allograft survival and rejection episodes. *J Clin Invest*. 2021;131:e146643.)

- Recurrent ANCA-vasculitis post transplantation has been successfully treated with mycophenolate mofetil, plasmapheresis, and rituximab.[47]
- Five-year graft survival is over 95% to 100% in patients with ESKD from ANCA-associated vasculitis.[45]
- Clinical recurrence of lupus nephritis post transplantation is rare if the patient had no disease activity before transplant.
- One study reported 5 of 12 patients with lupus nephritis as a cause for ESKD have recurrence of their lupus nephritis.[48]
- This study also reported a 5-year graft survival of 85%.[48]
- Like other glomerular diseases, induction with thymoglobulin reduced the risk of recurrence of lupus nephritis.
- Cyclophosphamide, corticosteroids, increased doses of mycophenolate and rituximab have been used to treat recurrent lupus nephritis.
- Recurrence of anti–glomerular basement membrane disease (anti-GBM) is very rare.
- One recent study examined 53 patients where recurrence occurred in only 1 patient giving a prevalence rate of 1.9%.[49]
- Recurrence of linear IgG staining of the GBM can occur in up to 50% of transplants. However, most remain asymptomatic.
- Treatment of recurrent anti-GBM is cyclophosphamide and plasmapheresis. One study reported rituximab was not an effective treatment.[50]

REFERENCES

1. Liu ZH. Nephrology in China. *Nat Rev Nephrol.* 2013;9:523-8.
2. ANZDATA Registry. *40th Report, Chapter 1: Incidence of End Stage Kidney Disease.* Australia and New Zealand Dialysis and Transplant Registry; 2018. Accessed April 13, 2023. http://www.anzdata.org.au
3. Evans K, Pyart R, Steenkamp R, et al. UK renal registry 20th annual report: introduction. *Nephron.* 2018;139(suppl 1):1-12.
4. Hariharan S, Adams MB, Brennan DC, et al. Recurrent and de novo glomerular disease after renal transplantation: a report from Renal Allograft Disease Registry (RADR). *Transplantation.* 1999;68(5):635-41.
5. Halloran PF, Pereira AB, Chang J, et al. Microarray diagnosis of antibody-mediated rejection in kidney transplant biopsies: an international prospective study (INTERCOM). *Am J Transplant.* 2013;13(11):2865-74.
6. Sellarés J, de Freitas DG, Mengel M, et al. Understanding the causes of kidney transplant failure: the dominant role of antibody-mediated rejection and nonadherence. *Am J Transplant.* 2012;12(2):388-99.
7. An JN, Lee JP, Oh YJ, et al. Incidence of post-transplant glomerulonephritis and its impact on graft outcome. *Kidney Res Clin Pract.* 2012;31(4):219-26.
8. Gourishankar S, Leduc R, Connett J, et al. Pathological and clinical characterization of the "troubled transplant": data from the DeKAF study. *Am J Transplant.* 2010;10(2):324-30.
9. Cosio FG, Cattran DC. Recent advances in our understanding of recurrent primary glomerulonephritis after kidney transplantation. *Kidney Int.* 2017;91(2):304-14.
10. Ivanyi B. A primer on recurrent and de novo glomerulonephritis in renal allografts. *Nat Clin Pract Nephrol.* 2008;4(8):446-57.
11. Bertelli R, Ginevri F, Caridi G, et al. Recurrence of focal segmental glomerulosclerosis after renal transplantation in patients with mutations of podocin. *Am J Kidney Dis.* 2003;41(6):1314-21.
12. Savin VJ, Sharma R, Sharma M, et al. Circulating factor associated with increased glomerular permeability to albumin in recurrent focal segmental glomerulosclerosis. *N Engl J Med.* 1996;334(14):878-83.
13. Hoyer JR, Vernier RL, Najarian JS, Raij L, Simmons RL, Michael AF. Recurrence of idiopathic nephrotic syndrome after renal transplantation. *Lancet.* 1972;2(7773):343-8.
14. Gallon L, Leventhal J, Skaro A, Kanwar Y, Alvarado A. Resolution of recurrent focal segmental glomerulosclerosis after retransplantation. *N Engl J Med.* 2012;366(17):1648-9.
15. Wei C, El Hindi S, Li J, et al. Circulating urokinase receptor as a cause of focal segmental glomerulosclerosis. *Nat Med.* 2011;17(8):952-60.
16. Wei C, Trachtman H, Li J, et al. Circulating suPAR in two cohorts of primary FSGS. *J Am Soc Nephrol.* 2012;23(12):2051-9.
17. Pescovitz MD, Book BK, Sidner RA. Resolution of recurrent focal segmental glomerulosclerosis proteinuria after rituximab treatment. *N Engl J Med.* 2006;354(18):1961-3.
18. Fornoni A, Sageshima J, Wei C, et al. Rituximab targets podocytes in recurrent focal segmental glomerulosclerosis. *Sci Transl Med.* 2011;3(85):85ra46.
19. Genovese G, Friedman DJ, Ross MD, et al. Association of trypanolytic ApoL1 variants with kidney disease in African Americans. *Science.* 2010;329(5993):841-5.
20. Ponticelli C, Glassock RJ. Posttransplant recurrence of primary glomerulonephritis. *Clin J Am Soc Nephrol.* 2010;5(12):2363-72.
21. Briganti EM, Russ GR, McNeil JJ, Atkins RC, Chadban SJ. Risk of renal allograft loss from recurrent glomerulonephritis. *N Engl J Med.* 2002;347(2):103-9.
22. Pascual J, Mezrich JD, Djamali A, et al. Alemtuzumab induction and recurrence of glomerular disease after kidney transplantation. *Transplantation.* 2007;83(11):1429-34.
23. Ponticelli C. Recurrence of focal segmental glomerular sclerosis (FSGS) after renal transplantation. *Nephrol Dial Transplant.* 2010;25(1):25-31.
24. Canaud G, Zuber J, Sberro R, et al. Intensive and prolonged treatment of focal and segmental glomerulosclerosis recurrence in adult kidney transplant recipients: a pilot study. *Am J Transplant.* 2009;9(5):1081-6.

25. Araya CE, Dharnidharka VR. The factors that may predict response to rituximab therapy in recurrent focal segmental glomerulosclerosis: a systematic review. *J Transplant.* 2011;2011:374213.
26. Alhamad T, Manllo Dieck J, Younus U, et al. ACTH gel in resistant focal segmental glomerulosclerosis after kidney transplantation. *Transplantation.* 2019;103(1):202-9.
27. Grupper A, Cornell LD, Fervenza FC, Beck LH Jr, Lorenz E, Cosio FG. Recurrent membranous nephropathy after kidney transplantation: treatment and long-term implications. *Transplantation.* 2016;100(12):2710-6.
28. Beck LH Jr, Bonegio RG, Lambeau G, et al. M-type phospholipase A2 receptor as target antigen in idiopathic membranous nephropathy. *N Engl J Med.* 2009;361(1):11-21.
29. Kattah A, Ayalon R, Beck LH Jr, et al. Anti-phospholipase A_2 receptor antibodies in recurrent membranous nephropathy. *Am J Transplant.* 2015;15(5):1349-59.
30. Quintana LF, Blasco M, Seras M, et al. Antiphospholipase A2 receptor antibody levels predict the risk of posttransplantation recurrence of membranous nephropathy. *Transplantation.* 2015;99(8):1709-14.
31. Larsen CP, Walker PD. Phospholipase A2 receptor (PLA2R) staining is useful in the determination of de novo versus recurrent membranous glomerulopathy. *Transplantation.* 2013;95(10):1259-62.
32. Sprangers B, Lefkowitz GI, Cohen SD, et al. Beneficial effect of rituximab in the treatment of recurrent idiopathic membranous nephropathy after kidney transplantation. *Clin J Am Soc Nephrol.* 2010;5:790-7.
33. Ponticelli C, Traversi L, Banfi G. Renal transplantation in patients with IgA mesangial glomerulonephritis. *Pediatr Transplant.* 2004;8(4):334-8.
34. Ortiz F, Gelpi R, Koskinen P, et al. IgA nephropathy recurs early in the graft when assessed by protocol biopsy. *Nephrol Dial Transplant.* 2012;27(6):2553-8.
35. Kiryluk K, Li Y, Scolari F, et al. Discovery of new risk loci for IgA nephropathy implicates genes involved in immunity against intestinal pathogens. *Nat Genet.* 2014;46(11):1187-96.
36. Berthelot L, Robert T, Vuiblet V, et al. Recurrent IgA nephropathy is predicted by altered glycosylated IgA, autoantibodies and soluble CD89 complexes. *Kidney Int.* 2015;88(4):815-22.
37. Von Visger JR, Gunay Y, Andreoni KA, et al. The risk of recurrent IgA nephropathy in a steroid-free protocol and other modifying immunosuppression. *Clin Transplant.* 2014;28(8):845-54.
38. Clayton P, McDonald S, Chadban S. Steroids and recurrent IgA nephropathy after kidney transplantation. *Am J Transplant.* 2011;11(8):1645-9.
39. Courtney AE, McNamee PT, Nelson WE, Maxwell AP. Does angiotensin blockade influence graft outcome in renal transplant recipients with IgA nephropathy? *Nephrol Dial Transplant.* 2006;21(12):3550-4.
40. Beckerman P, Bi-Karchin J, Park AS, et al. Transgenic expression of human APOL1 risk variants in podocytes induces kidney disease in mice. *Nat Med.* 2017;23(4):429-38.
41. Malone AF. APOL1 risk variants in kidney transplantation: a modulation of immune cell function. *J Clin Invest.* 2021;131(22):e154676.
42. Freedman BI, Pastan SO, Israni AK, et al. APOL1 genotype and kidney transplantation outcomes from deceased African American donors. *Transplantation.* 2016;100(1):194-202.
43. Reeves-Daniel AM, DePalma JA, Bleyer AJ, et al. The APOL1 gene and allograft survival after kidney transplantation. *Am J Transplant.* 2011;11(5):1025-30.
44. Zhang Z, Sun Z, Fu J, et al. Recipient APOL1 risk alleles associate with death-censored renal allograft survival and rejection episodes. *J Clin Invest.* 2021;131(22):e146643.
45. Gera M, Griffin MD, Specks U, Leung N, Stegall MD, Fervenza FC. Recurrence of ANCA-associated vasculitis following renal transplantation in the modern era of immunosupression. *Kidney Int.* 2007;71(12):1296-301.
46. Nachman PH, Segelmark M, Westman K, et al. Recurrent ANCA-associated small vessel vasculitis after transplantation: a pooled analysis. *Kidney Int.* 1999;56(4):1544-50.
47. Murakami C, Manoharan P, Carter-Monroe N, Geetha D. Rituximab for remission induction in recurrent ANCA-associated glomerulonephritis postkidney transplant. *Transpl Int.* 2013;26(12):1225-31.

48. Çeltİk A, Şen S, Tamer AF, et al. Recurrent lupus nephritis after transplantation: clinicopathological evaluation with protocol biopsies. *Nephrology*. 2016;21(7):601-7.
49. Coche S, Sprangers B, Van Laecke S, et al. Recurrence and outcome of anti-glomerular basement membrane glomerulonephritis after kidney transplantation. *Kidney Int Rep*. 2021;6(7):1888-94.
50. Sauter M, Schmid H, Anders HJ, Heller F, Weiss M, Sitter T. Loss of a renal graft due to recurrence of anti-GBM disease despite rituximab therapy. *Clin Transplant*. 2009;23(1):132-6.

15

Complement Disorders

Anuja Java

GENERAL PRINCIPLES

- Atypical hemolytic uremic syndrome (aHUS) is a thrombotic microangiopathy (TMA), characterized by the triad of microangiopathic hemolytic anemia, thrombocytopenia, and acute kidney injury.[1]
- C3 glomerulopathy (C3G) is a glomerulonephritis characterized by deposition of the C3 component within the glomerulus, in the absence or near absence of immunoglobulin deposits.[2]
- A diagnosis of C3G can only be made on immunofluorescence (IF), criterion on IF being presence of dominant C3 staining at least 2 orders of magnitude greater than any other immunoreactant (i.e., IgG, IgA, IgM, and C1q).
- C3G is further divided into C3 glomerulonephritis (C3GN) and dense deposit disease (DDD) based on electron microscopy.
- The major defect underlying the 2 diseases is a dysregulated complement system that often leads to overactivation with resultant organ damage.[3,4]
- The etiology of dysregulated complement system is a genetic variant in one of the complement proteins, identified in 40% to 60% of patients with aHUS and 20% to 30% patients with C3G.[3]
- Acquired deficiencies occur in 5% to 10% of patients with aHUS (e.g., factor H autoantibodies).
- Acquired factors are more common in C3G—C3 nephritic factor (~50%-80%), C5 nephritic factor (~50%).[2]
- Monoclonal gammopathy should be ruled out in patients with C3G who are >50 years; monoclonal immunoglobulins can impair complement regulation.[2]
- Disease penetrance is approximately 50%, suggesting that an environmental trigger is necessary in many cases.
- The risk of recurrence for both diseases after a kidney transplantation is high and depends on the underlying complement abnormality.[5,6]
- Reported recurrence rate of C3GN is greater than 50%; DDD is much higher and approaches approximately 80% to 100%, leading to allograft loss in ~50%.[2]

DIAGNOSIS

Clinical Manifestations and Laboratory Features—aHUS

- Microangiopathic hemolytic anemia (a nonimmune hemolytic anemia resulting from intravascular red cell fragmentation); laboratory findings include:
  - High lactate dehydrogenase
  - Low haptoglobin
  - Occasionally schistocytes on peripheral smear
  - Thrombocytopenia (due to consumption)

- Organ injury/end-organ ischemia occurs due to small-vessel thrombosis. Extrarenal manifestations may include stroke, seizures, myocardial infarction, hepatitis, pancreatitis, digital gangrene.
- Renal-limited TMA may only be diagnosed on a biopsy.
- In the pre-eculizumab era or if not treated timely, recurrence risk >50%; graft loss in 80% to 90% cases.[3]

Clinical Manifestations and Laboratory Features—C3G

- Varied—asymptomatic; hematuria, proteinuria; acute (could be rapidly progressive glomerulonephritis in some cases) or chronic kidney injury.[2]
- Extrarenal manifestations include acquired partial lipodystrophy and retinal drusen.
- Serum complement C3 levels are low in a majority of cases.
- Complement biomarker testing can be conducted to establish defect in the complement pathway (**Tables 15-1** and **15-2**).
- Within 10 years of diagnosis, 80% children and 30% to 50% adults reach end-stage kidney disease (ESKD).[2]

Genetic/Biomarker Testing in aHUS and C3G

- Should be considered as part of pre-and posttransplantation testing (**Figure 15-1**).
- Aids in diagnosis and can inform disease etiology.
- Provides prognostic information with regards to:
  - Risk of progression to ESKD
  - Risk of relapse
  - Risk of disease recurrence post transplantation

TABLE 15-1 Test Recommended for Pre- or PostTransplant Evaluation of aHUS/C3G

Class	Testing	Reasoning
Genetic screening	13-gene panel	Defines the genetic etiology
Complement functional assays	CH50 (classical), AP50 (alternative)	Identifies the pathway affected
Complement protein levels	C3, C4, FH, FI, FB, properdin, MCP (expression by flow cytometry)	Defines if there is a quantitative deficiency
Autoantibodies	FH autoantibodies; C3 and C5 nephritic factors; antiphospholipid evaluation	Establishes acquired defect
Plasma cell dyscrasia	SPEP, serum-free light chains	Monoclonal gammopathy as the driver of C3G (>50 y)

C3G, C3 glomerulopathy; FB, factor B; FH, factor H; FI, factor I; MCP, membrane cofactor protein; SPEP, serum protein electrophoresis.

TABLE 15-2 Tests to be Considered on a Case-by-Case Basis for C3G

Class	Testing	Reasoning
Complement split products	C3c, C3d, Ba, Bb, C5b-9	Presence supports increased complement activity/breakdown
Autoantibodies	FHAA, FBAA, C4 nephritic factor	Acquired factors

FBAA, factor B autoantibody; FHAA, factor H autoantibody.

- Risk of receiving a kidney from living related donors
- Patients with the following characteristics should be considered for genetic testing[6]:
  - History of TMA or C3G as cause of ESKD.
  - Significant family history of TMA/aHUS/C3G or unexplained kidney failure in patient and/or family members.
  - History of malignant hypertension (in younger population).
  - History of preeclampsia leading to ESKD.
  - "*De novo*" disease after kidney transplantation.
- Most centers test for the 15 common genes—*ADAMTS13, C3, CD46, CFB, CFH, CFHR1, CFHR2, CFHR3, CFHR4, CFHR5, CFI, DGKE, THBD, MMACHC,* and *PLG.*

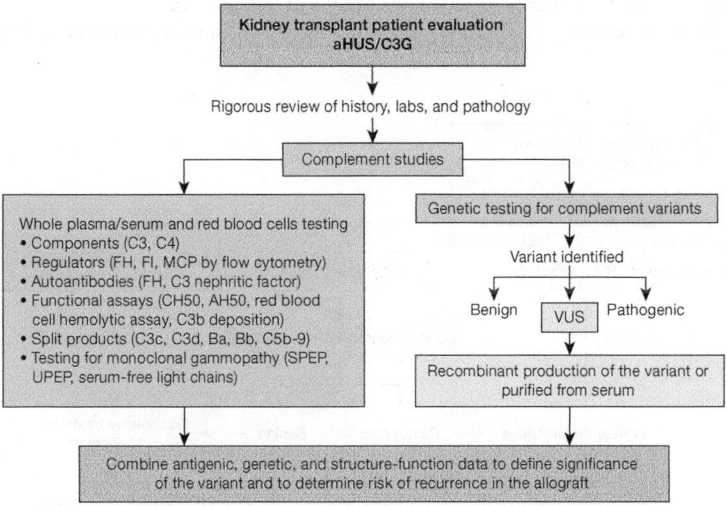

Figure 15-1. **Algorithm for aHUS and C3G Evaluation in Kidney Transplantation.** aHUS, atypical hemolytic uremic syndrome; C3G, C3 glomerulopathy; FH, factor H; FI, factor I; MCP, membrane cofactor protein; SPEP, serum protein electrophoresis; UPEP, urine protein electrophoresis; VUS, variant of uncertain significance.

- Variants are classified into 5 categories based on the guidelines established by the American College of Medical Genetics: Pathogenic, Likely pathogenic, Variant of Uncertain Significance (VUS), Likely benign, or Benign.[7]
- For variants reported as "VUS," specialized functional assays can be conducted to assess the significance of variants (**Figure 15-1**).

TREATMENT AND PROGNOSIS

Perioperative Management[6]

- Eculizumab (humanized monoclonal antibody directed against the terminal pathway protein C5) before transplantation should be considered in:
  - Patients with aHUS with a known pathogenic mutation in a complement protein (except those with a pathogenic MCP mutation because MCP is a membrane-bound protein and the allograft brings in the nonmutated MCP).
  - Biopsy-proven diagnosis of TMA in the native kidney in whom a genetic variant has not been identified but other etiologies of TMA have been excluded.
  - Recurrence in a prior allograft.
  - Persistent factor H autoantibody.
- Living unrelated donor transplant: we administer eculizumab at 900 mg intravenously 24 hours before transplantation and on days 7, 14, and 21 after transplantation, followed by 1,200 mg on week 5 and then every 2 weeks thereafter.
- Deceased-donor transplant: we administer eculizumab at 900 mg intravenously at the time of transplantation (on postoperative day 3 to allow for thymoglobulin completion) and continue 900 mg weekly for 3 additional doses, followed by 1,200 mg on week 5 and then every 2 weeks thereafter.
- The optimal duration of eculizumab therapy after kidney transplantation is unclear. At our center, we stratify the duration as outlined in **Figure 15-2**.
- There is no current US Food and Drug Administration–approved treatment of C3G.

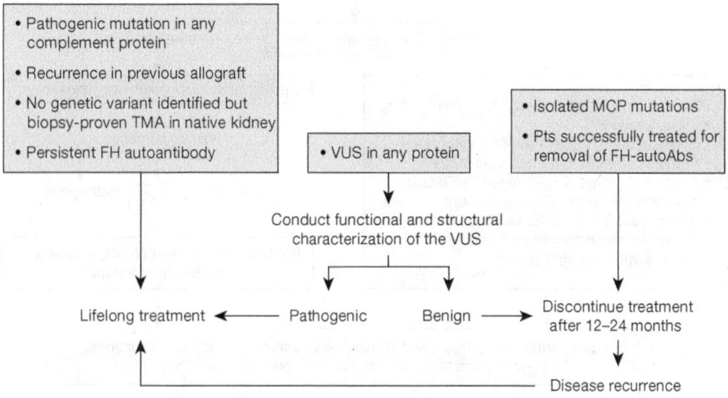

Figure 15-2. **Approach to eculizumab duration in kidney transplantation.** FH, factor H; MCP, membrane cofactor protein; TMA, thrombotic microangiopathy; VUS, variant of uncertain significance.

Vaccination and Antimicrobial Prophylaxis

- Both MenACWY (Menactra or Menveo) and MenB (Bexsero or Trumemba) vaccines should be administered before transplantation, in addition to Prevnar and Pneumovax.
- A booster dose of MenACWY vaccine should be administered every 5 years, for the duration of complement inhibitor therapy.
- Vaccines should be given at least 2 weeks before a living/planned transplant and before administering the first dose of the complement inhibitor.
- We also use antimicrobial prophylaxis (amoxicillin or ciprofloxacin) for the duration of eculizumab treatment to potentially reduce the risk for meningococcal disease.
- Suggestive symptoms of a bacteremia or septicemia should necessitate urgent investigation and antibiotic therapy.

Recurrence After Kidney Transplantation

- Patients with recurrent aHUS usually present within 1 year after transplantation and often within days to weeks due to the combined effect of multiple triggers for endothelial injury.[8]
- Potential triggers at the time of transplantation include:
    - Ischemia-reperfusion injury
    - Immunosuppressive drugs (calcineurin and mTOR inhibitors)
    - Antibody-mediated rejection (antigen-antibody complexes can activate the complement system)
- Infections (cytomegalovirus, BK virus, upper respiratory or gastroenteritis).
- The diagnosis of recurrent aHUS should be suspected in any kidney transplant recipient with an elevated serum creatinine, especially if hemolytic anemia and thrombocytopenia are present.
- Recurrence could also manifest with fever, confusion, headache, arrhythmia, myocardial infarction, and sudden cardiac death.
- Patients with renal-limited TMA may present with only an increased serum creatinine and abnormal urinalysis but without thrombocytopenia and hemolytic anemia.
- In recurrent aHUS, an allograft biopsy is not required to confirm the diagnosis of TMA (unless renal-limited TMA is suspected); the risk of bleeding may be prohibitive if thrombocytopenia is severe.
- A biopsy may be needed to exclude other causes of kidney failure/TMA (mentioned under triggers above), which can cause de novo TMA.
- Eculizumab should be initiated early to prevent recurrence of disease and to offer the best chance to recover kidney function in patients with recurrent disease.
- Recurrent C3G may present within days-weeks or, in some cases, several years after transplantation.[9]
- Patients may have elevated creatinine, hematuria, proteinuria, hypertension, or a combination of these.
- Diagnosis of recurrent C3G can only be made on a biopsy.
- Treatment of recurrent C3G includes optimal blood pressure control (<120/80 mm Hg) steroids, mycophenolate mofetil, and eculizumab (based on case reports and small trials).[10]
- Newer agents for C3G in trials include C3 inhibitor, factor B inhibitor, and factor D inhibitor.

TABLE 15-3 Posttransplant Monitoring for aHUS/C3G (Complete Blood Count, Renal Panel, Urinalysis, Lactate Dehydrogenase, Haptoglobin)

Immediate Posttransplant (During Hospitalization)	Daily; CH50 Prior to Eculizumab/Ravulizumab Administration for the 1st 4 Doses
Up to 6 mo	Weekly
6-12 mo	Biweekly
After 12 mo	Monthly

A biopsy should be obtained in addition to the above if there is any concern for recurrence.

SELECTION OF DONOR KIDNEY

- Living-related kidney transplant is relatively contraindicated (more in aHUS, less in C3G); consider with caution on a case-by-case basis.[11,12]
- Nephrectomy may trigger TMA in the genetically susceptible donor.
- Genetic and serological analysis should be performed in donors, but a negative mutational analysis does not guarantee freedom from risk.
- We may consider living donor transplants in patients who carry a known pathogenic mutation in a complement protein that is determined to be the cause of disease in the patient and if the donor tests negative for that mutation/serological abnormality.
- The recipient and the potential living donor should participate in decision-making after they understand the risks and benefits of this option.

POSTTRANSPLANT MONITORING

- The monitoring schedule including laboratory tests followed at our center is outlined in **Table 15-3**.
- Patients on eculizumab should be monitored for adverse reactions such as hypertension, headache, upper respiratory tract infection, urinary tract infection, nausea, vomiting, diarrhea, anemia, and leukopenia.

REFERENCES

1. Goodship TH, Cook HT, Fakhouri F, et al. Atypical hemolytic uremic syndrome and C3 glomerulopathy: conclusions from a "kidney disease—improving Global outcomes" (KDIGO) Controversies conference. *Kidney Int.* 2017;91(3):539-51.
2. Smith RJH, Appel GB, Blom AM, et al. C3 glomerulopathy—understanding a rare complement-driven renal disease. *Nat Rev Nephrol.* 2019;15(3):129-43.
3. Java A, Atkinson J, Salmon J. Defective complement inhibitory function predisposes to renal disease. *Annu Rev Med.* 2013;64:307-24.
4. Liszewski MK, Java A, Schramm EC, Atkinson JP. Complement dysregulation and disease: insights from contemporary genetics. *Annu Rev Pathol.* 2017;12:25-52.
5. Le Quintrec M, Zuber J, Moulin B, et al. Complement genes strongly predict recurrence and graft outcome in adult renal transplant recipients with atypical hemolytic and uremic syndrome. *Am J Transplant.* 2013;13(3):663-75.

6. Java A. Peri- and post-operative evaluation and management of atypical hemolytic uremic syndrome (aHUS) in kidney transplantation. *Adv Chronic Kidney Dis.* 2020;27(2):128-37.
7. Richards S, Aziz N, Bale S, et al. Standards and guidelines for the interpretation of sequence variants: a joint consensus recommendation of the American College of Medical Genetics and Genomics and the Association for molecular pathology. *Genet Med.* 2015;17(5):405-24.
8. Zuber J, Le Quintrec M, Sberro-Soussan R, Loirat C, Frémeaux-Bacchi V, Legendre C. New insights into postrenal transplant hemolytic uremic syndrome. *Nat Rev Nephrol.* 2011;7(1):23-35.
9. Regunathan-Shenk R, Avasare RS, Ahn W, et al. Kidney transplantation in C3 glomerulopathy: a case series. *Am J Kidney Dis.* 2019;73(3):316-23.
10. Gonzalez Suarez ML, Thongprayoon C, Hansrivijit P, et al. Treatment of C3 glomerulopathy in adult kidney transplant recipients: a systematic review. *Med Sci.* 2020;8(4):44.
11. Kurup M, Mandelbrot D, Garg N, Singh T. Living related donor kidney transplantation in atypical HUS: when should it Be considered? *Kidney360.* 2021;2(3):524-7.
12. Wong L, Moran S, Lavin PJ, Dorman AM, Conlon PJ. Kidney transplant outcomes in familial C3 glomerulopathy. *Clin Kidney J.* 2016;9(3):403-7.

16 Posttransplant Infections

Armaghan-e-Rehman Mansoor, Massini Merzkani, and Ige A. George

GENERAL PRINCIPLES

- Infections in renal transplant recipients are a leading cause of morbidity and mortality and account for up to 24% of deaths in the first year after transplant.[1]
- Posttransplant infections, including urinary tract infections (UTIs), pneumonias, wound infections, and cytomegalovirus (CMV) infections, in renal transplant recipients occur in 45% to 81% of patients.[2]
- Pretransplant donor and recipient risk assessment has a key role, with appropriate prophylactic vaccinations and anti-infectives being a cornerstone of posttransplant care.
- Community-acquired infections can have unusual clinical presentations and less severe symptoms. *Certain infections, such as UTIs, will be seen more commonly in* immunocompromised hosts following renal transplantation.
- Antimicrobial prophylaxis can influence the presentation of infectious syndromes and can impact drug resistance and empiric antimicrobial choice.
- Graft rejection, drug toxicities, and autoimmune phenomenon can mimic infections.

Risk Assessment for Infectious Diseases

- Risk and causes of infections are influenced by the "net state of immunosuppression"—a conceptual measure of factors contributing to a patient's risk for infection.
- Identify the following factors that influence infection risk:
  - Current and prior immunosuppression
  - Graft rejection
  - Mucocutaneous barrier integrity, i.e., indwelling catheters, drains
  - Underlying immune deficiency
  - Surgical site integrity and graft function
  - Comorbid conditions—diabetes mellitus, cirrhosis
  - Viral coinfections—CMV, Epstein-Barr virus (EBV), hepatitis C virus (HCV), hepatitis B virus (HBV)
  - Epidemiologic exposures and region-specific pathogens
  - Metabolic derangements—uremia, malnutrition, hyperglycemia
  - Neutropenia, lymphopenia
- Certain factors can confer a higher or lower infectious risk (**Table 16-1**).
- Infections can be derived from either donor or recipient, including reactivation of latent infections.

Donor and Recipient Screening

- Appropriate screening for both donor and recipient should be undertaken and interpreted. See **Table 16-2** for a list of routine screening recommended in the US and **Tables 16-3** and **16-4** for recommendations regarding prophylaxis and treatment of selected infections.

TABLE 16-1 Risk Factors for Infectious Complications

Higher Risk	Lower Risk
Induction therapy with lymphocyte-depleting agents, e.g., antithymocyte globulin, alemtuzumab	Appropriate anti-infective prophylaxis and vaccination
Early graft rejection, high risk of rejection	Good HLA match, immunologic tolerance
Anastomotic leak, bleeding, wound infection, poor wound healing	Technically successful surgery
Graft dysfunction	Immunologic tolerance

- Consider additional screening for recipients from an endemic region.
  - Strongyloides serology for recipients from endemic areas
  - Coccidioides serology for recipients from endemic areas
- Please see **Table 16-4** for antimicrobial prophylaxis for select infections including CMV, HBV, toxoplasmosis, strongyloides and coccidioides in renal transplant recipients.
- Donors with encephalitis or meningitis of unclear etiology should not be considered for organ donation given possibility of transmitting an unknown infectious agent. This is being studied.
- A brief summary on the treatment of syphilis and latent tuberculosis is provided in **Table 16-4**. It is important to check and monitor for drug interactions. Please also see the latent tuberculosis section later in this chapter.
- Use of T-lymphocyte-depleting agents such as **anti-thymocyte globulin** increases risk of community- and hospital-acquired bacterial infections; viral infections such as EBV, CMV, and BK virus; and fungal infections including endemic mycoses and molds.
- Use of cytotoxic T-lymphocyte antigen antagonists such as **belatacept** for prevention of graft rejection may increase risk of infections, especially in combination with other agents.

Infectious Entities in the Posttransplant Period

- The timeline of infections can be broadly divided into:
  - Early posttransplantation period (first month)
  - Intermediate posttransplantation period (1-6 months after transplant)
  - Late posttransplantation period (after 6 months)
- Please see **Table 16-5** for summary of infections by time period.

SURGICAL SITE INFECTIONS

- All patients should receive standard perioperative prophylaxis—IV cefazolin or vancomycin + aztreonam/aminoglycoside if history of severe β-lactam allergy.
- Perinephric collections or urinomas following ureterocystostomy can be a nidus.

TABLE 16-2 Pretransplant Screening Tests for Communicable Diseases

Infectious Agent	Test of Choice	Donor Test	Recipient Test	Recommendation	Comments
CMV	IgG antibody	+	–	Proceed, highest risk	See CMV section
		+	+	Moderate risk	
		–	–	Lowest risk	
EBV	EBV VCA IgG, IgM	±	+	Proceed	
		+	–	Proceed, higher risk	
Toxoplasma	IgG antibody	±	+	Proceed	TMP/SMX 6-12 mo
		+	–	Proceed, higher risk	TMP/SMX indefinitely
HBV		HBsAb +	±	Accept	
		HBsAg +	±	Reject	
		HBcAb +	HBsAb–	Accept	Lamivudine for prophylaxis
		HBcAb +	HBsAb+	Accept	Monitor for reactivation
HCV	HCV antibody	Positive	Positive	Accept	
		Positive	Negative	Accept	
HIV	HIV antibody	+	+	Being studied under clinical trials	
		+	–	Reject	
		–	+	Proceed if well controlled	
Syphilis	RPR	Positive	±	Accept	Treat
Latent tuberculosis	IGRA	N/A	IGRA+	Proceed	Treat

CMV, cytomegalovirus; EBV, Epstein-Barr virus; HBcAb, hepatitis B core antibody; HBsAb, hepatitis B surface antibody; HBsAg, hepatitis B surface antigen; HBV, hepatitis B virus; HCV, hepatitis C virus; IGRA, interferon-γ release assay; RPR, rapid plasma regain; TMP/SMX, trimethoprim/sulfamethoxazole; VCA, viral capsid antigen.

TABLE 16-3 Antimicrobial Prophylaxis for Select Infections in Renal Transplant Recipients

Infection	Indication for Prophylaxis	Dosage/Duration
CMV	See **Table 16-5** for detailed discussion of prophylaxis and treatment strategies	
HBV	Donor HBcAb + and recipient nonimmune	Antivirals for 1 y
	Donor HBcAb + and recipient immune	No prophylaxis needed
Toxoplasma	D+/R– (higher risk) or D–/R+	TMP-SMX Sulfa allergy: dapsone
Strongyloides	Recipient antibody positive	Ivermectin every 2 wk ×2
Coccidoides	Recipient antibody positive	Fluconazole lifelong

CMV, cytomegalovirus; D, donor; HBcAb, hepatitis B core antibody; HBV, hepatitis B virus; R, recipient; TMP/SMX, trimethoprim/sulfamethoxazole.

- Predominant organisms are *Staphylococcus aureus*, coagulase-negative *Staphylococci*, and enterococci. Gram-negative organisms including *Pseudomonas*, as well as yeast, can be implicated.
- Adequate drainage is essential for appropriate management in addition to antibiotics. Specimen should be sent for routine, acid-fast bacilli and fungal cultures.
- Empiric therapy should include coverage for *Staphylococci*, enterococcus, and gram-negative organisms including *Pseudomonas*.

BACTERIAL URINARY TRACT INFECTIONS

General Principles

- Bacterial UTIs are the most common posttransplant infection, with the highest incidence 3 to 6 months after transplant.

TABLE 16-4 Treatment for Select Infections in Renal Transplant Recipients

Infection	Treatment	Comments
Syphilis	IM benzathine Penicillin	Can consider subsequent RPR quarterly screening for 6 mo
Latent tuberculosis	Preferred: 3HP or 4R Alternative: 6H or 9H	Treatment can be instituted after transplant if emergent need for transplantation

3HP, 3 mo of once-weekly isoniazid (H) and rifapentine (P); 4R, 4 mo of daily rifampin (R); 6H, 6 mo of daily isoniazid (H); 9H, 9 mo of daily isoniazid (H); RPR rapid plasma regain.

TABLE 16-5 Timeline of Infections Following Renal Transplant

Time Period	Early Posttransplant Period (<1 mo)	Intermediate Posttransplant Period (1-6 mo)	Late Posttransplant Period (>6 mo)
Common causes of infection	Donor or recipient-derived infections, surgical complications, hospital-acquired infections	Reactivation of latent infections or opportunistic infections in absence or prophylaxis	Community-acquired infections, late reactivation of latent infections
Bacterial infections	Resistant hospital-acquired infections including MRSA, VRE, catheter-associated infections, wound and surgical site infections, *C. difficile* colitis, aspiration	*C. difficile* colitis, *M. tuberculosis*, nontuberculous mycobacteria, *Listeria*, *Nocardia*	Community-acquired bacteria including *Legionella*, pneumococcus, GI tract bacteria, *Nocardia*
Viral infections	Donor-derived infections such as HSV, WNV, LCMV, HIV	Herpesviruses (CMV, HSV), less likely with prophylaxis HCV, BK virus; respiratory viruses (adeno, RSV, influenza)	Community-acquired infections, late CMV after prophylaxis stopped, HBV, HCV, HSV, BK virus, EBV-associated PTLD
Fungal infections	Donor-derived infections, *Aspergillus*, *Candida*, *Cryptococcus*	PJP (without prophylaxis), endemic fungal infections (Histoplasma, Blastomyces, Coccidoides)	*Cryptococcus*, PJP, *Rhodococcus*, *Mucor*, atypical molds
Parasitic and protozoal infections	*Trypanosoma cruzi*, *Toxoplasma*	*Toxoplasma* (without prophylaxis), *Strongyloides*, *T. cruzi*	

CMV, cytomegalovirus; EBV, Epstein-Barr virus; GI, gastrointestinal; HBV, hepatitis B virus; HCV, hepatitis C virus; HSV, herpes simplex virus; LCMV, lymphocytic choriomeningitis virus; MRSA, methicillin-resistant *Staphylococcus aureus*; PJP, *Pneumocystis jirovecii* pneumonia; PTLD, posttransplant lymphoproliferative disorders; RSV, respiratory syncytial virus; VRE, vancomycin-resistant enterococcus; WNV, West Nile virus.

- Risk factors include female patients, older age, deceased-donor transplant, kidney-pancreas transplantation, prolonged urinary catheterization, ureteral stents, prolonged increased immunosuppressed state, and a history of recurrent UTI.
- Cumulative incidence of 17% at 6 months, 60% for women, 47% for men at 3 years.[3]
- The most common pathogen is *Escherichia coli*, although incidence of *Enterococcus* (including vancomycin-resistant enterococcus) is rising due to use of antibacterial prophylaxis.
- Consider atypical pathogens that may be overlooked in routine cultures:
  - *Mycoplasma hominis* can cause breakdown of ureterovesical anastomosis with subsequent graft loss.
  - *Corynebacterium urealyticum* may present with struvite stones, encrusted cystitis, alkaline urine, and apparent sterile pyuria.
- Significant localized discomfort may not be present due to denervated donor kidney; however, graft site tenderness may point to pyelonephritis.
- Prophylactic antibiotic regimens vary by transplant center. Our preferred regimen is to use trimethoprim/sulfamethoxazole (TMP/SMX), or cephalexin if sulfa allergy, for at least a period of 3 to 6 months depending on the institution protocols.
- Donor-derived bloodstream infections and UTIs are important entities in the early transplant period.
  - Directed antibiotic therapy based on donor data from the organ procurement organization is crucial in appropriate antibiotic selection. In some cases, this information may not be available prior to transplantation.
  - Duration of therapy is usually 7 days from date of transplantation for donor-derived UTI.

Diagnosis

- Urinalysis and urine culture should be obtained. In patients with systemic symptoms or concern for pyelonephritis, blood cultures should be obtained.
- Consider straight catheterization or collection from a newly placed urinary catheter if a mid-stream urine specimen cannot be obtained.

Treatment

- UTI can be classified as simple cystitis if symptoms are limited to the bladder and no indwelling catheters, nephrostomy tubes, or ureteral stents are present.
- Empiric therapy for complicated UTI/pyelonephritis includes coverage for *Pseudomonas*.
- Complications of UTIs include renal abscess, and adequate drainage is needed to achieve source control.
- Removal of stents and urinary catheters should be strongly considered.
- Longer therapy (14-21 days) should be considered for complicated UTIs (**Table 16-6**).
- Recurrent UTI should prompt evaluation of structural abnormality, presence of abscess, or prostatitis.

Asymptomatic Bacteriuria

- Defined as presence of greater than 10^5 CFU/mL without urinary or systemic symptoms.
- Treatment in the early posttransplant period is controversial, with no data to suggest an impact on mortality or graft function. American Society of Transplantation

TABLE 16-6 Management of Asymptomatic Bacteriuria and Urinary Tract Infections

Classification	Diagnosis	Treatment Considerations
Asymptomatic bacteriuria	In first 2 mo post transplant, consider if same pathogen on >1 cultures	Empiric therapy is not recommended, base therapy on susceptibilities. Recommended duration is 5 d
Simple cystitis	Localized symptoms without presence of hardware or indwelling catheters	Amoxicillin-clavulanate, oral 3rd-generation cephalosporin, ciprofloxacin, or levofloxacin. Treat for 5-7 d
Pyelonephritis or complicated UTI	Systemic symptoms, flank or allograft pain, bloodstream infection with the same organism as in urine	Include antipseudomonal coverage—cefepime, piperacillin-tazobactams, carbapenem. 14-21 d of therapy recommended. Image for source control
Recurrent UTI	>2 UTIs in a 12-mo period	Evaluate for unaddressed source, i.e., ureteral stent, nephrostomy, indwelling catheter, or voiding dysfunction, infected cysts in native kidney

UTI, urinary tract infection.

(AST) guidelines suggest considering treatment for 5 days if the same uropathogen is isolated in consecutive specimen in the first 2 months.[4]

- Treatment is not recommended beyond the early transplant period.

POSTTRANSPLANT PNEUMONIA

- Etiology of pneumonia in the immediate posttransplant period is usually nosocomial. Pathogens include *S. aureus, Streptococcus,* and gram-negative bacteria including *Pseudomonas.*
- *Pneumocystis jirovecii* pneumonia (PJP) is rare due to the use of prophylaxis at least 6 to 12 months after transplant depending on transplant center's practices.
- Empiric therapy for patients with signs or symptoms of a lower respiratory tract infection should be promptly initiated and include coverage for *Pseudomonas* and methicillin-resistant *Staphylococcus aureus* (MRSA).
- Consider CT of the chest in initial evaluation, especially in high-acuity settings or patients with a high net state of immunosuppression.
- Sputum culture is recommended in patients reporting sputum production.
- Expanded evaluation for pneumonia due to opportunistic organisms should be considered based on presenting symptoms, current antimicrobial prophylaxis, and exposure history, especially if a lack of response to initial antibiotic therapy is noted. This includes serologic testing, fungal biomarkers, multiplex polymerase chain reaction (PCR) for viral infections, and consideration for bronchoalveolar lavage.

INVASIVE FUNGAL INFECTIONS

- *Candida* is the most common cause of infections, followed by *Aspergillus*. The highest risk of candidal infections is in the early postoperative period.
- *Cryptococcus* infections can present with atypical manifestations. All patients with *Cryptococcus* should be evaluated for central nervous system (CNS) disease regardless of neurological symptoms.
- Renal transplantation is a risk factor for endemic mycoses, more commonly seen in recipients from endemic areas, and can have more severe presentation. Infections via donors have been reported for endemic mycoses.
- Azoles including fluconazole and voriconazole are strong inducers of CYP3A4, which can impact immunosuppression. Tacrolimus dose and levels should be carefully monitored while on these medications.
- Guidelines for prophylaxis vary by institution. We routinely use 1 month of azole prophylaxis for kidney recipients and 6 months for kidney/pancreas recipients.

CYTOMEGALOVIRUS

General Principles

- CMV disease is associated with increased risk of allograft nephropathy and death.
- CMV prevention strategies vary by center (**Table 16-7**). These strategies include:
  - Prophylaxis—preferred in recipients with intermediate or high risk for CMV.
  - Preemptive treatment—Interval PCR testing and initiation of treatment upon detection of active infection in high- or intermediate-risk recipients.

TABLE 16-7 A Prophylactic Management Strategy for CMV

Risk Category	High Risk (CMV D+/R–):	Intermediate Risk (CMV R+)	Low Risk (CMV D–/R–):
Antiviral of choice—Note that renal dosing cutoffs for ganciclovir and valganciclovir are different	Valganciclovir per the following renal dosing: CrCl > 60 mL/min: 900 mg PO q24h CrCl 40-59 mL/min: 450 mg PO q24h CrCl <40 mL/min: 450 mg PO every M/W/F	Valganciclovir per the following renal dosing: CrCl > 40 mL/min: 450 mg PO q24h CrCl <40 mL/min: 450 mg PO every M/W/F	Acyclovir 200 mg PO q12h
Timing of prophylaxis	Start POD7 or discharge Continue to 9 mo	Start POD7 or discharge Continue to 3 mo	Continue to 3 mo

CMV, cytomegalovirus; CrCl, creatinine clearance; D, donor; M/W/F, Monday/Wednesday/Friday; POD, postoperative day; R, recipient.

- The greatest risk for CMV infection is transplantation from seropositive donors to seronegative recipients (D+/R–), followed by (D+/R+).
- See **Table 16-7** for prophylactic management strategy for CMV.

Diagnosis

- The most common presentation is a constitutional mononucleosis-like syndrome—fever, malaise, cytopenias with detectable viremia.
- Invasive disease can present as colitis, hepatitis, pneumonitis. Rare presentations include encephalitis, adrenalitis. Spectrum of CMV infection is shown in **Table 16-8**.
- Invasive disease may occur without viremia, e.g., in CMV colitis. Colonoscopy and biopsy help establish the diagnosis.

Treatment

- The initial therapy of choice for mild disease is IV ganciclovir or PO valganciclovir.
- Consider reducing immunosuppression, especially antimetabolites.
- Treatment is continued until symptoms resolve and viremia is undetectable for at least 2 serial tests. Care should be made to use the same assay for evaluation of viremia, as there is significant interassay variability.
- Once symptoms and viremia resolve, some clinicians extend therapy for 1 to 3 months in severe disease as secondary prophylaxis. Of note, international consensus guidelines do not recommend secondary prophylaxis because of uncertain efficacy.[5]
- If there is no clinical or virological improvement 2 weeks after starting therapy, consider CMV resistance, mediated by UL97 (resistance to ganciclovir) and UL54 (ganciclovir, cidofovir, foscarnet).
- Treatment alternatives include foscarnet, cidofovir, maribavir.
- Maribavir is a novel oral agent that inhibits CMV DNA replication, encapsidation, and nuclear egress via UL97 kinase.[6] It has been approved for refractory and resistant CMV infections and can be considered in the following situations:
  - Suspected or documented ganciclovir-resistant CMV
  - Refractory CMV infection or disease (failure to achieve >1 $\log^{10}$ decrease in CMV DNA after at least 10 days of therapy at induction dosing)
  - Safety concerns with (val)ganciclovir, foscarnet, or cidofovir
- CMV T-cell therapy is early but promising.

TABLE 16-8 Spectrum of CMV Infection in Renal Transplant Recipients

Classification	Description	Diagnostics
Acute CMV infection/viremia	CMV replication in blood, regardless of signs/symptoms	CMV PCR + CMV IgM + if primary infection
CMV syndrome	Viremia + signs/symptoms, without evidence of tissue-invasive disease	CMV PCR+
CMV disease	End-organ disease—pneumonitis, enteritis, colitis, retinitis, nephritis, meningitis	Histopath+ CMV PCR+/–

CMV, cytomegalovirus; PCR, polymerase chain reaction.

EPSTEIN-BARR VIRUS AND POSTTRANSPLANT LYMPHOPROLIFERATIVE DISORDER

General Principles

- Usually seen within 1 year of transplant.
- Patients with primary EBV infection, young age, CMV infection or those receiving antilymphocyte antibodies are at higher risk.
- Incidence is low in kidney recipients (1%-2%) compared with other organs (up to one-third in lung).

Diagnosis

- Presents as mononucleosis syndrome with fever and adenopathy.
- It is associated with posttransplant lymphoproliferative disorder, which is characterized by B-cell infiltration of organs. Can affect transplant organ and CNS.

Treatment

Decreasing immunosuppression is the mainstay of management. Antivirals have in vitro activity but are not usually clinically effective. Rituximab has been used.

HERPES SIMPLEX VIRUS

General Principles

- Solid organ transplant (SOT) recipients are more likely to shed virus, have more frequent and severe presentation of disease, and have atypical presentation.
- Infection is typically from reactivation and seen within 1 month post transplant if not given prophylaxis.
- Serostatus of all recipients must be checked. Seropositive individuals must receive prophylaxis if not already receiving CMV prophylaxis.
- Prophylactic agents include acyclovir, valacyclovir, ganciclovir, valganciclovir.
- Letermovir (agent used for CMV prophylaxis, primarily in stem cell transplant) does not have activity against herpes simplex virus (HSV).
- Ongoing prophylaxis should be given for patients with history of HSV recurrence or with a history of shingles who have not received the Shingrix vaccination post transplant.
- Continued suppression is associated with less resistance than intermittent therapy.

Diagnosis

- Presents usually with vesicular or ulcerative lesions in the orolabial, genital, perianal region.
- Visceral disease can occur: esophagitis, hepatitis, pneumonitis.
- PCR of lesions or tissue specimen is test of choice.

Treatment

- Limited mucosal disease can be treated with oral acyclovir or valacyclovir. Ganciclovir also has coverage.
- IV acyclovir is treatment of choice for disseminated or visceral disease.
- Consider HSV resistance in patients not improving with appropriate treatment. Treatment options include foscarnet, cidofovir. HSV resistance testing should be sent.

ADENOVIRUS

General Principles

- Adenovirus is associated with renal allograft nephropathy and hemorrhagic cystitis.
- Can present with hematuria, dysuria, and fever. Extrarenal manifestations include pneumonia, gastroenteritis, and orchitis.
- Asymptomatic viremia is common; therefore, routine screening is not recommended.
- PCR is highly sensitive. Detection at >1 site is predictive of disseminated disease. Serial quantitative testing may be helpful to determine when to start therapy.
- Histopathology remains the gold standard for diagnosis.

Treatment

- Reduction of immunosuppression should be the initial approach, if possible.
- Cidofovir is the preferred antiviral agent. Intravenous hydration and probenecid can reduce risk of nephrotoxicity.
- Therapy should be continued until resolution of symptoms and documentation of negative samples from sites that were originally positive.
- Intravenous immunoglobulin may be of benefit in select patients with hypogammaglobulinemia.

BK POLYOMAVIRUS

General Principles

- Primary BK infection occurs early in life in the first decade. The virus then establishes in renal and urothelial cells.
- Monthly screening for BK virus PCR in the blood is recommended for the first 9 to 12 months. The AST recommends bimonthly screening through 2 years.
- If positive, consider preemptive decrease in immunosuppression.
- Disease usually occurs as unexplained rise in serum creatinine within 1 year of transplant.
- One-third of patients with high-grade BK viruria can progress to nephropathy.

Diagnosis

- The best screening method is BK virus PCR in blood, as BK virus is present in plasma in almost all cases. Viruria has lower specificity for nephropathy.
- Definitive diagnosis is made by histology showing BK-virus-associated cytopathic changes and SV40 staining.

Treatment

- Treatment involves reducing immunosuppression. Therapy with cidofovir has been used with limited evidence of efficacy. The use of ciprofloxacin and leflunomide has been discouraged due to lack of demonstrated efficacy.
- New studies showing BK T-cell therapy are promising in those who have been refractory to standard treatment.

SARS-COV-2 INFECTION (COVID-19)

- COVID-19 can present with more severe symptoms in transplant recipients. Acute kidney injury and graft loss have been reported. Direct viral toxicity, cytokine-induced tubular damage, hypovolemia, and reduction of immunosuppression may be contributory.

- Living donors, and recipients, should be encouraged to use preventive strategies.
- Donors and recipients should be strongly encouraged to be fully vaccinated and boosted for COVID-19.
- Renal transplant recipients may have a lower immune response to vaccination.
- Precise risk of COVID-19 infection from living or deceased donor is unclear. Infections from transplanted organs have so far been reported only in lung transplant recipients.
- The AST currently recommends screening for all donors and real-time PCR for SARS-CoV-2 infection from a respiratory specimen in all deceased donors. Testing of nonrespiratory sites is not currently recommended.
- Donors with a history of resolved COVID-19 infection and positive PCR testing beyond 21 days after onset of symptoms are unlikely to transmit infection and can be considered potential donors.
- Guidance regarding donor and recipient selection and treatment considerations is likely to evolve in the future.

HEPATITIS C VIRUS

General Principles

- HCV infection is associated with higher rates of proteinuria, chronic rejection, glomerular disease, and posttransplant diabetes.
- Genotype 1 is the most common worldwide and in the US.
- Transmission is most often parenteral, less commonly from mucosal surfaces.
- A significant proportion of new infections progress to chronic disease without treatment.
- All donors and recipients should be screened for HCV antibody (HCV Ab). See interpretation and recommendations regarding further screening in **Table 16-9**.
- For donors with positive HCV Ab, an HCV RNA, hepatitis B surface antigen (HBsAg), and total hepatitis B core antibody (HBcAb) are to be obtained. HCV genotype is recommended. Further testing interval for recipient is determined by result of HCV RNA (see **Table 16-9**).

Treatment

- If recipient screening reveals positive HCV RNA, treatment is recommended—this may be instituted after transplantation, especially if an HCV^+ donor is considered.
- Early management of HCV infection is recommended following transplant. Treatment should be instituted with a direct acting antiviral (DAA). See **Table 16-10** for treatment options based on genotype.
- Unexplained elevations in liver enzymes during or after DAA therapy should prompt investigation for immune-mediated dysfunction and assessment of HBV infection.
- Note that calcineurin inhibitors, e.g., cyclosporine, tacrolimus, can have drug-drug interactions with DAAs (glecaprevir/pibrentasvir, elbasvir/grazoprevir). Drug levels should be monitored while on DAA therapy.

HIV INFECTION

General Principles

- HIV-positive recipients have 2 to 4 higher rates of acute rejection compared with HIV-negative counterparts. This may be from drug-drug interactions or dysregulated immune system from HIV infection.
- Opportunistic infections are rare (<10%). Most patients experience typical infections.

TABLE 16-9 Interpretation and Evaluation of HCV Donor Screening

Donor HCV Antibody	Recipient HCV Antibody	Screening Recommendations	Interpretation
Negative	Negative	Additional screening not needed	-
Positive	Negative	Donor HCV RNA negative	Monitor HCV RNA. Stop if negative by 6 mo. If PCR positive, therapy with DAA should be considered
Positive	Negative	Donor HCV RNA positive	Monitor HCV RNA closely until positive PCR detected. If PCR positive, therapy with DAA
Negative	Positive	Recipient HCV RNA negative	If no prior history of HCV treatment, recheck in 3 mo. If repeat test is negative, no additional testing needed If prior history of therapy, additional testing may be warranted
Negative	Positive	Recipient HCV RNA positive	Consider treatment with DAA. Timing of treatment would need to be coordinated in relation to transplant

DAA, direct acting antiviral; HCV, hepatitis C virus; PCR, polymerase chain reaction.

- Recurrent HIV-associated nephropathy has been reported even with undetectable viral load, which may be asymptomatic.
- HIV-positive donor to HIV-positive recipient transplantation is being investigated.
- Patients with HBV or HCV coinfection may need additional evaluation for treatment considerations and drug-drug interactions.

TABLE 16-10 Therapeutic Options for Management of Treatment-Naive HCV Infection

Recommended Regimens		
Glecaprevir + pibrentasvir	12 wk	All genotypes
Ledipasvir + sofosbuvir	12 wk	Genotype 1, 4-6 only
Sofosbuvir + velpatasvir	12 wk	All genotypes
Alternative Regimen		
Elbasvir + grazoprevir	12 wk	Genotype 1 or 4 without baseline NS5A mutations

Pretransplant Considerations

- Recipient must have well-controlled disease on a stable antiretroviral regimen, viral load <20 copies/mL during the 4 months pretransplant, with CD4 > 200 cells/mL.
- History of opportunistic infections (e.g., PJP pneumonia, *Mycobacterium tuberculosis*) is not a contraindication as long as appropriate treatment has been provided with no evidence of active disease.
- Careful evaluation of antiretroviral therapy, immunosuppression, and prophylaxis should be made to prevent drug-drug interactions (**Table 16-11**). Boosted protease inhibitor regimens (cobicistat, ritonavir) should be avoided unless no alternative is present.
- Patients receiving boosted protease inhibitors need marked reduction in doses of calcineurin inhibitors and mammalian target of rapamycin inhibitors.

Posttransplant Considerations

- HIV viral load and CD4+ T-cell counts should be followed 1 month post transplant, and every 2 to 3 months afterward per American Society of Transplantation guidelines.
- Consider genotypic resistance testing in patients with ongoing viremia.

SYPHILIS

- Positive donor syphilis testing is not a contraindication to transplantation.
- Recipients are typically treated as latent syphilis of unknown duration with 3 weekly doses of 2.4 million units of benzathine penicillin G.

LATENT TUBERCULOSIS

- Active tuberculosis must be ruled out before treatment is initiated.
- In patients with latent tuberculosis diagnosed prior to transplant, treatment is recommended with one of the regimens given in **Table 16-4**.
- Indeterminate interferon-γ release assay results are not uncommon—risk stratification and treatment strategy, if indicated, need to be individualized.

TABLE 16-11 Notable Drug-Drug Interactions in Renal Transplant Recipients Receiving Antiretroviral Therapy for HIV Infection

	Calcineurin Inhibitors	Glucocorticoids	mTOR Inhibitors
NRTIs		No interaction expected	
NNRTIs	↓	↓	↓
Boosted PIs	↑↑↑	↑↑	↑↑↑
INSTIs		No interaction expected	
CCR5 antagonists		No interaction expected	
Fusion inhibitors		No interaction expected	

↑ reflects increased serum values; ↓ reflects decreased serum values.
CCR5, cysteine-cysteine chemokine receptor 5; INSTI, integrase strand transfer inhibitor; mTOR, mechanistic target of rapamycin; NRTI, nucleoside reverse transcriptase inhibitor; NNRTI, nonnucleoside reverse transcriptase inhibitor; PI, protease inhibitor.

CLOSTRIDIUM DIFFICILE COLITIS

General Principles

- Antibiotics, proton pump inhibitor use, and abdominal surgery are key risk factors.
- Management includes supportive therapy with fluid and electrolyte repletion, initiation of contact precautions, good hand hygiene, and discontinuation of unnecessary antibiotics.
- Establish severity of disease—fulminant disease is defined by hypotension, shock, ileus, megacolon, perforation, colonic ischemia, gastrointestinal bleeding requiring resuscitation with blood.

Treatment

- Fidaxomicin is the preferred initial regimen for nonfulminant disease due to lower likelihood of recurrence compared with oral vancomycin.
- If fidaxomicin is unable to be obtained upon discharge, it is acceptable to complete treatment with PO vancomycin in most instances. PO or PR vancomycin and IV metronidazole are used in fulminant disease—Infectious Disease consultation should be strongly considered.

TOXOPLASMA

Prophylaxis

- All patients should have *Toxoplasma* serostatus confirmed.
- Prophylactic options include TMP/SMX, atovaquone, or inhaled pentamidine.
- In highest-risk patients (D+/R–), consider 1 year of prophylaxis.
- Dapsone (used for PJP prophylaxis) does NOT have prophylactic activity against toxoplasmosis.
- Follow renal function and electrolytes closely on TMP/SMX.

Treatment

- Infections are rare and typically secondary to reactivation. Symptoms include fever, adenopathy, chorioretinitis, pneumonitis, usually within 3 months of transplant.
- Treatment involves sulfadiazine and pyrimethamine.

INFECTIOUS DISEASE MIMICS IN RENAL TRANSPLANT RECIPIENTS

- Calcineurin inhibitors are associated with posterior reversible encephalopathy syndrome (PRES). PRES presents with seizures and confusion and can mimic encephalitis. It also commonly presents with white matter edema most prominent in posterior cerebral hemispheres.
- Acute graft-versus-host disease is a rare but potentially devastating complication after SOT:
  - Presents with skin rash, diarrhea, pancytopenia usually in the first 8 weeks after transplant.
  - Diagnosis by clinical and pathological evidence, supported by HLA studies.

ROUTINE VACCINATIONS IN RENAL TRANSPLANT RECIPIENTS

- Appropriate vaccinations are an important component of reducing the risk of infection following transplantation.
- See **Table 16-12** for recommendations regarding routine vaccinations before and after transplantation.

TABLE 16-12 Routine Adult Vaccines in Renal Transplant Recipients

Vaccine	Recommended Before Transplant	Recommended After Transplant	Monitor Vaccine Titers
Influenza	Yes	Yes	No
(not live attenuated)	No	No	No
Hepatitis B	Yes	Yes	Yes
Hepatitis A	Yes	Yes	Yes
Tetanus	Yes	Yes	No
Pertussis (Tdap)	Yes	Yes	No
Pneumovax	Yes	Yes	Yes
PCV13	Yes	Yes	Yes
Menactra	Yes	Yes	No
Rabies	Yes	Yes	No
HPV	Yes	Yes	No
Shingrix	Yes	Yes	No
Smallpox	No	No	No

PCV, pneumococcal conjugate vaccine; Tdap, tetanus, diphtheria, pertussis.

REFERENCES

1. Singh N, Haidar G, Limaye AP. *Infections in solid-organ transplant recipients*. In: Bennett JE, Dolin R, Blaser MJ, eds. *Mandell, Douglas, and Bennett's Principles and Practice of Infectious Diseases*. 9th ed. Elsevier; 2020. 308-3672-3697. https://www.clinicalkey.com/#!/browse/book/3-s2.0-C2016100010X
2. Ljungman P, Boeckh M, Hirsch HH, et al. Definitions of cytomegalovirus infection and disease in transplant patients for use in clinical trials. *Clin Inf.* 2017;64(1):87-91.
3. Abbott KC, Swanson SJ, Richter ER, et al. Late urinary tract infection after renal transplantation in the United States. *Am J Kidney Dis.* 2004;44(2):353-62.
4. Goldman JD, Julian K. Urinary tract infections in solid organ transplant recipients: guidelines from the American Society of transplantation infectious diseases community of practice. *Clin Transplant.* 2019;33(9):e13507.
5. Kotton CN, Kumar D, Caliendo AM, et al. The third international consensus guidelines on the management of cytomegalovirus in solid-organ transplantation. *Transplantation.* 2018;102(6):900-31.
6. Avery RK, Alain S, Alexander BD, et al. Maribavir for refractory cytomegalovirus infections with or without resistance post-transplant: results from a phase 3 randomized clinical trial. *Clin Infect Dis.* 2022;75(4):690-701.

17 Posttransplant Malignancy

Mohamed M. Ibrahim, Neha Mehta-Shah, and Rowena Delos Santos

GENERAL PRINCIPLES

The long-term use of immunosuppressive medications in solid organ transplant helps mitigate allograft rejection; however, it increases the overall risk of malignancy compared with immunocompetent individuals.

Epidemiology

- The overall posttransplant malignancy incidence varies between 2% and 31%; however, it reached as high as 34% to 50% in kidney transplant recipients followed for more than 20 years.[1]
- Studies have demonstrated an increased risk of cancer among kidney transplant recipients when compared with an age- and gender-matched general population or in patients undergoing dialysis.[2] See **Table 17-1**.
- Skin cancers are the most frequent posttransplant malignancy, occurring in up to 8% of recipients and accounting for more than 40% of all posttransplant malignancies.[3]
- Cancer-related death is 1 of the 3 leading causes of death in solid organ transplant recipients, which also include cardiovascular disease and infections.
- The type of posttransplant malignancy can vary according to the organ transplanted, for example, lung transplant recipients have a 2-fold increase in non-Hodgkin lymphoma (NHL) compared with kidney, liver, and heart transplant recipients.[4]
- The difference of pattern of malignancy in cancer transplant can be due to the amount of lymphoid tissue that is transplanted within the lung, as well as the intensity and duration of immunosuppression.[4]
- Post transplant, there is an overall 2- to 4-fold elevated risk of malignancy.
  - An extensive cohort study involving 175,732 solid organ transplant recipients (included 58.4% kidney, 21.6% liver, 10% heart, and 4% lung) in the US showed an incidence of 1,375 per 100,000 person-years, representing a standardized incidence ratio (SIR) of 2.1.[1]
  - Risk was increased for 32 different malignancies, some related to known infections (anal cancer, Kaposi sarcoma) and others unrelated (melanoma, thyroid, and lip cancers).[1]
  - The cancers with the highest relative risk in transplant population include Kaposi sarcoma (SIR 61.5), lip (SIR 16.8), nonmelanomatous skin (SIR 13.9), liver (SIR 11.6), vulvar (SIR 7.6), NHL (SIR 7.5), and anal cancer (SIR 5.8).[1]
  - The risk of breast and prostate cancers was lower in the transplant population compared with the general population (SIR 0.85 and SIR 0.92, respectively), and the risk of cervical cancer was not increased (SIR 1.03).[1]
- Lung cancer is most common in lung transplant recipients (SIR 6.13), but it is also increased in heart recipients (SIR 2.67) compared with kidney (SIR 1.46) and liver (SIR 1.95) transplant recipients.[1]
- It has been suggested that the elevated incidence of lung cancer in lung and heart transplant recipients could be due to the high incidence of tobacco use among this transplant population.[5]

TABLE 17-1 Standardized Incidence Ratio of Posttransplant Malignancies

Malignancy	SIR
Higher Risk	
Kaposi sarcoma	61.5
Lip cancer	16.8
Nonmelanomatous skin cancer	13.9
Liver	11.6
Vulvar	7.6
Non-Hodgkin lymphoma	7.5
Anal cancer	5.8
Lung cancer	6.13 (lung recipients) 1.95 (liver recipients) 1.46 (kidney recipients)
Kidney cancers overall	10.77 (kidney recipients) No increased risk (liver recipients)
Renal cell carcinoma	6.7 (kidney recipients) 1.5-2.9 (other organ recipients)
Same Risk	
Cervical cancer	1.03
Lower Risk	
Breast cancer	0.85
Prostate cancer	0.92

SIR, standardized incidence ratio.
Data from Sargen MR, Cahoon EK, Yu KJ, et al. Spectrum of nonkeratinocyte skin cancer risk among solid organ transplant recipients in the US. *JAMA Dermatol.* 2022;158:414-25; Manickavasagar R, Thuraisingham R. Post renal-transplant malignancy surveillance. *Clin Med (Lond).* 2020;20:142-5; Wheless L, Jacks S, Mooneyham Potter KA, Leach BC, Cook J. Skin cancer in organ transplant recipients: more than the immune system. *J Am Acad Dermatol.* 2014;71:359-65; Hofmann P, Benden C, Kohler M, Schuurmans MM. Smoking resumption after heart or lung transplantation: a systematic review and suggestions for screening and management. *J Thorac Dis.* 2018;10:4609-18; Kasiske BL, Klinger D. Cigarette smoking in renal transplant recipients. *J Am Soc Nephrol.* 2000;11:753-9; and Wang Y, Lan GB, Peng FH, Xie XB. Cancer risks in recipients of renal transplants: a meta-analysis of cohort studies. *Oncotarget.* 2018;9:15375-85.

- Smoking cessation more than 5 years before transplantation reduced the relative risk of graft failure by 34% (relative risk 0.66; 95% confidence interval [CI], 0.52-0.85; $P < .001$).[6]
- Smoking cessation less than 5 years before transplantation did not reduce the risk of cancer.
- The adjusted relative risk for lung malignancies with smoking with greater than 25 pack-years was 8.48 (95% CI, 1.64-43.92; P 0.011).

- In contrast, smoking had no statistically significant effect on nonlung malignancies.[7]
- Incidence and risk of posttransplant malignancy are always increased regardless of transplanted organ type, recipient age, or gender.
- The incidence of kidney cancers is higher in kidney transplant recipients (SIR: 10.77; 95% CI, 6.40-18.12; $P < .001$).[7]
- There is no significant relationship between renal transplantation and risk of liver cancer if follow-up duration was less than 8 years.[7]
- De novo posttransplant malignancies are associated with worse outcomes when compared with the same malignancies in the general population.[8]
- Prolonged dialysis in end-stage renal disease can lead to acquired cystic disease, which has the potential for malignant transformation.
- The incidence of renal cell carcinoma (RCC) in native kidneys is reported to be 1.6% to 4.2%.
- RCC is reported to be most common in kidney transplant recipients (SIR 6.7) compared with other organ transplant recipients (SIR 1.5-2.9); this finding can suggest that intrinsic renal defects associated with end-stage renal disease are as significant as impaired immunosurveillance in cancer pathogenesis.[9]

Risk Factors

Several risk factors have been linked to the increased incidence of posttransplant malignancy.[10]

- Intensity and duration of immunosuppression
- Oncogenic viral infections (e.g., Epstein-Barr virus [EBV], human herpes virus 8 [HHV-8])
- Ultraviolet radiation (sun exposure)
- Donor-derived malignancy: rare
- Length of pretransplant dialysis was reported as a contributing factor.

Immunosuppression

- Immunosurveillance protects the cells from undergoing malignant transformation through CD41 and CD81T cells.
- With improved immunosuppressive regimens, the survival of organ transplants has significantly prolonged with lower rejection rates; however, this has caused alterations of the natural immunosurveillance process.
- Lymphocytes-depleting agents used for induction of immunosuppression, such as antithymocyte globulin and alemtuzumab (anti-CD52), impose a higher risk of posttransplant malignancies.[11]
- Depleting agents have been linked to a higher risk of posttransplant lymphoproliferative disorder (PTLD), melanoma, colorectal cancer, and thyroid cancer.[11]
- Patients treated for rejection episodes during the first year posttransplantation have higher risk of malignancy when depleting agents are used.
- Nondepleting immunosuppressive agents such as basiliximab and daclizumab have not been consistently associated with an increased risk of posttransplant malignancies.[12]

Calcineurin Inhibitors

- Maintenance immunosuppressive agents, such as calcineurin inhibitors (CNIs) act through inhibition of interleukin-2 production, which interferes with the activation and proliferation of T cells and hence immunosurveillance.[13]

- CNIs also increase the expression of 2 regulators that play a key role in angiogenesis and tumor progression: vascular endothelial growth factor (VEGF) and transforming growth factor b1.[12]
- CNIs have also been linked to increased production of interleukin-6, which stimulates B-cell activation. This can cause increased viral replication of oncogenic viruses such as EBV, human papilloma virus (HPV), and HHV-8.[13]
- A dose-dependent effect has been reported for CNIs. The low-dose regimens were associated with fewer malignant disorders, but more demonstrated more frequent rejection.

Azathioprine

- Azathioprine (AZA) is a purine analogue that interferes with DNA replication and inhibits T-cell proliferation.[13]
- AZA interrupts DNA synthesis and can inhibit the DNA repair process that occurs following mutations caused by sun (ultraviolet radiation) exposure.[12]
- A meta-analysis that utilized AZA demonstrated a significant increase in the risk of skin squamous cell skin carcinoma (SCC) in AZA-exposed patients when compared with no exposure to AZA (odds ratio 1.56).[14]

Mycophenolic Acid and Mycophenolate Mofetil

- Mycophenolic acid (MPA) and mycophenolate mofetil (MMF) are more recent antimetabolites that have largely replaced the use of AZA.
- MPA and MMF block the synthesis of purine through inhibiting the inosine monophosphate dehydrogenase enzyme.
- Studies comparing AZA and MPA demonstrated that transplant recipients treated with AZA were twice as likely to develop SCC (OR 2.67). The use of MPA was associated with a lower risk of SCC (OR 0.45).[15]
- Interestingly, some tumors have elevations of the enzyme inosine monophosphate dehydrogenase, suggesting that MMF/MPA may have antiproliferative effects through inhibition of this enzyme.[15]
- Overall, the use of MMF/MPA is associated with fewer episodes of rejection and subsequently mitigating the need to use depleting agents for rejection episodes, and thus causing relative reduced malignancy risk.[15]

Mammalian Target of Rapamycin Inhibitors

- Mammalian target of rapamycin (mTOR) inhibitors include everolimus and sirolimus.
- Both mTOR inhibitors prevent T-cell activation and replication. Sirolimus also inhibits angiogenesis through reduction of VEGF and decrease in the response of vascular endothelial cells to stimulation by VEGF.
- A reported meta-analysis of more than 20 randomized trials of kidney transplant alone or simultaneous pancreas/kidney transplants demonstrated that sirolimus was associated with a 40% reduction in the risk of malignancy (adjusted hazard ratio 0.6) and 56% reduction in the risk of nonmelanomatous skin cancer (hazard ratio 0.44) compared with controls.[16]
- Sirolimus, however, was found to be associated with an increased mortality risk when compared with controls (hazard ratio 1.43), mainly due to increased cardiovascular and infection-associated death.[16]

Belatacept

- Belatacept, is a costimulation blocker of T cells. A study comparing belatacept with cyclosporine demonstrated increased risk of PTLD with almost 50% showing central nervous system involvement in the belatacept arms in the EBV-seronegative transplant recipients.
- The use of belatacept is not recommended in organ transplant recipients who are EBV immunoglobulin G–negative due to the PTLD risk.

Oncogenic Viral Infections

- Oncogenic viruses alter the cell cycle causing uncontrolled proliferation and compromise the apoptosis process of infected cells.[17]
- Almost all posttransplant malignancies with a significantly increased relative risk have viral associations (**Table 17-2**).
- Several viral infections,[18] when chronic, are recognized to be mediators of certain malignancies post transplantation.

Human Herpes Virus 8

- HHV-8 has been related to all forms of Kaposi sarcoma. Almost all organ transplant recipients with Kaposi sarcoma were found to be seropositive against the virus.
- Reported incidence of Kaposi sarcoma post transplant was 8.8 per 100,000 person-years, with a median time from transplantation diagnosis of 1.49 years.[19]
- HHV-8 infection alone does not cause the development of Kaposi sarcoma, because the intensity of immunosuppression is an important factor.
- In immunocompetent individuals, Kaposi sarcoma is a localized skin disease with low risk for dissemination.
- In immunocompromised individuals, Kaposi sarcoma can be aggressive and can involve the viscera.[20]

Human Papillomavirus

- In SCC post transplantation, HPV was found in about 90% of the diagnosed cases.[21]
- Different strains of HPV have been associated with tumors post transplantation.
  - Benign cutaneous strains: HPV 1 and 2
  - Oncogenic mucosal strains: HPV 16 and 18
  - Nononcogenic mucosal strains: HPV 6 and 11
- The role of HPV in posttransplant malignancy remains to be not fully understood.

Merkel Cell Polyomavirus

- Merkel cell carcinoma is a neuroendocrine tumor that has a high incidence of recurrence.
- Merkel cell polyomavirus can be detected in about 80% of Merkel cell carcinoma.[22]

Ultraviolet Radiation

Ultraviolet radiation (sun exposure), especially in fair-skinned patients, is an established risk factor for causing skin cancers, mainly SCC and basal cell carcinoma.[23]

Donor-Derived Malignancy

- Despite being rare, impaired immunosurveillance in the recipient can cause donor-derived malignancies to occur; this can result in metastatic disease.

TABLE 17-2 Oncogenic Viruses and Associated Malignancies

Virus	Associated Malignancy
HHV-8	Kaposi sarcoma
EBV	PTLD, nasopharyngeal cancers
Hepatitis B or C	Hepatocellular carcinoma
Merkel cell polyomavirus	Merkel cell carcinoma
Hepatitis B or C	Hepatocellular carcinoma
Merkel cell polyomavirus	Merkel cell carcinoma

- Donor-derived malignancies that have been reported include colon cancer, breast cancer, lung cancer, kidney cancer, prostate cancer, liver cancer, malignant melanoma, Kaposi sarcoma, and glioblastoma multiforme.
- Living kidney donors usually receive age-appropriate screening for breast, colon, prostate, and cervical cancer prior to donation.
- Donor-derived malignancies with minimal risk of transmission include local nonmelanomatous skin cancers, cervical carcinoma in situ, and resected solitary RCC less than 1.0 cm.[24]

CANCER SCREENING

- Posttransplant malignancy imposes high mortality and unfavorable outcomes, which makes cancer screening a crucial process in early detection of premalignant and early malignant lesions.
- Cancer screening begins in the pretransplant evaluation phase and should continue regularly post transplant.

Pretransplant Cancer Screening

- Colorectal, breast, prostate, and cervical cancer screening for organ transplant candidates follows general screening guidelines.
  - Colorectal cancer: it has been reported that the prevalence of colorectal polyps in candidates of kidney transplant is 24% to 33%; thus, pretransplant screening is important.[25]
  - Prostate cancer: even though the utility of prostate cancer screening in pretransplant evaluation remains controversial, due to the low specificity of the prostate-specific antigen, some transplant centers may elect to use it for screening purpose.
  - Cervical cancer: several reports demonstrated that the benefits of HPV vaccine outweigh the harms. Even though vaccination after transplantation may be less effective, it is likely beneficial in the transplant population and should be encouraged before transplantation if possible.[26]
  - Skin cancer: screening is recommended for candidates with history of skin cancer or uncertain skin lesions on examination.
- Waiting time ranges between no delay and 2 years for cancers with low risk of recurrence such as successfully treated nonmelanomatous skin cancers, localized solitary RCC less than 1.0 cm, testicular cancer, noninvasive cervical carcinoma, thyroid cancer, noninvasive bladder carcinoma, and early-stage colorectal cancers and lymphomas.[27]
- Cancers mandating longer waiting periods before transplantation include breast cancer, malignant melanoma, colorectal cancer, and SCC with lymph node involvement (3-5 years).
- Patients with metastatic cancers are not eligible for transplantation.

Posttransplant Cancer Screening

The data to support posttransplant cancer screening are not abundant; thus, most recommendations are derived from guidelines available on the general population[28] (**Table 17-3**).

Cervical Cancer

- Screening post transplant has not been studied sufficiently.
- Recommendations stemmed from the HIV populations and immunosuppressed patients undergoing treatment of lupus.

TABLE 17-3 Posttransplant Cancer Screening

Malignancy	Screening Method	Frequency
Skin cancer	Physical examination by physician	Annual, or more frequent if high risk
Cervical cancer	Papanicolaou smear cytology, cotesting with HPV for high-risk populations or after the age of 30 years	Annual to every 3 y
Breast cancer	Mammogram starting at age of 40 years	Annual
Colorectal carcinoma	Colonoscopy	Starting at the age of 50 y, every 5-10 y
Renal cell carcinoma of native kidneys	Surveillance ultrasonography or CT	Every 3-6 y if highly suspicious

Data from Kasiske BL, Vazquez MA, Harmon WE, et al. Recommendations for the outpatient surveillance of renal transplant recipients. American Society of Transplantation. *J Am Soc Nephrol.* 2000;11(suppl 15):S1-86.

- Initiation of cervical cancer screening with cytology only should begin within 1 year of onset of sexual activity but no later than 21 years of age. Cotesting with HPV for high-risk populations, or after the age of 30 years.
- Cervical cancer screening should continue throughout a woman's lifetime.
- Before the age of 30 years, if the initial cytology screening is normal, testing should be repeated yearly.
- If 3 consecutive cytology screenings are normal, follow-up cervical cytology should be every 3 years, and cotesting with HPV is not recommended in this setting.
- After the age of 30 years frequency of testing remains the same, but cotesting for HPV may be added.
- Positive results should be treated as in the general population.

Skin Cancer

- For screening, annual full-body skin examination is recommended.
- More periodic examinations may be needed in patients with a history of skin cancer.
- All transplant recipients should be advised to practice preventive precautions, including avoiding sun exposure with regular use of sunscreen, hats, and protective clothes.

Renal Cell Carcinoma

- Kidney transplant recipients are at a higher risk of developing RCC in native kidneys.
- Microscopic hematuria and urine cytology are not reliable markers for nonfunctioning native kidneys.
- Surveillance ultrasonography or CT scanning can be done periodically yearly or every 3 to 6 years, if indicated.
- It has been reported that the overall prevalence of RCC varies between 4.8% and 19% among those diagnosed with acquired cystic kidney disease.
- Four or more cysts should be present for the diagnosis of acquired cystic disease.[29]

Posttransplant Lymphoproliferative Disorder

- EBV polymerase chain reaction test for donor-positive recipient-negative mismatched patients should be considered in the prevention of early PTLD.
- Early detection of EBV viremia followed by treatment and reduction of immunosuppression may reduce the incidence of PTLD.[30]

Kaposi Sarcoma

Screening for HHV-8 antibody before transplant can be helpful to identify patients at risk of developing posttransplant Kaposi sarcoma.[20]

MANAGEMENT OF POSTTRANSPLANT MALIGNANCY

- At the time of posttransplant malignancy diagnosis, reduction of immunosuppression should be considered as the first step.
- The increased risk of rejection should be balanced against the risk of cancer spread and recurrence.
- Reducing or altering the maintenance immunosuppression depends on the treatment plan.
  - Maintenance immunosuppression may be held during chemotherapy and resumed at lower dose after treatment course is completed.[31]
  - AZA, MPA/MMF may be held temporarily or indefinitely depending on the risk of recurrence.
  - Lower target CNIs levels may be advised, if there is high risk of recurrence or spread of malignancy.[31]
  - In the case of Kaposi sarcoma, reduction of immunosuppression and the use of mTOR inhibitors should be considered as the initial step; this is because Kaposi sarcoma is a highly vascularized disease and it is thought that HHV-8 replication depends on the mTOR pathway. Thus, the change from a CNI to mTOR inhibitor has been associated with tumor regression.[32]

Posttransplant Lymphoproliferative Disorders

GENERAL PRINCIPLES

- Organ transplant recipients have a significantly higher risk for developing PTLDs, which include Hodgkin lymphoma (HL) and NHL.
- NHL is the most common hematologic malignancy in organ transplant recipients, with 5- to 15-fold higher risk than in the general population.
- The incidence of PTLD varies by the transplanted organ (heart, lung > liver, kidney), which is likely due to the amount of lymphoid tissue within the allograft and the intensity of immunosuppression.[33]
- Since EBV is considered an oncogenic virus, the donor-positive recipient-negative mismatched patients and EBV seronegative status are strongly associated with PTLD development.[17]
- The degree of T-cell immunosuppression, time post transplantation, recipient age, and ethnicity are risk factors.
- Early PTLD: malignancy occurring within the first 2 years post transplantation and is commonly EBV-positive.[34]
- Late PTLD: malignancy occurring after 2 years of transplantation with a higher proportion of EBV-negative cases.[4]

- The 5-year incidence of PTLD ranges between 0.7% and 9.0% after solid organ transplantation per the Scientific Registry of Transplant Recipients data.[35]
- The intensity, duration, and type of immunosuppression have been associated with PTLD.
  - Sirolimus: has anti-EBV proliferation effects in vivo; however, the use of sirolimus has not been associated with decreased PTLD risk clinically. On the contrary, registry data suggested that it may be associated with higher risk of PTLD.[16]
  - Belatacept: a costimulation blocker of T cells, increases the risk of PTLD, especially in the central nervous system (CNS). It is contraindicated for use in EBV-seronegative kidney recipients.
- PTLD can be recipient-derived and also donor derived.
  - Recipient-derived: multisystem involvement
  - Donor-derived: usually localized to the allograft tissue
- PTLD presents clinically with the following:
  - Constitutional symptoms, such as fever, weight loss, fatigue, lymphadenopathy
  - Symptoms related to dysfunction of the involved organs
- Laboratory findings in PTLD can include the following:
  - Unexplained anemia, thrombocytopenia, leukopenia
  - Elevated serum lactate dehydrogenase
  - Hypercalcemia and hyperuricemia

DIAGNOSIS

- The 2008 World Health Organization (WHO) classification of PTLD is used to stratify NHL and HL after tissue diagnosis.[36]
- If tissue diagnosis is not possible (e.g., in CNS lesions), then serum and cerebral spinal fluid analysis for EBV viral load, radiologic data, and brain biopsy can be used to make a diagnosis in select circumstances.
- CT and positron emission tomography scans can be used for staging and monitoring of response to therapy.
- Screening: there is no specific screening modality currently validated for PTLD. Some centers use EBV viral load for screening, because high viral load has been associated with PTLD.
- Prophylaxis: chemoprophylaxis for PTLD is controversial because antiviral agents, such as acyclovir and ganciclovir, did not demonstrate efficacy in preventing the development of EBV viremia clinically.

TREATMENT

- Treatment options for PTLD depend on several factors.
  - The WHO classification
  - The histopathology of PTLD including CD20 status
  - Location and staging of disease
- Treatment strategies include the following:
  - Reduction of immunosuppression
  - Monoclonal antibodies (against CD20 or other antigens)
  - Chemotherapeutic agents
  - Radiation
- Reduction of immunosuppression should always be the initial intervention for early diagnosis.

- Systemic therapy should be considered for PTLD.
  - Immunotherapy alone (e.g., rituximab): An anti-B-cell antibody that is used in CD20-positive B-cell NHLs including PTLD.
  - Chemoimmunotherapy regimens: Anthracycline-based regimens used for curative intent for NHLs are commonly used for PTLD. These can be based on the "CHOP" regimen (cyclophosphamide, hydroxydaunorubicin or doxorubicin, oncovin or vincristine, and prednisone).
- Patients achieving PTLD remission may experience transplanted organ failure.
- It is unclear whether retransplantation is safe in patients with persistently high EBV viral load.

Checkpoint Inhibitors and Posttransplant Malignancy

- Checkpoint inhibitor antibodies are lifesaving treatments against many tumors.
- The use of checkpoint inhibitor antibodies has resulted in significant improvements and demonstrated significant clinical benefits in tumor regression and prolonged stabilization of non–small cell lung cancer, melanoma, and renal cell cancer.[37]
- The benefits of treatment versus the potential risk of allograft rejection and loss should be considered carefully. Rejection reportedly developed at a median of 24 days after initiation of checkpoint inhibitor antibodies according to one study, and 80% of all rejection episodes occurred within the first 60 days following initiation.[38]
- The mechanism of checkpoint inhibitors and site of action of different checkpoint inhibitor antibodies are illustrated in **Figure 17-1**.

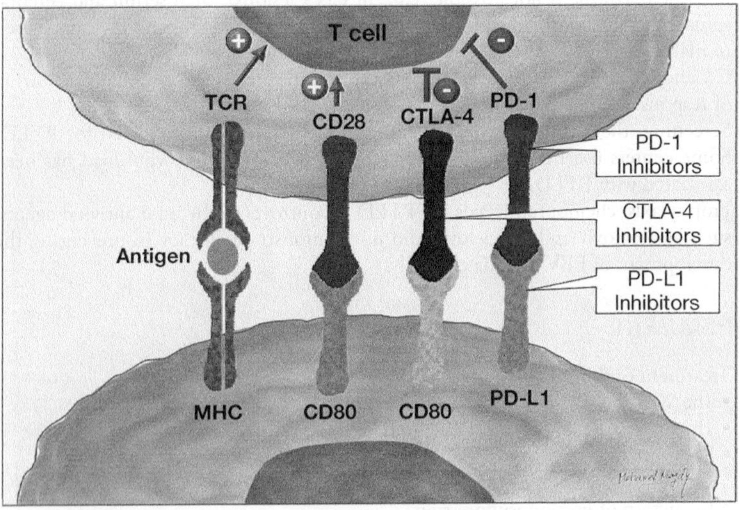

Figure 17-1. **Mechanism of checkpoint inhibitors.** (Reproduced with permission from Ibrahim MM, Alhamad T. Checkpoint inhibitors in kidney transplant recipients and the potential risk of rejection. In: Aziz F, Parajuli S. (eds). *Complications in Kidney Transplantation*. Springer, Cham; 2022. Figure 2. https://doi.org/10.1007/978-3-031-13569-9_36)

- There are no specific recommendations to manage recipients receiving checkpoint inhibitors.
- Current suggested strategies include the following:
  - Holding checkpoint inhibitors during acute kidney injury with possible reintroduction after creatinine has normalized.
  - Increasing or restarting corticosteroids.
- Maintenance immunosuppression during checkpoint inhibitor therapy:
  - Use dual therapy of low calcineurin inhibitor dose and prednisone.
  - May consider switching to everolimus and higher-dose prednisone.
- Limited studies so far demonstrate poor outcomes of kidney transplant recipients with metastatic cancer receiving checkpoint inhibitors.[37]

REFERENCES

1. Sargen MR, Cahoon EK, Yu KJ, et al. Spectrum of nonkeratinocyte skin cancer risk among solid organ transplant recipients in the US. *JAMA Dermatol.* 2022;158(4):414-25.
2. Manickavasagar R, Thuraisingham R. Post renal-transplant malignancy surveillance. *Clin Med.* 2020;20(2):142-5.
3. Wheless L, Jacks S, Mooneyham Potter KA, Leach BC, Cook J. Skin cancer in organ transplant recipients: more than the immune system. *J Am Acad Dermatol.* 2014;71(2):359-65.
4. Quinlan SC, Pfeiffer RM, Morton LM, Engels EA. Risk factors for early-onset and late-onset post-transplant lymphoproliferative disorder in kidney recipients in the United States. *Am J Hematol.* 2011;86(2):206-9.
5. Hofmann P, Benden C, Kohler M, Schuurmans MM. Smoking resumption after heart or lung transplantation: a systematic review and suggestions for screening and management. *J Thorac Dis.* 2018;10(7):4609-18.
6. Kasiske BL, Klinger D. Cigarette smoking in renal transplant recipients. *J Am Soc Nephrol.* 2000;11(4):753-9.
7. Wang Y, Lan GB, Peng FH, Xie XB. Cancer risks in recipients of renal transplants: a meta-analysis of cohort studies. *Oncotarget.* 2018;9(20):15375-85.
8. Doycheva I, Amer S, Watt KD. De novo malignancies after transplantation: risk and surveillance strategies. *Med Clin North Am.* 2016;100(3):551-67.
9. Dharia A, Boulet J, Sridhar VS, Kitchlu A. Cancer screening in solid organ transplant recipients: a focus on screening liver, lung, and kidney recipients for cancers related to the transplanted organ. *Transplantation.* 2022;106(1):e64-5.
10. Sprangers B, Nair V, Launay-Vacher V, Riella LV, Jhaveri KD. Risk factors associated with post-kidney transplant malignancies: an article from the Cancer-Kidney International Network. *Clin Kidney J.* 2018;11(3):315-29.
11. Lim WH, Turner RM, Chapman JR, et al. Acute rejection, T-cell-depleting antibodies, and cancer after transplantation. *Transplantation.* 2014;97(8):817-25.
12. Mukherjee S, Mukherjee U. A comprehensive review of immunosuppression used for liver transplantation. *J Transplant.* 2009;2009:701464.
13. Suthanthiran M, Morris RE, Strom TB. Immunosuppressants: cellular and molecular mechanisms of action. *Am J Kidney Dis.* 1996;28(2):159-72.
14. Jiyad Z, Olsen CM, Burke MT, Isbel NM, Green AC. Azathioprine and risk of skin cancer in organ transplant recipients: systematic review and meta-analysis. *Am J Transplant.* 2016;16(12):3490-503.
15. Coghill AE, Johnson LG, Berg D, Resler AJ, Leca N, Madeleine MM. Immunosuppressive medications and squamous cell skin carcinoma: nested case-control study within the Skin Cancer after Organ Transplant (SCOT) cohort. *Am J Transplant.* 2016;16(2):565-73.
16. Knoll GA, Kokolo MB, Mallick R, et al. Effect of sirolimus on malignancy and survival after kidney transplantation: systematic review and meta-analysis of individual patient data. *BMJ.* 2014;349:g6679.

17. Krump NA, You J. Molecular mechanisms of viral oncogenesis in humans. *Nat Rev Microbiol.* 2018;16(11):684-98.
18. Vajdic CM, van Leeuwen MT. Cancer incidence and risk factors after solid organ transplantation. *Int J Cancer.* 2009;125(8):1747-54.
19. Mbulaiteye SM, Engels EA. Kaposi's sarcoma risk among transplant recipients in the United States (1993-2003). *Int J Cancer.* 2006;119(11):2685-91.
20. Dow DE, Cunningham CK, Buchanan AM. A review of human herpesvirus 8, the Kaposi's sarcoma-associated herpesvirus, in the pediatric population. *J Pediatric Infect Dis Soc.* 2014;3(1):66-76.
21. Chockalingam R, Downing C, Tyring SK. Cutaneous squamous cell carcinomas in organ transplant recipients. *J Clin Med.* 2015;4(6):1229-39.
22. Pietropaolo V, Prezioso C, Moens U. Merkel cell polyomavirus and Merkel cell carcinoma. *Cancers (Basel).* 2020;12(7):1774.
23. Armstrong BK, Kricker A. The epidemiology of UV induced skin cancer. *J Photochem Photobiol B.* 2001;63(1-3):8-18.
24. Nalesnik MA, Woodle ES, Dimaio JM, et al. Donor-transmitted malignancies in organ transplantation: assessment of clinical risk. *Am J Transplant.* 2011;11(6):1140-7.
25. AlAmeel T, Bseiso B, AlBugami MM, AlMomen S, Roth LS. Yield of screening colonoscopy in renal transplant candidates. *Can J Gastroenterol Hepatol.* 2015;29(8):423-6.
26. Kidney Disease: Improving Global Outcomes Transplant Work G. KDIGO clinical practice guideline for the care of kidney transplant recipients. *Am J Transplant.* 2009;9:S1-155.
27. Kasiske BL, Cangro CB, Hariharan S, et al. The evaluation of renal transplantation candidates: clinical practice guidelines. *Am J Transplant.* 2001;1(suppl 2):3-95.
28. Kasiske BL, Vazquez MA, Harmon WE, et al. Recommendations for the outpatient surveillance of renal transplant recipients. American Society of Transplantation. *J Am Soc Nephrol.* 2000;11(suppl 15):S1-86.
29. Doublet JD, Peraldi MN, Gattegno B, Thibault P, Sraer JD. Renal cell carcinoma of native kidneys: prospective study of 129 renal transplant patients. *J Urol.* 1997;158(1):42-44.
30. Martin SI, Dodson B, Wheeler C, Davis J, Pesavento T, Bumgardner GL. Monitoring infection with Epstein-Barr virus among seromismatch adult renal transplant recipients. *Am J Transplant.* 2011;11(5):1058-63.
31. Otley CC, Berg D, Ulrich C, et al. Reduction of immunosuppression for transplant-associated skin cancer: expert consensus survey. *Br J Dermatol.* 2006;154(3):395-400.
32. Stallone G, Schena A, Infante B, et al. Sirolimus for Kaposi's sarcoma in renal-transplant recipients. *N Engl J Med.* 2005;352(13):1317-23.
33. Penn I. Cancers complicating organ transplantation. *N Engl J Med.* 1990;323(25):1767-9.
34. Schober T, Framke T, Kreipe H, et al. Characteristics of early and late PTLD development in pediatric solid organ transplant recipients. *Transplantation.* 2013;95(1):240-6.
35. Kotton CN, Huprikar S, Kumar D. Transplant infectious diseases: a review of the scientific registry of transplant recipients published data. *Am J Transplant.* 2017;17(6):1439-46.
36. Swerdlow SH, Campo E, Pileri SA, et al. The 2016 revision of the World Health Organization classification of lymphoid neoplasms. *Blood.* 2016;127(20):2375-90.
37. Venkatachalam K, Malone AF, Heady B, Santos RD, Alhamad T. Poor outcomes with the use of checkpoint inhibitors in kidney transplant recipients. *Transplantation.* 2020;104(5):1041-7.
38. Murakami N, Mulvaney P, Danesh M, et al. A multi-center study on safety and efficacy of immune checkpoint inhibitors in cancer patients with kidney transplant. *Kidney Int.* 2021;100(1):196-205.

18 Pregnancy After Transplant

Rowena Delos Santos

END-STAGE RENAL DISEASE NEGATIVELY AFFECTS FEMALE REPRODUCTIVE ABILITY

- Discuss with patients who are of reproductive age BEFORE transplant that they may become fertile again after transplant.
- Have this conversation multiple times while undergoing evaluation and before actual transplantation to plan ahead for contraception and conception.
- End-stage renal disease (ESRD) leads to hypothalamic-pituitary-ovarian (HPO) dysregulation.[1]
  - Uremia leads to high prolactin, follicle stimulating hormone (FSH), and luteinizing hormone (LH).
  - Decreased estradiol and progesterone leads to lack of LH surge and anovulation in women.
  - Low testosterone, high LH, with associated low spermatogenesis.
  - Manifestations of reproductive dysregulation are summarized in **Table 18-1**.
  - Pregnancy rates in women on dialysis can be as low as <1% to 7%.[2]
- Transplant corrects HPO axis dysregulation.
  - Normalization can occur within weeks posttransplant.
  - Pregnancy rate can be up to 22.7% post transplant.[3,4]
  - Pregnancy rate 30/1,000 in transplant females versus 100/1,000 in general population.[3,4]
  - Live birth rate 19/1,000 in transplant females versus 70/1,000 in general population.[3,4]

TABLE 18-1 Manifestations of Female and Male Reproductive Dysregulation

Female Manifestations	Male Manifestations
Anovulatory cycles	Impaired gonadal testosterone production
Amenorrhea	Impaired spermatogenesis
Early menopause	Erectile dysfunction
Very low conception rate 0.44%-7% with high risk of maternal and fetal complications[1]	

Data from Holley JL, Schmidt RJ. Changes in fertility and hormone replacement therapy in kidney disease. *Adv Chronic Kidney Dis.* 2013;20:240-5.

CONTRACEPTION POST KIDNEY TRANSPLANT

- Discuss contraception plans with patients preferably before transplantation.
- Discuss fetotoxicity of certain transplant medications and need for effective contraception to prevent pregnancy. See **Table 18-2** for the Centers for Disease Control and Prevention's summary of different contraception methods and unintended pregnancies in first year of use.[1,4-6]
- Restart contraception or start it when out of window of deep vein thrombosis risk.

Uncomplicated Post–Kidney Transplant Patient

- Defined as patients without history of rejection, chronic allograft dysfunction, or vasculopathy.
- Contraceptives and intrauterine devices (IUDs) considered to have favorable risk-benefit profile.

Complicated Post–Kidney Transplant Patient

- Defined as patients with history of rejection, acute or chronic allograft failure, or vasculopathy.
- Avoid estrogen-containing contraceptives, new IUDs, and continuing IUDs (copper and levonorgestrel) in complicated post–kidney transplant patients. There is a risk of failure of the use of IUD alone.
- Progestin-only methods are recommended.

TABLE 18-2 CDC Summary of Different Contraception Methods and Unintended Pregnancies in First Year of Use[5,6]

Highly Effective (<1 Pregnancy/100 Women in a year)	Highly Effective (<1 Pregnancy/100 Women in a year)	Moderately Effective (6-12 Pregnancies/100 Women in a year)	Least Effective (≥18 Pregnancies/100 Women in a Year)
Permanent sterilization	Implanted devices	Injectable hormone	Male condom
Female tubal ligation	Implants	Oral contraceptive pill	Female condom
Male vasectomy	IUD (copper or hormonal)	Patch	Withdrawal
		Ring	Sponge
		Diaphragm	Spermicide
			Calendar fertility monitoring

CDC, Centers for Disease Control and Prevention; IUD, intrauterine device.
Data from Klein CL, Josephson MA. Post-transplant pregnancy and contraception. *Clin J Am Soc Nephrol.* 2022;17:114-20; and Summary of Classifications for Hormonal Contraceptive Methods and Intrauterine Devices. *US Medical Eligibility Criteria (US MEC) for Contraceptive Use.* Reviewed March 27, 2023. Accessed October 6, 2022. https://www.cdc.gov/reproductivehealth/contraception/mmwr/mec/appendixk.html.

Emergency Contraception in Kidney Transplant Patients

Levonorgestrel 1.5 mg orally given once within 3 days from unprotected sex or ulipristal 30 mg orally given once within 5 days from unprotected sex.

TIMING OF PREGNANCY

- In the US, the recommendation is to wait 1 year post transplant before attempts at conception.[7]
- Rejection is possible when conception/birth occur within 1 year of transplant.

FACTORS ASSOCIATED WITH BETTER OUTCOMES FOR PREGNANCY IN KIDNEY TRANSPLANT

- No history of rejection
- Serum Cr < 1.5 mg/dL
- No or minimal proteinuria
- No infections
- On stable doses of immunosuppression. If switch in immunosuppression occurs for the purposes of prepregnancy planning, then allow 6 months stability on new regimen before attempts at conception.

IMMUNOSUPPRESSIVE MEDICATIONS IN PREGNANCY AND POST PARTUM

Please see a summary of immunosuppressive medications in pregnancy and the postpartum period in **Table 18-3**.[1,5,7]

Calcineurin Inhibitors

Tacrolimus

- No cases of birth defects related to tacrolimus; well tolerated during pregnancy.
- Need to increase frequency of testing to assure levels are within goal as pregnancy progresses due to several factors:
  - Increased enzymatic activity of cytochrome P450 isoenzymes through pregnancy.
  - Expansion of blood volume up to 20% and fall in red blood cell concentration.
  - Increased unbound fraction in plasma during pregnancy.
  - Albumin changes by 1% to 13% during pregnancy.
- May need to increase dose of tacrolimus by 20% to 25% during pregnancy to achieve goal trough levels.
- Minimal (1%) excretion of tacrolimus in breast milk; typically undetectable in baby.

Cyclosporine

- No cases of birth defects related to cyclosporine; well tolerated during pregnancy.
- Levels need to be tested frequently as pregnancy progresses similar to tacrolimus.
- More excreted via breastmilk compared with tacrolimus but usually undetectable in baby.

TABLE 18-3 Maintenance Immunosuppressive Medications for Kidney Transplant in Pregnancy and Postpartum

	Medication Class	Use during Pregnancy	Exposure in Breast Milk
Tacrolimus	Calcineurin inhibitor (CNI)	Yes	Minimal excretion, undetectable in baby
Cyclosporine	CNI	Yes	More excretion compared with tacrolimus, typically undetectable in baby
Mycophenolate	Antimetabolite	No	No data on safety during breastfeeding
Azathioprine	Antimetabolite	Yes	Undetectable in breast milk
Prednisone	Corticosteroid	Yes	Minimal exposure in breast milk
Sirolimus	Mammalian target of rapamycin inhibitor (mTOR)	No	No data on safety during breastfeeding
Everolimus	mTOR	No	No data on safety during breastfeeding
Belatacept	Costimulation blockade	Not enough safety data	No data on safety during breastfeeding

Antimetabolites

Mycophenolate Mofetil/Mycophenolate Sodium

- Contraindicated in pregnancy; miscarriage rate in women who underwent transplantation on mycophenolate is 28% to 64% compared with 13% to 24% in the general transplant population not on mycophenolate. REMS (Risk Evaluation and Mitigation Strategy) issued in 2012.[7,8]
- Birth defects in 14% of pregnancies before 2nd trimester, 32% during 2nd trimester. Birth defects include cleft lip/palate, microtia, hypoplastic nails, shortened 5th finger.[7,8]
- No reports of increased congenital defects with father exposed to drug.
- Should stop mycophenolate 6 weeks prior to attempts at conception.
- No safety data on mycophenolate in breastfeeding.

Azathioprine

- Generally considered safe in pregnancy; reports of congenital malformations in utero in animals exposed to azathioprine, but no confirmed data in humans.
- Mother metabolizes azathioprine and metabolites, leading to minimal amounts in fetus.
- Low and rare risk of leukopenia and thrombocytopenia.
- Azathioprine undetectable in breast milk.

Corticosteroids

- Prolonged high doses of steroids have been associated with fetal adrenal suppression, not reported in transplant patients at low doses.
- Minimal excretion of prednisone in breast milk.

Mammalian Target of Rapamycin Inhibitors Sirolimus and Everolimus

- In animal studies there is some association with increased fetal mortality, delayed skeletal ossification, growth retardation.
- May lead to decreased spermatogenesis and decreased spermatozoa motility.
- Recommend discontinuing 6 months prior to attempts at conception (switch to azathioprine if able), as there are not enough data to support its safety in posttransplant pregnant patients.
- No data on mammalian target of rapamycin (mTOR) inhibitors and presence in breastmilk.

Costimulation Blockade (Belatacept)

Not enough data to guarantee safety of this drug with pregnancy.

MALE TRANSPLANT RECIPIENTS

- Exposure of male transplant recipients to calcineurin inhibitor, mycophenolate, azathioprine, prednisone does not appear to lead to adverse outcomes for their female partners' pregnancies regarding birth weight, gestational age at birth, birth defects.
- Not enough data regarding male transplant recipients on belatacept and pregnancy outcomes for their female partners.
- Sirolimus/everolimus mTOR inhibitors may lead to decreased sperm counts and motility, lower pregnancy rates. Male transplant recipients should be counseled regarding this possibility.

PREGNANCY AND ALLOGRAFT OUTCOMES

Pregnancy Outcomes

- Female kidney transplant patients outcomes and general population outcomes differ for maternal and fetal outcomes. These data are summarized in **Table 18-4**.[3,9-11]
- The live birth rate in the general population is higher compared with kidney transplant patients.
- Preterm birth, extreme prematurity, small for gestational age, stillbirths, and neonatal death are lower in the general US population compared with the kidney transplant patient population.[3,9-11]
- Rates of preeclampsia and diabetes are higher in patients with transplant compared with the general population of pregnant individuals.[3,9-11]

Allograft Outcomes During and Post Pregnancy

- Rejections can occur during pregnancy between 4% and 9%.[9,10]
- Transplant Pregnancy Registry data between 1967 and 2016 showed rejection rate during pregnancy of 0.9% to 1%.[5,8]
- Several factors affect this rejection and allograft loss—length of time post transplant at the time of pregnancy, history of rejections, history of infections, proteinuria present.

TABLE 18-4 Pregnancy Rates and Outcomes and Complications in Transplant Compared With General Population

Pregnancy Rates and Outcomes	General US Population	Kidney Transplant Population
Live birth rate (%)	88	70-80
Preterm birth, <37 wk gestation (%)	8-12	22-52
Extreme prematurity, <32 wk gestation (%)	1-2	17
Mean gestational age at birth (weeks)	38.7	34.9
Small for gestational age (%)	9-16	24
Miscarriage (%)	10-15	15.4
Stillbirths (%)	0.6	5
Neonatal death (%)	1.3	3.8
Mean birth weight (grams)	3,389	2,470
Maternal Complications		
Hypertension (%)	5-8	24
Preeclampsia (%)	3.8	11-30
Gestational diabetes (%)	3.9	8
Cesarean section delivery (%)	31.8	62.6

- Postpregnancy allograft loss is variable (**Table 18-5**).[9,10] For perspective—median survival for a deceased donor allograft is about 12 years and nearly 20 years for a living donor allograft.[12]

Children Born to Female Transplant Recipients

- There are a few small studies looking at children of females who underwent transplantation.[13,14]
- Children of females who underwent transplantation (on calcineurin inhibitors, azathioprine, prednisone) who are born preterm and small for gestational age tend to catch up in their height and weight by 12 months of age.[13]
- Neurological development and intelligence of children of females who underwent transplantation appear to be similar to children of females who did not undergo transplantation.[13,14]

TABLE 18-5 Postpregnancy Allograft Loss

Years Post Pregnancy	Allograft Loss Rate (%)
1	6
2	6-9
3	6
5	7
6	10
10	19

REFERENCES

1. Holley JL, Schmidt RJ. Changes in fertility and hormone replacement therapy in kidney disease. *Adv Chronic Kidney Dis.* 2013;20(3):240-5.
2. Jesudason S, Grace BS, McDonald SP. Pregnancy outcomes according to dialysis commencing before or after conception in women with ESRD. *Clin J Am Soc Nephrol.* 2014;9(1):143-9.
3. Gill JS, Zalunardo N, Rose C, Tonelli M. The pregnancy rate and live birth rate in kidney transplant recipients. *Am J Transplant.* 2009;9:1541-9.
4. Centers for Disease Control and Prevention. *Reproductive Health: Maternal and Infant Health.* 2022. Accessed October 6, 2022. https://www.cdc.gov/reproductivehealth/maternalinfanthealth/index.html
5. Klein CL, Josephson MA. Post-transplant pregnancy and contraception. *Clin J Am Soc Nephrol.* 2022;17(1):114-20.
6. *US Medical Eligibility Criteria (US MEC) for Contraceptive Use.* 2020. Accessed October 6, 2022. https://www.cdc.gov/reproductivehealth/contraception/mmwr/mec/appendixk.html
7. McKay DB, Josephson MA, Armenti VT, et al. Reproduction and transplantation: report on the AST consensus conference on reproductive issues and transplantation. *Am J Transplant.* 2005;5(7):1592-9.
8. Transplant Pregnancy Registry International. 2022. Accessed October 6, 2022. https://www.transplantpregnancyregistry.org/
9. Deshpande NA, James NT, Kucirka LM, et al. Pregnancy outcomes in kidney transplant recipients: a systematic review and meta-analysis. *Am J Transplant.* 2011;11:2388-404.
10. Shah S, Venkatesan RL, Gupta A, et al. Pregnancy outcomes in women with kidney transplant: metaanalysis and systematic review. *BMC Nephrol.* 2019;20(1):24.
11. van Buren MC, Schellekens A, Groenhof TKJ, et al. Long-term graft survival and graft function following pregnancy in kidney transplant recipients: a systematic review and meta-analysis. *Transplantation.* 2020;104(8):1675-85.
12. Poggio ED, Augustine JJ, Arrigain S, Brennan DC, Schold JD. Long-term kidney transplant graft survival—making progress when most needed. *Am J Transplant.* 2021;21(8):2824-32.
13. Schreiber-Zamora J, Szpotanska-Sikorska M, Drozdowska-Szymczak A, et al. Neurological development of children born to mothers after kidney transplantation. *J Matern Fetal Neonatal Med.* 2019;32(9):1523-7.
14. Kociszewska-Najman B, Szpotanska-Sikorska M, Mazanowska N, Wielgos M, Pietrzak B. The comparison of intelligence levels of children born to kidney or liver transplant women with children of healthy mothers. *J Matern Fetal Neonatal Med.* 2018;31(23):3160-5.

19

Posttransplant Diabetes Mellitus

Petra Krutilova, Kristin Progar, and Maamoun Salam

GENERAL PRINCIPLES

- In the US, almost 50% of patients with end-stage renal disease have diabetes mellitus (DM).[1]
- In 22% of kidney transplant recipients, DM is the primary cause of the prior-to-transplant kidney disease.[1]
- Approximately 90% of kidney transplant recipients experience hyperglycemia in the first few weeks post transplant due to a variety of stressors such as inflammation, use of high doses of steroids, infections, and use of enteral or parenteral nutrition. If hyperglycemia persists 6 weeks after kidney transplantation in an individual with no prior diagnosis of diabetes, posttransplantation diabetes mellitus (PTDM) diagnosis is made.
- PTDM is a common complication after kidney transplantation and is associated with increased morbidity, mortality, and healthcare costs.
- This chapter reviews the terminology, epidemiology, risk factors, clinical implications, and management of PTDM.

Definitions

- **Posttransplantation diabetes mellitus (PTDM):** describes newly diagnosed diabetes after transplantation and includes patients who may have had undiagnosed pretransplant diabetes. It does not include patients with transient posttransplant hyperglycemia. It is the preferred term and was adopted by the international consensus meeting on PTDM in 2014. This diagnosis should be made at least 6 weeks after transplantation, when patients are stable, on their maintenance immunosuppressive therapy, with stable renal function, and in the absence of infection.[2]
- **New-onset diabetes after transplantation (NODAT):** an older term that has been replaced by PTDM. It describes the pathophysiological consequences of transplantation on glucose metabolism. It assumes patients did not have diabetes prior to transplant. The term NODAT does not include patients who may have had unrecognized diabetes prior to transplant, which makes this term misleading as screening for undiagnosed diabetes before transplant is not always included in pretransplant evaluation.[2]
- **Transient posttransplant hyperglycemia:** occurs in the immediate/early posttransplant period, typically due to postsurgical stress and administration of high-dose glucocorticoids or as a consequence of acute infection or treatment of rejection.[3] It usually resolves within the first few weeks after transplantation. These patients should not be diagnosed with PTDM.[2]
- **Other terms** including *posttransplantation hyperglycemia* or *diabetes after transplantation* are not recommended.

Epidemiology

- The literature describing the incidence and prevalence of PTDM reports wide variations in rates that range from 4% to 40%, which is partly due to the lack of consistent criteria for its diagnosis and therefore must be interpreted in the context of the definition used, time from transplant, study population, and immunosuppressive agents used.[4-6]
- Studies using the 2014 guidelines criteria report a prevalence of PTDM of 10% to 30% in kidney transplant recipients.[1]
- Compared with kidney transplant recipients, the incidence of PTDM is higher in non-kidney transplant recipients: 20% to 30% in heart transplant, 20% to 40% in liver transplant, and 20% to 40% in lung transplant.[1] The progress in management of kidney transplant recipients results in fewer episodes of rejection, decreased use of steroids, and lower doses of calcineurin inhibitors. These changes, among others, translated into reduction of the 1-year-prevalence of PTDM from 10% in 2007 to under 4% in 2016 and a reduction in the 5-year-incidence of PTDM from 16% in 2007 to 10% in 2012.[6,7]

Pathophysiology

- PTDM shares many pathophysiological mechanisms with pretransplant type 2 diabetes (T2DM), but the pathogenesis of PTDM has some distinct features.[4] **Figure 19-1** shows the common pathways in T2DM and posttransplant diabetes.[4]
- PTDM occurs due to a combination of impaired insulin sensitivity in peripheral tissues, impaired insulin-mediated suppression of hepatic glucose output, abnormal insulin production in the setting of β-cell dysfunction, lack of glucagon suppression with hyperglycemia, hypertriglyceridemia, obesity, and inflammation. Alterations in the incretin axis between the gut and pancreas have also been proposed as a factor contributing to PTDM.[1]
- Immunosuppressive medications affect the pancreatic β cells' function and the peripheral tissues insulin sensitivity by multiple pathways promoting the development of PTDM.[4] See **Figure 19-2**.

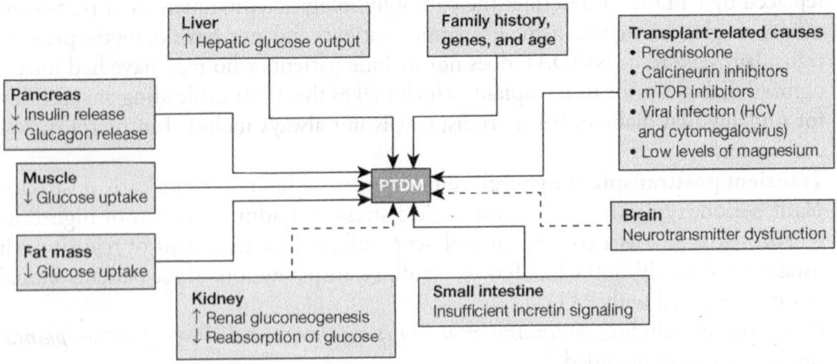

Figure 19-1. **Common pathways in type 2 diabetes mellitus and posttransplant diabetes mellitus (PTDM).** (Reproduced with permission from Jenssen T, Hartmann A. Post-transplant diabetes mellitus in patients with solid organ transplants. *Nat Rev Endocrinol.* 2019;15:172-88.)

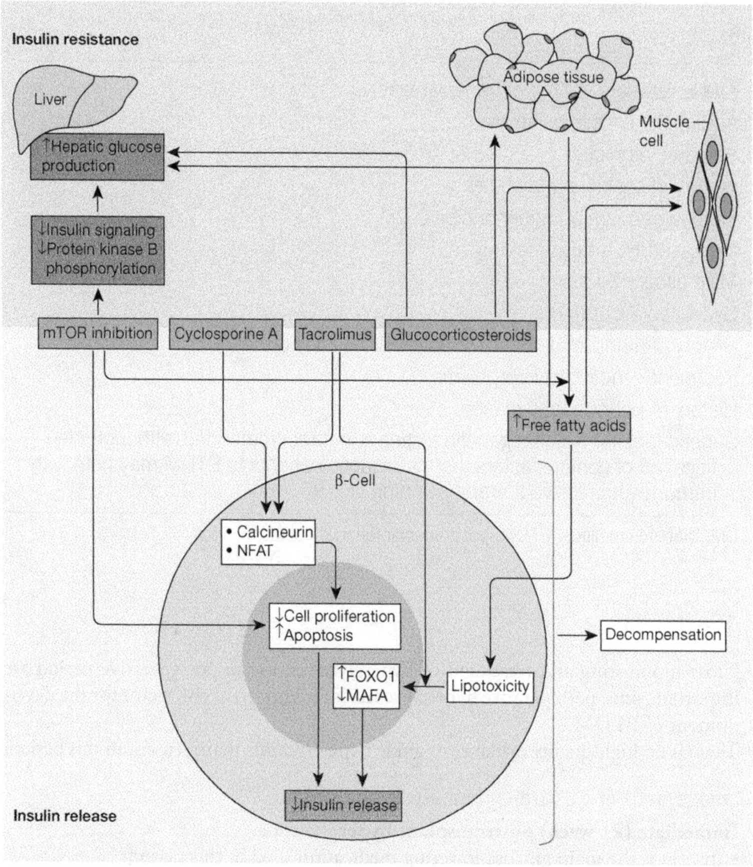

Figure 19-2. **Pathways of immunosuppressive therapy that induce the development of posttransplant diabetes mellitus.** FOXO1, forkhead box protein O1; MAFA, transcription factor MafA; NFAT, nuclear factor of activated T cells. (Reproduced with permission from Jenssen T, Hartmann A. Post-transplant diabetes mellitus in patients with solid organ transplants. *Nat Rev Endocrinol.* 2019;15:172-88.)

Risk Factors

- Risk factors for PTDM are similar to those that increase the risk of diabetes before transplantation and also include some nonmodifiable (**Table 19-1**)[4,8,9] and modifiable (**Table 19-2**) transplant-related risk factors.
- Identification of modifiable risk factors during pretransplantation evaluation is crucial for timely PTDM screening and treatment planning.

DIAGNOSIS

The diagnosis of PTDM can be made (at least) 6 weeks after transplantation using the same American Diabetes Association (ADA) diabetes and prediabetes diagnostic criteria as for nontransplant patients.[19] See **Table 19-3**.

TABLE 19-1	Nonmodifiable Posttransplantation Diabetes Mellitus Risk Factors
Age ≥ 40 years at time of transplantation	
African American, Asian race	
Hispanic ethnicity	
History of gestational diabetes	
First degree family history of type 2 DM	
Increased HLA mismatching	
Male allograft donor	
Deceased allograft donor	
History of autosomal dominant polycystic kidney disease	
Recipient genetic polymorphisms	
History of prior transplantation	
Genetic factors: Routine genetic testing is not recommended, although identification of genetic factors that predispose patients to PTDM may help with immunosuppressive therapy planning.	

DM, diabetes mellitus; PTDM, posttransplantation diabetes mellitus.

TREATMENT

- Close monitoring and treatment of hyperglycemia in the postoperative period are important since perioperative hyperglycemia is an important risk factor for the development of PTDM.
- There is no high-quality evidence to guide hyperglycemia management in this period.

Management of Posttransplant Hyperglycemia

- **Immediate (<1 week) posttransplant hyperglycemia**
  - Insulin is the main glucose-lowering medication used in this period.
  - Patients with blood glucose >140 mg/dL should be treated with insulin, as this approach showed a decreased risk of PTDM compared with patients treated with oral glucose-lowering agents.[1]
  - Critically ill patients with hyperglycemia (≥180 mg/dL) should be treated with standard IV insulin infusion protocol. The recommended optimal glycemic target is 140 to 180 mg/dL.
  - Stable patients can be treated with SC insulin regimens tailored individually with glycemic targets of <140 mg/dL for fasting blood glucose and <180 mg/dL for random blood glucose.
  - More intensive blood glucose control (with tighter blood glucose targets, 70-110 mg/dL) has not been shown to be beneficial among patients undergoing kidney transplantation and led to higher rates of hypoglycemia.[20]
  - Washington University School of Medicine in St. Louis, Division of Endocrinology uses a formula to estimate insulin doses to treat steroid-induced hyperglycemia. It suggests that 0.1 U/kg of extra insulin is needed to cover every 20 mg of prednisone (or equivalent) over 20 mg. This formula goes up to a dose of 100 mg of prednisone. In case of a dose >100 mg, more insulin may be needed. The effect below

TABLE 19-2 Modifiable Posttransplantation Diabetes Mellitus Risk Factors

Immunosuppressive Agents		
Drug Type	**Mechanism**	**Notes**
Glucocorticoids • Dexamethasone • Methylprednisolone • Prednisone	• Enhance gluconeogenesis and lipolysis • Reduce glycogen synthesis • Reduce skeletal muscle glucose uptake • Stimulate appetite • Cause increase in central and visceral adiposity	• Impact is dose dependent: High doses used in the immediate posttransplant period have much greater impact than chronic low-dose glucocorticoids used in maintenance immunosuppression protocols. However, complete withdrawal increases the risk of acute rejection and reinstitution of treatment at higher doses.[10] • The use of other antirejection agents allows steroid avoidance where glucocorticoids are withdrawn at ≤7 d from transplant. Although this approach resulted in increased mild biopsy-confirmed acute rejection, it provided less insulin dependency at 5 y (3.7% vs. 11.6%) while maintaining similar long-term renal allograft survival and function.[11]
Calcineurin inhibitors (CNIs) • Cyclosporine (CSA) • Tacrolimus	• Increase islet cell apoptosis, swelling, and vacuolation • Decrease transcriptional regulation of insulin expression	• Impact is dose dependent • Tacrolimus is more diabetogenic (33.6%) compared with CSA (26%)[12,13] • Tacrolimus level >15 ng/mL is strongly associated with PTDM. Target goals are transplant center dependent. A typical goal of 5-15 ng/mL is frequently used, with even lower target later in the posttransplant period.[14] • Effect is similar between extended- and immediate-release formulations.[14]

(Continued)

TABLE 19-2 Modifiable Posttransplantation Diabetes Mellitus Risk Factors (Continued)

mTOR inhibitors (mTORis) • Sirolimus (rapamycin) • Everolimus	• Reduce β-cell mass through apoptosis • Antiproliferative effect on pancreatic duct cells • Reduce insulin signal transduction	• Conversion to mTORi from CNI is associated with worsening insulin resistance and increased incidence of acute rejection[15] • Effect is similar between sirolimus and everolimus[15]
Other agents	• Azathioprine, mycophenolate, and belatacept do not play a major role in PTDM[16]	
Preoperative impaired glucose tolerance and perioperative hyperglycemia • Risk seems to be highest among patients who require insulin in the immediate postoperative period[15] • Perioperative hyperglycemia might help identifying patients at increased risk for PTDM[15]		
Obesity • BMI ≥ 30 kg/m^2 [14,16] • Central obesity: the location of adipose tissue around the center of the body is more important than the total mass[4] • Weight gain after transplant is very common (steroid use, improved appetite, fewer dietary restrictions), which leads to increase in insulin resistance[1]		
Infections: Hepatitis C, CMV • Patients with HCV are 4 times likely to develop PTDM due to HCV-induced islet cell dysfunction and increased insulin resistance in setting of liver dysfunction.[17] • HCV treatment prior to transplantation may decrease the incidence of PTDM.[17]		
Hypomagnesemia • Low magnesium levels (commonly seen with CNI use) impact insulin signaling. Studies evaluating magnesium supplementation were inconclusive.[18]		
Several other factors including vitamin D deficiency or the use of statins are under investigation for their possible effect on development of PTDM.		

BMI, body mass index; CMV, cytomegalovirus; HCV, hepatitis C virus; mTORi, mammalian target of rapamycin inhibitor; PTDM; posttransplantation diabetes mellitus.

20 mg of prednisone is much more variable. Steroids mainly cause postprandial hyperglycemia; hence, the extra insulin required can be administered by increasing the rapid-acting mealtime insulin dose or by using a single dose of neutral protamine Hagedorn (NPH) at the same time as steroids administration. NPH peak

TABLE 19-3 Criteria for Posttransplant Diabetes and Prediabetes

	Posttransplant Diabetes	Posttransplant Prediabetes	
Oral glucose tolerance (OGTT)	≥200 mg/dL	140 and 199 mg/dL **Impaired glucose tolerance** (IGT)	• Measures 2-h plasma glucose level after a glucose load of 75 g • Considered the gold standard for the diagnosis of PTDM • Allows the diagnosis of IGT, which is an independent risk factor for long-term PTDM • Use is limited by inconvenience and cost
Fasting plasma glucose (FPG)	≥126 mg/dL	100 and 125 mg/dL **Impaired fasting glucose**	• Fasting is defined as no caloric intake for at least 8 hours • An abnormal fasting blood glucose should be confirmed on another day
Hemoglobin A1C	≥6.5%	5.7%-6.4%	• Done at least 3 or more months post transplantation[17] • A normal HbA1C in the first 12 mo is not reliable and does not exclude PTDM due to multiple variables in this period of time affecting RBC life span including kidney disease–associated anemia, reduced erythropoiesis by immunosuppressive therapy, erythropoietin analogues use, posttransplant blood transfusion, and inflammation[1] • An abnormal A1C (5.7% or higher) in the early posttransplant period or with anemia indicates a possible PTDM, which should be investigated using other methods like OGTT

(Continued)

TABLE 19-3 Criteria for Posttransplant Diabetes and Prediabetes (Continued)

	Posttransplant Diabetes	Posttransplant Prediabetes	
Random plasma glucose	≥200 mg/dL + Symptomatic hyperglycemia	-	• Symptoms include polyuria, polydipsia, and unexplained weight loss

PTDM diagnosis should not be made within the first 6 wk after transplantation to avoid labeling kidney transplant recipients with PTDM in the setting of transient hyperglycemia

The diagnosis of PTDM has no "end date": a patient diagnosed with diabetes at any time after kidney transplantation can be still classified as PTDM[2]

Screening for PTDM

All kidney transplant recipients should be routinely screened for PTDM after transplantation by one of the following methods[2,4]:

- *FPG:* measured weekly during the first 4 wk post transplant, then at 3 and 6 mo post transplant, then yearly
- *Hb A1C*: can be checked at 3 mo post transplant (not sooner) followed by repeat measurement every 3 mo in the first year and then yearly thereafter
- *OGTT*: might be reserved for patients with A1C of >5.7% as it will detect PTDM in 90% of these individuals compared with only 50% if administered to all transplant recipients
- *Afternoon glucose monitoring*: used mainly in the first few weeks post transplant. Readings of ≥200 mg/dL are concerning for PTDM and warrant further testing. This approach has not been validated for diagnosis of PTDM.

PTDM, posttransplantation diabetes mellitus.

effect and duration of action mimic the effect of steroids on glycemia. **Tables 19-4** and **19-5** show the general Washington University School of Medicine guidelines to estimate insulin doses.[21]

- **Early (1-6 weeks) posttransplant hyperglycemia**
  - The total daily dose of insulin in the immediate posttransplant period can provide guidance for posthospitalization hyperglycemia management[2] (**Table 19-6**).
  - Prior to discharge, patients should receive proper nutritional and diabetes education that should include self-monitoring of blood glucose, insulin administration, storage of insulin, troubleshooting, and hypoglycemia detection and management.
  - In patients on oral agents or basal insulin only, checking blood glucose once or twice per day—before breakfast (fasting) and in the afternoon/evening before dinner—is typically recommended.
  - Patients on multiple doses of insulin will need more frequent monitoring—4 times per day including fasting, premeal, and bedtime or the use of continuous glucose monitoring systems.
  - Recommended glycemic targets: preprandial capillary plasma glucose 80 to 130 mg/dL, peak postprandial capillary plasma glucose <180 mg/dL.

TABLE 19-4 General Insulin Dosing Suggestions

Patient Population	Total Daily Dose (units/kg)
Insulin sensitive	
No history of DM, BG > 180	0.2
H/o pancreatectomy	0.2
AKI/CKD/ESKD/ESLD	0.3
Malnourished/elderly	0.3
T1DM	0.4
T2DM—insulin naïve, BMI < 30	0.3-0.4
Insulin resistant	
T2DM—insulin naïve, BMI ≥ 30	0.4-0.5
T2DM—insulin experienced	0.5-0.6
T2DM on steroids	0.5+

AKI, acute kidney injury; BG, blood glucose; BMI, body mass index; CKD, chronic kidney disease; DM, diabetes mellitus; ESKD, end-stage kidney disease; ESLD, end-stage liver disease; T1DM, type 1 diabetes mellitus; T2DM, type 2 diabetes mellitus.

TABLE 19-5 Steroid-Induced Hyperglycemia Insulin Dosing

1. Convert steroids to prednisone dose equivalent: prednisone 20 mg = methylprednisolone 16 mg = dexamethasone 3 mg
2. For patient on >100 mg of prednisone, consider Endocrinology Diabetes consult
3. For patients on 40-100 mg of prednisone, use the following recommendations as initial regimen
4. Clinical judgment in insulin dosing is essential, monitor BG trends closely

Insulin naïve, prednisone dose <40 mg	Insulin resistant, prednisone dose >40 mg but <100 mg
→ If on prednisone or methylprednisolone once daily, start NPH 10 units with steroids → If on dexamethasone or other steroid dosed multiple times daily, start rapid-acting insulin (lispro) 3-5 units with meals plus correction scale → Adjust dose by 10%-20% daily to meet BG goals	$\frac{(\textit{prednisone equivalent}\,(mg) - 20)}{20} \times 0.1\ \textit{units} \times \textit{weight}\,(kg)$ → Max. initial dose of NPH – 20 units for insulin naïve or 40 units for experienced → Add this dose to patient's basal-bolus regimen

BG, blood glucose; NPH, neutral protamine Hagedorn.

TABLE 19-6 Early (1-6 wk) Posttransplant Hyperglycemia Management

Total Daily Dose of Insulin in the Immediate posttransplant Period	Insulin Therapy & Consideration	
≥20 units • Patient typically requires insulin therapy after hospital discharge. • Use one or more of the following insulins:	**Intermediate-acting insulin:** **Neutral Protamine Hagedorn (NPH) insulin** Duration of action: 8-12 h	• Once daily, administered same time as steroids dose • Initial dose is 5-10 units or based on steroids-induced hyperglycemia equation as above • The timing of NPH peak matches the timing of steroids-induced hyperglycemia in the afternoon • Adjust dose based on afternoon glucose levels
	Basal insulin: Detemir/Glargine Duration of action: Detemir: 18-24 h Glargine: 20-24 h	• Used in patients with more persistent hyperglycemia, including fasting hyperglycemia • Once daily dosing • Morning dosing may be preferred, which allows the peak effect of these insulins (if present) to happen during the daytime when steroids peak effect is expected. Also, this approach may reduce nighttime hypoglycemia when steroids effect starts fading away.
	Rapid-acting insulin: Aspart/Lispro Duration of action: 4 h	• Used either as a fixed dose before each meal, might need a higher dose for lunch and dinner, or as a sliding scale insulin to correct hyperglycemia
	• Regimen should be tailored individually based on glucocorticoids dose, allograft function, concurrent infection, nutritional source, appetite/food intake. • The duration of insulin treatment depends on patient's response to therapy and subsequent blood glucose monitoring. • Patients whose insulin requirements decrease to <20 units per day can typically be transitioned to oral hypoglycemic agents.	
<20 units	• Can be usually treated with oral hypoglycemic agents only. • Use of agents that have a low risk of hypoglycemia and have low or no renal excretion is preferred.	

Management of PTDM

- In the absence of randomized controlled trials, the management of PTDM follows similar principles as used for treatment of T2DM with some transplant-specific adjustments.
- Management strategies aim to improve β-cell function and decrease insulin resistance.

Lifestyle Modifications

- In all kidney transplant recipients with PTDM, we start with lifestyle interventions focusing on dietary modification, weight loss, and exercise.
- Weight gain after kidney transplantation is very common as a consequençe of the use of steroids and improved appetite due to uremic anorexia resolution, so counseling on appropriate weight gain management is crucial.[1]
- Studies examining the effects of lifestyle modification in the transplant population are limited; however, lifestyle changes are likely beneficial based on data in nontransplant patients with T2DM where a combination of exercise and weight loss improves insulin resistance and β-cell function.

Pharmacologic Therapy

- Medical therapy is challenging due to paucity of available studies in this patient population, frequent interactions between glucose-lowering and immunosuppressive agents, need for frequent dose adjustments due to changing kidney function, and medication side effects.
- Therapy should begin with oral hypoglycemic agents. If adequate glycemic control cannot be achieved, patients should be started on insulin therapy.
- It is important to remember that calcineurin inhibitors and mammalian target of rapamycin inhibitors are metabolized and eliminated via cytochrome P450 3A4/5 and permeability glycoprotein, so drugs that inhibit/induce or competitively compete for elimination can significantly alter their levels. In addition, medications that delay gastric emptying may affect absorption of immunosuppressive agents; however, this has yet to be demonstrated in clinical studies.
- **Adjustment of immunosuppression**
  - Immunosuppression is one of the most important modifiable risk factors for PTDM.
  - Renal transplant providers may consider adjustment of immunosuppressive therapy in order to reverse or ameliorate glycemic control, on a case-by-case basis, while maintaining reasonable risk and benefit assessment.[22]
- **Noninsulin agents**
  - Pharmacological agents for treatment of T2DM have expanded significantly over the past few years, but their role in improving outcomes in PTDM is not well understood because most studies evaluating these medications in PTDM are small, single center, and noncontrolled.[23]
  - Drug selection should be based on efficacy, side effects, potential drug-drug interactions, renal function, and cost.
  - **Table 19-7** shows different types of glucose-lowering agents, their mechanisms of action, main side effects, and considerations when used for patients with reduced renal function.[3,25,26]
- **Insulin therapy**
  - Many patients with PTDM will require initiation of insulin, especially those with blood glucose >200 mg/dL.

TABLE 19-7 Noninsulin Therapy for Posttransplantation Diabetes Mellitus

Medication	Mechanism	A1C Reduction/ Limitations/Side Effects/ Notes	Use in Reduced Renal Function
DPP-4 inhibitors Sitagliptin Linagliptin Saxagliptin Alogliptin Vildagliptin	• Inactivate DPP-4, an enzyme responsive for deactivation of glucose-dependent insulinotropic polypeptide and GLP-1 • Cause a glucose-dependent increase in insulin release • Reduce postprandial hepatic glucose production	• Expected A1C reduction 0.5%-0.8% • Low risk for hypoglycemia • Associated with pancreatitis (rare). Do not start if Hx of pancreatitis is present. Stop if pancreatitis developed[24] • Sitagliptin might increase cyclosporine level and may prolong the QT interval • Avoid Saxagliptin in patients with heart failure	• Require dose adjustment with kidney dysfunction (except for linagliptin)
GLP-1 receptor agonists Exenatide IR (SC bid) Liraglutide (SC once daily) Exenatide ER (SC once weekly) Dulaglutide (SC once weekly) Semaglutide (SC once weekly) Lixisenatide (SC once daily) **GLP1/GIP agonists** Tirzepatide	• Enhance glucose-dependent insulin secretion and inhibit β-cell apoptosis • Reduce postprandial hepatic glucose production • Decrease glucagon secretion • Delay gastric emptying promoting satiety and appetite suppression contributing to weight loss	• Expected A1C reduction 0.9%-1.4% • Associated with pancreatitis (rare). Do not start if Hx of pancreatitis is present. Stop if pancreatitis develops. • Do not use if personal or family history of medullary thyroid cancer or MEN type 2 is present • Associated with nausea, vomiting, diarrhea, abdominal pain (dose limiting, may worsen with concomitant mycophenolate administration) • Associated with decrease in cardiovascular events in the general population • Emerging data suggest that these drugs might be a safe and effective option for treatment of PTDM	• Do not use: Exenatide if eGFR <30 (careful if <45) Lixisenatide if eGFR <15 (careful if <30) • Other agents should be used with caution in renal impairment given potential GI side effects, which may lead to dehydration and worsening of renal function

TABLE 19-7 Noninsulin Therapy for Posttransplantation Diabetes Mellitus (Continued)

Medication	Mechanism	A1C Reduction/ Limitations/Side Effects/ Notes	Use in Reduced Renal Function
SGLT2 inhibitors Canagliflozin Dapagliflozin Empagliflozin Ertugliflozin	• Inhibit glucose absorption in the proximal tubule causing glycosuria, weight loss, and improved glycemic control	• Expected A1C reduction 0.6%-1.0% • Associated with increased urination/ urgency, hypotension, bone fractures, yeast and urinary tract infections • Associated with euglycemic ketoacidosis, especially in patient with insulin insufficiency/deficiency • Associated with AKI due to afferent arteriole vasoconstriction coupled with volume loss due to its diuretic effect • Decrease in albuminuria, hyperlipidemia, risk of kidney failure, and cardiovascular events in patients with CKD observed • SGLT2 inhibitors are used on a case-by-case basis due to paucity of data in transplant patients and concern for infection. Overall, we elect to avoid these agents until 6 mo post transplant. • Theoretical interaction through competitive elimination via P-glycoprotein with mTORi and CNI agents (not clinically significant)	• Dose adjustment necessary based on eGFR • Usually not recommended for eGFR <30-45 (case-by-case basis)

(Continued)

TABLE 19-7 Noninsulin Therapy for Posttransplantation Diabetes Mellitus (Continued)

Medication	Mechanism	A1C Reduction/ Limitations/Side Effects/ Notes	Use in Reduced Renal Function
Biguanides Metformin	• Decrease hepatic glucose release • Decrease intestinal absorption of glucose • Improve insulin sensitivity (glucose uptake and utilization)	• A1C reduction of 0.8%-1.0% • Associated with nausea, diarrhea, bloating, and abdominal pain, which may worsen with mycophenolate • Extended-release formulation might help with GI side effects • Avoid use in congestive heart failure, cirrhosis, and renal failure due to possible increased risk of lactic acidosis • No significant interactions with immunosuppressive agents	• Start if eGFR ≥60 • OK to continue if eGFR is 45-60 • Do not start if eGFR 30-45 • Contraindicated/ stop if < 30
Sulfonylureas Glimepiride Glipizide Glyburide	• Stimulate pancreatic secretion of insulin independent of glucose levels	• A1C reduction of 0.7%-1.0% • Associated with hypoglycemia, weight gain, and photosensitivity • Glipizide or glimepiride are preferred in CKD due to a lower risk of hypoglycemia • Glipizide and glyburide have been associated with increased cyclosporine levels	• Dose adjustment is necessary based on eGFR
Glinides Repaglinide Nateglinide	• Increase insulin secretion from pancreas in glucose-dependent fashion	• A1C reduction 0.5%-1.0% • Associated with hypoglycemia, weight gain • Needs to be taken within 30 min of a meal • Daily dosing of 2-3 times might limit use • Cyclosporine may increase repaglinide levels, dose limit 6 mg/d	• No dose adjustment is necessary with impaired renal function • Titrate dose carefully

TABLE 19-7 Noninsulin Therapy for Posttransplantation Diabetes Mellitus (Continued)

Medication	Mechanism	A1C Reduction/ Limitations/Side Effects/ Notes	Use in Reduced Renal Function
α-Glucosidase inhibitors Acarbose Miglitol	• Delay digestion and absorption of carbohydrates leading to lower postprandial hyperglycemia	• A1C reduction 0.6%-0.9% • Associated with flatulence, diarrhea, abdominal pain, elevations in AST/ALT • Take with meals • Avoid use in patients with history of IBD	• Not recommended if CrCl <25 or creatinine >2 mg/dL
Thiazolidine-diones Pioglitazone Rosiglitazone	• Decrease insulin resistance (muscle and fat tissue) • Do not increase pancreatic insulin secretion	• A1C reduction 0.7%-1.1%, used as an adjunctive therapy • Associated with fluid retention, edema, weight gain, bone loss, anemia, bladder cancer, macular edema • May worsen immunosuppression-associated bone loss • Delayed onset of action 4-12 wk • Activation of proliferator-activated receptor γ (PPARγ) increases sodium reabsorption leading to fluid retention. Do not use with advanced heart failure or hepatic dysfunction. • Rosiglitazone is not used in transplant patient	• No dose adjustment is necessary with impaired renal function • Titrate dose carefully

A1C, hemoglobin A1C; AKI, acute kidney injury; ALT, alanine transaminase; AST, aspartate aminotransferase; CKD, chronic kidney disease; CNI, calcineurin inhibitor; CrCl; creatinine clearance; DDP4, dipeptidyl peptidase 4; eGFR, estimated glomerular filtration rate; GI, gastrointestinal; GIP, gastric inhibitory polypeptide; GLP-1, glucagon-like peptide-1; IBD, inflammatory bowel disease; mTORi, mammalian target of rapamycin inhibitor; PTDM, posttransplantation diabetes mellitus; SGLT2: sodium glucose transporter 2.

- We initiate insulin therapy if oral agents have not been effective or have caused unacceptable side effects.
- Diurnal glucose patterns differ among patients who are receiving glucocorticoids and even with small doses of prednisone (5 mg/d in the morning.) We typically observe a late-afternoon or early-evening peak in blood glucose, requiring higher mealtime insulin doses with lunch and dinner.
- There are little data regarding insulin therapy among kidney transplant recipients. We use the same approach as in the early posttransplant period (see Early posttransplant hyperglycemia section).

Other Nonpharmacologic Therapies

- There are no studies evaluating the efficacy of diabetes technology (including continuous glucose monitors [CGMs] and insulin pumps) in kidney transplant recipients.
- CGMs have been successfully used to examine glycemic control and variability after kidney transplantation.[27,28]
- These devices play an increasingly important role in the management of hyperglycemia in patients with type 1 and type 2 diabetes and provide less invasive glucose measurements and more comprehensive glycemic data than conventional metrics.
- CGMs and insulin pumps have the potential to improve metabolic outcomes and quality of life in patients after kidney transplantation, and we recommend their use based on case-by-case approach.

MONITORING

- Glycemic control targets in kidney transplant recipients are similar to those in nontransplant patients with diabetes. The ADA suggests a reasonable A1C target of <7%. However, this target could be loosened to <8% based on duration of diabetes, comorbidities, hypoglycemia risk, and life expectancy.[19] The Kidney Disease: Improving Global Outcomes (KDIGO) guidelines recommend an A1C goal of 7% to 7.5% in PTDM.[22]
- Factors affecting A1C validity (anemia, blood transfusions, erythropoietin replacement, chronic renal disease, etc.) should be always considered, and alternative methods to evaluate glycemic control might need to be used.
- When A1C accuracy is questioned while evaluating for glycemia, providers should use other markers of glycemic control, including self-monitoring of blood glucose using multiple daily glucose checks (fasting, preprandial, and bedtime), glycated albumin, and fructosamine. The last 2 markers reflect glycemia over 2 to 3 weeks but can be falsely low in situations associated with rapid serum protein turnover such as nephrotic syndrome.
- CGM devices can also be used to evaluate glycemic control when A1C is not reliable. Current general population targets for CGM use are[29]
  - time in range (70-180 mg/dL) of more than 70%
  - time below range (<70 mg/dL) of less than 4%
  - time above range (>180 mg/dL) of less than 26%
- Patients should undergo regular screening for kidney disease, retinopathy, neuropathy, and diabetic foot disease.
- In addition, patients with PTDM require tight control of other cardiovascular risk factors, such as smoking cessation, dyslipidemia management, and blood pressure control.

OUTCOME AND PROGNOSIS

- PTDM is associated with poor outcomes, including a higher risk of microvascular and macrovascular complications, which may develop at an accelerated rate within 3 years post transplant.[1,30] PTDM is associated with a 60% increase in posttransplantation myocardial infraction, increased risk of cerebrovascular accidents, and aortic and lower extremity arterial disease.[1]
- PTDM can negatively affect long-term patient survival, with cardiovascular mortality being the main cause for decreased survival rates. The effect of PTDM on mortality remains lower than that of pretransplant diabetes.[31,32]
- PTDM is associated with decreased long-term graft survival, with a 3.7 relative risk of graft loss.[33] While the effect of PTDM on graft survival is mainly driven by the associated increased mortality, graft failure without death can still occur due to diabetic nephropathy and/or graft rejection.[8,34]
- PTDM is associated with increased risk for infections, mainly urinary tract infections; pneumonia; and cytomegalovirus infections.

CONCLUSION

- Transient hyperglycemia, impaired glucose tolerance, and diabetes are commonly encountered after kidney transplantation. These conditions are associated with increased morbidity and mortality.
- Graft and patient survival after kidney transplant have significantly improved over time, with advances in immunosuppression, surgical techniques, and management of infectious complications.
- Early identification and management of posttransplant diabetes and prediabetes are crucial to improving patients' survival and quality of life.

REFERENCES

1. Martinez Cantarin MP. Diabetes in kidney transplantation. *Adv Chronic Kidney Dis.* 2021;28(6):596-605.
2. Sharif A, Hecking M, de Vries AP, et al. Proceedings from an international consensus meeting on posttransplantation diabetes mellitus: recommendations and future directions. *Am J Transplant.* 2014;14(9):1992-2000.
3. Galindo RJ, Fayfman M, Umpierrez GE. Perioperative management of hyperglycemia and diabetes in cardiac surgery patients. *Endocrinol Metab Clin North Am.* 2018;47(1):203-22.
4. Jenssen T, Hartmann A. Post-transplant diabetes mellitus in patients with solid organ transplants. *Nat Rev Endocrinol.* 2019;15(3):172-88.
5. Porrini EL, Díaz JM, Moreso F, et al. Clinical evolution of post-transplant diabetes mellitus. *Nephrol Dial Transplant.* 2016;31(3):495-505.
6. Hart A, Smith JM, Skeans MA, et al. OPTN/SRTR 2017 Annual data report: kidney. *Am J Transplant.* 2019;19(suppl 2):19-23.
7. Matas AJ, Smith JM, Skeans MA, et al. OPTN/SRTR 2013 Annual data report: kidney. *Am J Transplant.* 2015;15(suppl 2):1-34.
8. Kasiske BL, Snyder JJ, Gilbertson D, Matas AJ. Diabetes mellitus after kidney transplantation in the United States. *Am J Transplant.* 2003;3(2):178-85.
9. Malik RF, Jia Y, Mansour SG, et al. Post-transplant diabetes mellitus in kidney transplant recipients: a multicenter study. *Kidney360.* 2021;2(8):1296-307.

10. Serrano OK, Kandaswamy R, Gillingham K, et al. Rapid discontinuation of prednisone in kidney transplant recipients: 15-year outcomes from the University of Minnesota. *Transplantation*. 2017;101(10):2590-8.
11. Woodle ES, First MR, Pirsch J, et al; Astellas Corticosteroid Withdrawal Study Group. A prospective, randomized, double-blind, placebo-controlled multicenter trial comparing early (7 day) corticosteroid cessation versus long-term, low-dose corticosteroid therapy. *Ann Surg*. 2008;248(4):564-77.
12. Torres A, Hernández D, Moreso F, et al. Randomized controlled trial assessing the impact of tacrolimus versus cyclosporine on the incidence of posttransplant diabetes mellitus. *Kidney Int Rep*. 2018;3(6):1304-15.
13. Vincenti F, Friman S, Scheuermann E, et al; DIRECT Diabetes Incidence after Renal Transplantation: Neoral C Monitoring Versus Tacrolimus Investigators. Results of an international, randomized trial comparing glucose metabolism disorders and outcome with cyclosporine versus tacrolimus. *Am J Transplant*. 2007;7(6):1506-14.
14. Maes BD, Kuypers D, Messiaen T, et al. Posttransplantation diabetes mellitus in FK-506-treated renal transplant recipients: analysis of incidence and risk factors. *Transplantation*. 2001;72(10):1655-61.
15. Sulanc E, Lane JT, Puumala SE, Groggel GC, Wrenshall LE, Stevens RB. New-onset diabetes after kidney transplantation: an application of 2003 International Guidelines. *Transplantation*. 2005;80(7):945-52.
16. Faucher Q, Jardou M, Brossier C, Picard N, Marquet P, Lawson R. Is intestinal dysbiosis-associated with immunosuppressive therapy a key factor in the pathophysiology of post-transplant diabetes mellitus? *Front Endocrinol*. 2022;13:898878.
17. Fabrizi F, Martin P, Dixit V, Bunnapradist S, Kanwal F, Dulai G. Post-transplant diabetes mellitus and HCV seropositive status after renal transplantation: meta-analysis of clinical studies. *Am J Transplant*. 2005;5(10):2433-40.
18. Shivaswamy V, Boerner B, Larsen J. Post-transplant diabetes mellitus: causes, treatment, and impact on outcomes. *Endocr Rev*. 2016;37(1):37-61.
19. American Diabetes Association. Standards of medical care in diabetes-2022 abridged for primary care providers. *Clin Diabetes*. 2022;40(1):10-38.
20. Wallia A, Schmidt K, Oakes DJ, et al. Glycemic control reduces infections in post-liver transplant patients: results of a prospective, randomized study. *J Clin Endocrinol Metab*. 2017;102(2):451-9.
21. Baranski TJ, McGill JB, Silverstein JM, eds. *The Washington Manual Subspecialty Consult Series. Endocrinology Subspecialty Consult*. 4th ed. Wolters Kluwer/Lippincott Williams & Wilkins; 2020.
22. Kasiske BL, Zeier MG, Chapman JR, et al. KDIGO clinical practice guideline for the care of kidney transplant recipients: a summary. *Kidney Int*. 2010;77(4):299-311.
23. Lo C, Toyama T, Oshima M, et al. Glucose-lowering agents for treating pre-existing and new-onset diabetes in kidney transplant recipients. *Cochrane Database Syst Rev*. 2020;8(8):CD009966.
24. Lee M, Sun J, Han M, et al. Nationwide trends in pancreatitis and pancreatic cancer risk among patients with newly diagnosed type 2 diabetes receiving dipeptidyl peptidase 4 inhibitors. *Diabetes Care*. 2019;42(11):2057-64.
25. Vanhove T, Remijsen Q, Kuypers D, Gillard P. Drug-drug interactions between immunosuppressants and antidiabetic drugs in the treatment of post-transplant diabetes mellitus. *Transplant Rev (Orlando)*. 2017;31(2):69-77.
26. Tsapas A, Avgerinos I, Karagiannis T, et al. Comparative effectiveness of glucose-lowering drugs for type 2 diabetes: a systematic review and network meta-analysis. *Ann Intern Med*. 2020;173(4):278-86.
27. Aouad LJ, Clayton P, Wyburn KR, Gracey DM, Chadban SJ. Evolution of glycemic control and variability after kidney transplant. *Transplantation*. 2018;102(9):1563-8.
28. Jin HY, Lee KA, Kim YJ, et al. The degree of hyperglycemia excursion in patients of kidney transplantation (KT) or liver transplantation (LT) assessed by continuous glucose monitoring (CGM): pilot study. *J Diabetes Res*. 2019;2019:1757182.

29. Battelino T, Danne T, Bergenstal RM, et al. Clinical targets for continuous glucose monitoring data interpretation: recommendations from the international consensus on time in range. *Diabetes Care*. 2019;42(8):1593-603.
30. Burroughs TE, Swindle J, Takemoto S, et al. Diabetic complications associated with new-onset diabetes mellitus in renal transplant recipients. *Transplantation*. 2007;83(8):1027-34.
31. Sumrani N, Delaney V, Ding Z, et al. Posttransplant diabetes mellitus in cyclosporine-treated renal transplant recipients. *Transplant Proc*. 1991;23(1 pt 2):1249-50.
32. Lim WH, Lok CE, Kim SJ, et al. Impact of pretransplant and new-onset diabetes after transplantation on the risk of major adverse cardiovascular events in kidney transplant recipients: a population-based cohort study. *Transplantation*. 2021;105(11):2470-81.
33. Miles AM, Sumrani N, Horowitz R, et al. Diabetes mellitus after renal transplantation: as deleterious as non-transplant-associated diabetes? *Transplantation*. 1998;65(3):380-4.
34. Cole EH, Johnston O, Rose CL, Gill JS. Impact of acute rejection and new-onset diabetes on long-term transplant graft and patient survival. *Clin J Am Soc Nephrol*. 2008;3(3):814-21.

20 ABO-, HLA-Incompatible Transplantation and Paired Exchange

Rowena Delos Santos

ABO-Incompatible Kidney Transplantation

GENERAL PRINCIPLES

- ABO blood group antigens include A and B, and lack of A and B (O blood group). Individuals can be blood group A, B, AB, and O. Another part of blood group antigens includes Rhesus (Rh) factor. Transplant focuses on the major blood groups and not necessarily the Rh factor, so (Rh+ and Rh−) will be grouped together.[1] Blood transfusions take into consideration the Rh factor. **Table 20-1** gives ABO blood group frequency and antibodies in the US.[2]
- ABO blood group antigens are expressed on red blood cells, lymphocytes, platelets, and endothelial and epithelial cells of the body.
- Naturally occurring antibodies against ABO blood group antigens exist such that blood group A makes antibodies against B antigens, blood group B makes antibodies against A antigens, blood group AB makes no antibodies, and blood group O makes antibodies against blood groups A and B.[1]
- Red blood cell (RBC) agglutination uses serial dilutions using patient serum incubated with RBC of appropriate type looking for macroscopic agglutination of RBC to detect IgM isoagglutinins. Anti-human globulin to heavy chain IgG is used to measure IgG antibodies and measure agglutination.[1]
- Antibodies against blood group antigens are reported out as an anti-A and/or anti-B isoagglutinin titer, which can range from 1:2 to >1:256.
- Isoagglutinin titer testing is in part subjective due to reader/observer variation. For example, an anti-A isoagglutinin titer of 1:32 could be lower 1:16 or higher 1:64.

TABLE 20-1 ABO Blood Group Frequency in the US, Naturally Occurring Antibodies Against Other Blood Group Antigens[2]

	A	B	AB	O
Frequency of blood type in the US (%)				
• African American	26	19	4.3	51
• Asian	27.5	25.4	7.1	40
• Caucasian	40	11	4	45
• Hispanic	31	10	2.2	57
Naturally occurring antibodies against blood group antigens	B	A	None	A and B

Data from Facts About Blood and Blood Types. American Red Cross. Accessed April 8, 2023. https://www.redcrossblood.org/donate-blood/blood-types.html.

GOALS AND OUTCOMES

- Blood group incompatibility is usually an absolute contraindication to transplantation.
- Performing ABO-incompatible transplants would normally lead to hyperacute or severe acute antibody-mediated rejection (AMR) from preformed anti-A and/or anti-B antibodies, with complement activation, coagulation cascade activation leading to ischemic injury.
- ABO-incompatible transplantation was pioneered due to lack of available deceased donors and difficulty of expanding the donor pool.
- Goal of ABO-incompatible transplant is to prepare a recipient to accept and not reject a kidney transplant from a donor with an incompatible blood type, i.e., decrease risk from ABO-incompatible barrier.
- Slightly higher risk of graft/patient loss in the first year after transplant but comparable with ABO compatible afterward.[3] Please see **Table 20-2**.
- Lower 1-year patient survival in ABO incompatible appears mainly related to infection-related mortality.[3]
- Uncensored allograft survival within 1 year of transplant was 96% in ABO-incompatible compared with 98% in ABO-compatible transplant.[3]
- Higher biopsy-proven acute rejection in ABO incompatible compared with ABO compatible within the first year post transplant (24% vs. 17%, respectively), with more AMR.[3]
- More viral-related, BK and cytomegalovirus, infections as well as nonviral infections in ABO incompatible compared with ABO compatible.
- Bleeding risk is increased in ABO incompatible compared with ABO compatible.
- Most complications are within the first year, and the allograft survival of those who are past 1 year for ABO incompatible is comparable with ABO compatible.
- No significant difference between cancer risks for ABO-incompatible and ABO-compatible transplantation. The risk for cancer is higher than in the general population.

TABLE 20-2 ABO-Incompatible Kidney Transplant Outcomes

	ABO Incompatible	ABO Compatible
1-y Patient survival (%)	98	99
1-y Allograft survival (%) uncensored	96	98
Bleeding (%)	11	4
Severe nonviral infections (%)	12	6
BK infection (%)	14	8
CMV infection (%)	22	19
Biopsy-proven acute rejection (%)	24	17
Antibody-mediated rejection (%)	10	2

CMV, cytomegalovirus.
Data from Annelies E. de Weerd, Michiel G.H. Betjes. ABO-incompatible kidney transplant outcomes. A meta-analysis. *Clin J Am Soc Nephrol*. 2018;13(8):1234-43.

PREPARATION FOR ABO-INCOMPATIBLE TRANSPLANTATION

Titers

- Centers will typically set an isoagglutinin cutoff titer acceptable to attempt an ABO-incompatible transplant.
- For instance, our center chooses a titer of ≤1:128.
- Prior to the planned transplant, centers will follow protocols to prepare the recipient, with goal of reaching a lower isoagglutinin titer that the center deems acceptable to perform a transplant.[3]
- Isoagglutinin titer goal for transplant is center specific; we aim for levels of ≤1:8.

Therapies

- B-cell-depleting therapies such as anti-CD20 antibody such as rituximab that depletes B cells, which can turn into plasma cells that produce anti-A or anti-B antibodies.[4-6]
- Splenectomy was previously used in ABO-incompatible protocols, but less so now.[4] Splenectomy has been used in cases of refractory AMR.
- Removal of circulating ABO antibodies with therapeutic plasma exchange (plasmapheresis, done in the US) or immunoadsorption (done in Europe and Japan).[4-6] Each session typically decreases the isoagglutinin titer by 1 dilution. Example: with a starting titer of 1:32, it would take 2 plasmapheresis treatments to get down to desired titer, i.e., 1:32 → 1:16 → 1:8.
- Immunomodulation with IV immunoglobulin—given typically after plasmapheresis treatments to replace lost immunoglobulin during plasmapheresis and to potentially block receptors on anti-A and anti-B plasma cells to prevent antibody rebound post plasmapheresis.[4-6]
- Timing of treatments is dependent on center-specific protocols.

Washington University Guidelines

- General guidelines of Washington University Transplant Center are summarized in **Figure 20-1**.
- Evaluation, education, and explanation of risks and benefits of ABO-incompatible transplant.
- Four weeks prior to planned surgery, patient receives rituximab and final crossmatch is completed. The rationale for early crossmatch is that rituximab will lead to false-positive flow crossmatch.
- After rituximab, patients are started on antimetabolite, acyclovir and sulfamethoxazole/trimethoprim, to maintain a degree of immune suppression and for infection prophylaxis.
- Two weeks before surgery, a repeat isoagglutinin titer is performed to determine the number of therapeutic plasma exchanges that need to be done prior to surgery.
- We do therapeutic plasma exchanges; 1 to 1.5 × plasma volume exchanged per treatment. We usually use albumin replacement and give intravenous immunoglobulin (IVIg) following each treatment.
- We do daily testing of isoagglutinin titer to determine that treatments are decreasing titer appropriately. In addition, we test international normalized ratio and fibrinogen daily.
- If blood products are required during treatment, the packed RBCs should match the recipient blood type. **If fresh frozen plasma (FFP) is required**, we use **DONOR-type FFP or AB-type FFP**, as these will lack anti-A and/or anti-B antibodies.

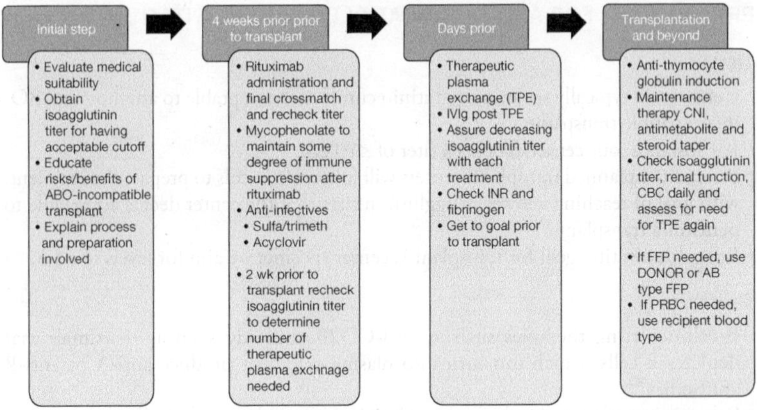

Figure 20-1. **Steps for ABO-incompatible transplantation.** CBC, complete blood count; CNI, calcineurin inhibitor; FFP, fresh frozen plasma; INR, international normalized ratio; IVIg, intravenous immunoglobulin; PRBC, packed red blood cell.

- We use anti-thymocyte globulin for induction. Our typical dose if 5 mg/kg.
- For maintenance immunosuppression, we prescribe calcineurin inhibitor (tacrolimus), antimetabolite (mycophenolate), and corticosteroid (prednisone).
- Isoagglutinin titers are checked daily after transplantation to assure that titers remain low.
- Further treatments with plasmapheresis with or without rituximab might be needed based on the titer level.

A2 INTO B OR O BLOOD TYPE

- Two types of antigens exist for A blood type, A1 and A2 (non-A1).
- The A2 blood type is expressed less on cells and less immunogenic than A1.
- United Network of Organ Sharing (UNOS) allows for A2 into B or O blood types for patients whose centers determine they are eligible based on isoagglutinin titer testing. There are center-specific protocols for transplanting these ABO-incompatible organs.[7,8]

NOTES IN TRANSPLANT PATHOLOGY

- Protocol biopsies of ABO-incompatible transplants C4d staining is positive in peritubular capillaries but without other histologic evidence of AMR such as glomerulitis and peritubular capillaritis.[9,10]
- C4d staining alone in the absence of an inflammatory/histologic reaction may suggest transplant accommodation for ABO-incompatible transplant.[9,10]

HLA-Incompatible Transplantation

GENERAL PRINCIPLES

- HLA incompatibility does not refer to HLA mismatches in A, B, DR between donor and recipient. HLA incompatibility refers to the presence of preexisting HLA antibodies within a recipient against potential donors.

- HLA antibodies arise due to a sensitizing event:
  - Blood transfusion
  - Pregnancy
  - Transplant
- Not all sensitizing events will lead to development of antibodies, but these do pose a risk for developing potential HLA antibodies.
- Approximately 11% of the US transplant waiting list is sensitized with calculated panel reactive antibody (cPRA) level of ≥80%.[11] See **Table 20-3**.
- Waiting times for patients with higher cPRA levels can be longer due to difficulty finding a compatible donor. Patients with high cPRA levels have added points that will prioritize them on the wait-list due to greater difficulty finding a compatible donor.[12] See **Table 20-4**.
- HLA incompatibility with resulting positive complement-dependent cytotoxicity (CDC) crossmatch is normally a contraindication to transplantation.
- If transplanted with preexisting anti-HLA antibodies and positive CDC crossmatch, result will be hyperacute rejection via AMR.
- Performed less frequently with increasing use of paired kidney donor exchange (see paired kidney donor exchange section below).

OUTCOMES

- Due to difficulty in finding compatible matches for patients with high cPRA and existing HLA antibodies, attempts at transplanting patients through this barrier have been done.
- Risk of clinical AMR after an HLA-incompatible transplant with presence of donor-specific antibody (DSA) can be between 30% and 40%.[13]
- The 1- and 5-year allograft outcomes with sensitized, CDC crossmatch-positive versus crossmatch-negative recipients (CDC+/FXM+ vs. CDC−/FXM+) showed 1-year allograft survival 82.4% versus 96.7% and 5-year allograft survival 64.9% versus 72.7%.[14]
- Differences between class I and class II DSAs and survival.
- Class I DSA with resulting AMR in the first year had higher graft loss in the first year post transplant but lower rates of graft loss in subsequent years, similar to the FXM- group.
- Class II DSA had less AMR and graft loss in the first year but higher graft loss in subsequent years compared with the class I DSA group; more chronic transplant glomerulopathy changes on biopsy.

TABLE 20-3 Calculated Panel Reactive Antibody Category and Representation on Waiting List

Calculated Panel Reactive Antibody	Number (%) of Total on Wait-list (*N* = 89,903)
0%	53,404 (59.4%)
1%-19%	11,965 (13.3%)
20%-79%	16,608 (18.5%)
80%-97%	4,770 (5.3%)
98%-100%	5,355 (5.9%)

Data from Organ Procurement & Transplantation Network. OPTN data on organ donation, waitlist and transplant activity dates from 1988, the first full year of OPTN data collection. Retrieved from https://optn.transplant.hrsa.gov/data/view-data-reports/build-advanced/.

TABLE 20-4 Additional Points for cPRA Categories for Prioritization of Kidney Donor Organs in High-cPRA Candidates on UNOS Deceased Donor Waiting List

cPRA (%)	Additional Points for Wait-List Candidate
0-19	0
20-29	0.08
30-39	0.21
40-49	0.34
50-59	0.48
60-69	0.81
70-74	1.09
75-79	1.58
80-84	2.46
85-89	4.05
90-94	6.71
95	10.82
96	12.17
97	17.3
98	24.4
99	50.09
100	202.1

cPRA, calculated panel reactive antibody; UNOS, United Network for Organ Sharing. Adapted with permission from Israni AK, Salkowski N, Gustafson S, et al. New national allocation policy for deceased donor kidneys in the united states and possible effect on patient outcomes. *J Am Soc Nephrol*. 2014;25(8):1842-8.

- The incidence of AMR is higher in HLA-incompatible transplants (47%) compared with ABO-incompatible transplants (14%).[15] See **Table 20-5**.
- Patients with clinical AMR have 80% death censored graft survival at 1 year and 69% at 5 years compared with non-AMR patients with death censored graft survival of 97% at 1 year and 93% at 5 years.[15]
- Patient survival of HLA-incompatible living donor kidney recipients at 8 years post transplant is 13.6% higher than matched patients who remained on wait-list and received deceased donor transplant.[15]
- Survival of HLA-incompatible living donor kidney recipients at 8 years post transplant is 32.6% higher than matched patient controls who remained on wait-list and did not receive a deceased donor transplant.[16]
- Despite less favorable outcomes, desensitization may be an option for some patients such as those with high cPRA > 98%, those who have tried kidney paired donation but have not been matched with a HLA-compatible donor, and those who are highly sensitized and have been on the waiting list for several years.[16]
- Patients need to be counseled extensively on risks and benefits of undergoing desensitization.[16]

TABLE 20-5 Antibody-Mediated Rejection Incidence and Proportion That are Subclinical

Total Population 2,316	Incidence of AMR ($n = 219$)	Clinical AMR ($n = 142$)	Subclinical AMR ($n = 77$)
Total patients	9.5%	6.1%	3.3%
Deceased donor compatible	1.7%	1.6%	0.1%
Deceased donor HLA incompatible	44.7%	28.2%	16.5%
Living donor compatible	0.7%	0.2%	0.5%
Living donor ABO incompatible	13.6%	11.1%	2.5%
Living donor HLA incompatible	47.4%	29.3%	18.1%

AMR, antibody-mediated rejection.
Data from Orandi BJ, Chow EH, Hsu A, et al. Quantifying renal allograft loss following early antibody-mediated rejection. *Am J Transplant.* 2015;15(2):489-98.

THERAPIES

- Goal is to attain a negative CDC crossmatch or negative flow crossmatch that is considered acceptable per center protocol for the intended recipient prior to transplant.
- Different protocols exist at select centers that perform desensitization for kidney transplant.
- Course takes weeks to months depending on whether living or deceased donor is being planned.
- Various procedures and agents are used in desensitization protocols. Some of these therapies are similar to those done for ABO-incompatible transplant, see **Table 20-6**.
- Some procedures and agents are used regularly (plasmapheresis, IVIg, rituximab), others are used for refractory cases (eculizumab, tocilizumab, splenectomy) or are under investigation (daratumumab, imlifidase, isatuximab, ixazomib, clazakizumab, carfilzomib). Note that a majority of these medications are used off-label.[17,18]

Kidney Paired Donor Exchange

GENERAL PRINCIPLES

- The Charlie Norwood Living Organ Donation Act of 2007 amended the original National Organ Transplant Act (NOTA) and made kidney paired donation allowable.[19]
- Advent of kidney paired donor exchange allows transplantation while avoiding ABO and HLA incompatibility.
- Donors who would have donated to their desired recipient instead would donate to a different person whom they are paired.

TABLE 20-6 Procedures and Treatments With Doses Used in HLA Desensitization Protocols for Select Patients

Treatment/Procedure	Purpose in Desensitization	Doses Found in Various Protocols
Plasmapheresis or immunoadsorption (Europe or Japan only)	Remove already present HLA alloantibodies	Treatments between 3 and 10 sessions depending on alloantibody titers
IV immunoglobulin	Immune modulatory; various inhibitory effects on immune system	Variable doses, anywhere between 100 mg/kg and 2 g/kg each administration, multiple doses
Anti-CD20 antibody	B-cell depletion; inhibits antibody production	Rituximab: Single or multiple doses 375 mg/m^2[a]
Proteosome inhibitors	Inhibit proteasomes leading to apoptosis of plasma cells thus decreases antibody production	Bortezomib 1.3 mg/m^2[a] Others with similar mechanism: carfilzomib[a] and ixazomib[a]
Anti-CD38 antibody	Leads to cell apoptosis of plasma cells	Daratumumab 8-16 mg/kg[a] also isatuximab[a]
Complement inhibitor	C5 complement inhibitor, prevents membrane attack complex from forming	Eculizumab 900 mg[a]
Interleukin-6 inhibitor	Inhibits IL-6 receptor, anti-inflammatory effect	Tocilizumab 8 mg/kg[a] monthly also clazakizumab[a]
Cysteine protease	Cleaves IgG heavy chain making IgG ineffective	Imlifidase[a]
Splenectomy	Removes stored lymphocytes	Done less often

[a]Many of above medications are used off-label.
Data from Marfo K, Lu A, Ling M, Akalin E. Desensitization protocols and their outcome. *Clin J Am Soc Nephrol.* 2011;6:922-36; and Durlik M. New approach to desensitization in solid organ transplantation-imlifidase. *Front Immunol.* 2021;1:951360. doi:10.3389/frtra.2022.951360.

- Donors donate on behalf of their recipient, with the knowledge that their recipient will have a living donor transplant with an exchange.
- There are a minimum of 2 donor-recipient pairs but can be multiple pairs. See **Figure 20-2**. The left side indicates the incompatible pairs (due to either ABO or HLA incompatibility), and the right panel shows the exchanges between pairs that result in compatible matches.

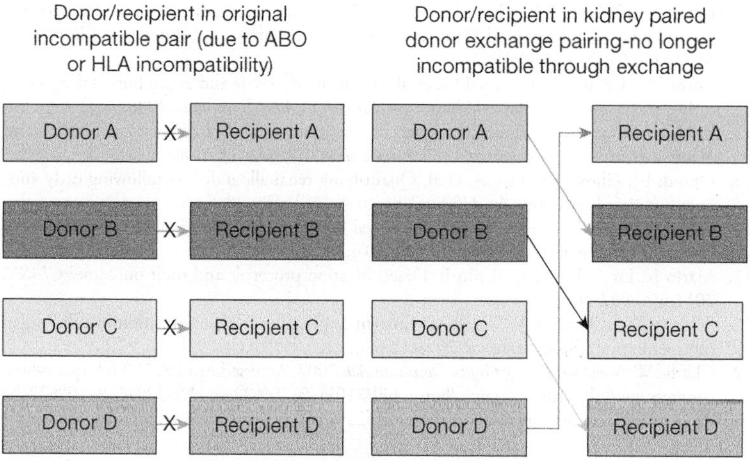

Figure 20-2. **Illustration of kidney paired donor exchange.**

REFERENCES

1. Denomme GA. The structure and function of the molecules that carry human red blood cell and platelet antigens. *Transfus Med Rev.* 2004;18(3):203-31.
2. American Red Cross. 2023. Accessed April 8, 2023 https://www.redcrossblood.org/donate-blood/blood-types.html
3. de Weerd AE, Betjes MGH. ABO-incompatible kidney transplant outcomes. A meta-analysis. *CJASN.* 2018;13(8):1234-43.
4. Montgomery RA, Locke JE, King KE, et al. ABO incompatible renal transplantation: a paradigm ready for broad implementation. *Transplantation.* 2009;87(8):1246-55.
5. Shirakawa H, Ishida H, Shimizu T, et al. The low dose of rituximab in ABO-incompatible kidney transplantation without a splenectomy: a single-center experience. *Clin Transplant.* 2011;25(6):878-84.
6. Sonnenday CJ, Warren DS, Cooper M, et al. Plasmapheresis, CMV hyperimmune globulin, and anti-CD20 allow ABO-incompatible renal transplantation without splenectomy. *Am J Transplant.* 2004;4(8):1315-22.
7. Bryan CF, Nelson PW, Shield CF, et al. Long-term survival of kidneys transplanted from live A2 donors to O and B recipients. *Am J Transplant.* 2007;7(5):1181-4.
8. Williams WW, Cherikh WS, Young CJ, et al. First report on the OPTN National variance: allocation of A2/A2 B deceased donor kidneys to blood group B increases minority transplantation. *Am J Transplant.* 2015;15(12):3134-42.
9. Haas M, Rahman MH, Racusen LC, et al. C4d and C3d staining in biopsies of ABO- and HLA-incompatible renal allografts: correlation with histologic findings. *Am J Transplant.* 2006;6(8):1829-40.
10. Haas M, Segev DL, Racusen LC, et al. C4d deposition without rejection correlates with reduced early scarring in ABO-incompatible renal allografts. *JASN (J Am Soc Nephrol).* 2009;20(1):197-204.
11. Lentine KL, Smith JM, Hart A, et al. OPTN/SRTR 2020 annual data report: kidney. *Am J Transplant.* 2022;22(suppl 2):21-136.

12. Israni AK, Salkowski N, Gustafson S, et al. New National allocation policy for deceased donor kidneys in the United States and possible Effect on patient outcomes. *JASN (J Am Soc Nephrol)*. 2014;25(8):1842-8.
13. Burns JM, Cornell LD, Perry DK, et al. Alloantibody levels and acute humoral rejection early after positive crossmatch kidney transplantation. *Am J Transplant*. 2008;8(12):2684-94.
14. Bentall A, Cornell LD, Gloor JM, et al. Five-year outcomes in living donor kidney transplants with a positive crossmatch. *Am J Transplant*. 2013;13(1):76-85.
15. Orandi BJ, Chow EH, Hsu A, et al. Quantifying renal allograft loss following early antibody-mediated rejection. *Am J Transplant*. 2015;15(2):489-98.
16. Orandi BJ, Luo X, Massie AB, et al. Survival benefit with kidney transplants from HLA-incompatible live donors. *N Engl J Med*. 2016;374(10):940-50.
17. Marfo K, Lu A, Ling M, Akalin E. Desensitization protocols and their outcome. *CJASN*. 2011;6(4):922-36.
18. Schinstock C, Tambur A, Stegall M. Current approaches to desensitization in solid organ transplantation. *Front Immunol*. 2021;12:686271.
19. Charlie W. *Norwood Living Organ Donation Act*. 2007. Accessed April 8, 2023. https://www.congress.gov/bill/110th-congress/house-bill/710?q=%7B%22search%22%3A%5B%22charlie+norwood+living+organ+donation+act%22%5D%7D&s=3&r=4

21 Pediatric Kidney Transplantation

Raja S. Dandamudi and Vikas R. Dharnidharka

GENERAL PRINCIPLES

- According to the US Renal Data System database, the adjusted incidence and prevalence of end-stage kidney disease (ESKD) in the pediatric population in 2019 was 11 and 75 individuals per million in the general population.[1]
- Within the pediatric range, the prevalence of ESKD increased with age. African American children had the highest prevalence of ESKD. The prevalence of ESKD was nearly 50% higher in boys than in girls, since obstructive uropathies are more common in boys.[1]
- Rates of preemptive wait-listing are higher in children when compared with adults. In 2019, 13.7% of children who initiated dialysis had been preemptively wait-listed, whereas corresponding values were 8.9%, 6.8%, 4.9%, and 0.8% in patients aged 18 to 44, 45 to 64, 65 to 74, and ≥75 years.[1]
- Based on the 2020 Annual Data Report of the US Organ Procurement and Transplantation Network (OPTN) and the Scientific Registry of Transplant Recipients (SRTR) data, around 800 kidney transplants are performed in children below 18 years of age annually in the US.[2]
  - The number of prevalent pediatric candidates on the kidney transplant waiting list has been increasing steadily, and 1,083 pediatric candidates were added to the kidney transplant waiting list in 2020 bringing prevalent pediatric candidates to 2,637 in 2020.
  - Stratifying by age, 12 to 17 years are the largest proportion of those waiting (59.5%) in 2020 followed by younger than 6 years (21.1%) and 6 to 11 years (19.4%).
  - Multiorgan listing and transplant is uncommon, and only 1.6% of pediatric candidates were awaiting multiorgan transplant at the end of 2020. Kidney-liver transplants are the most common multiorgan transplants.
  - The gender distribution remained stable over the years with approximately 60% male recipients.
  - The racial distribution was notably different for deceased and living donor transplant recipients; 67.8% of living donor recipients and 35.8% of deceased donor recipients were white, whereas 7.5% of living donor recipients and 22.7% of deceased donor recipients were black.
  - About 95% deceased donor recipients received kidney from a donor with Kidney donor profile index (KDPI) < 35%.
  - About 94.3% pediatric kidney transplant recipients received some form of induction immunosuppression in 2020.
  - For maintenance immunosuppression, a regimen with tacrolimus, mycophenolate mofetil (MMF), and steroids was used in 54.1% patients, followed by tacrolimus and MMF in 36.8%.
  - Approximately 22% of children with newly diagnosed ESKD in North America receive a preemptive transplant, and around 80% of children receive any type of kidney transplant within 3 years of renal replacement therapy initiation.

- Seventy-four percent of prevalent patients with ESKD in 2019 in the 1- to 17-year age group utilized kidney transplant as kidney replacement therapy modality.
- Analysis of the North American Pediatric Renal Trials and Collaborative Studies database over 30 years (1987-2017) demonstrated[3] the following:
  - Decrease in the percentage of white recipients.
  - The 13- to 17-year age group remained the most common age group over the years.
  - Living donor transplants peaked at 64% in 2001, and then there is a steady decline to only 31.5% in 2017.
  - See **Figure 21-1**.

ETIOLOGY OF KIDNEY FAILURE AND INDICATIONS

- Renal aplasia/hypoplasia/dysplasia, obstructive uropathy, reflux nephropathy, focal segmental glomerulosclerosis (FSGS), or another type of chronic glomerulonephritis are the 5 most common primary causes of kidney failure in children receiving a kidney transplant.

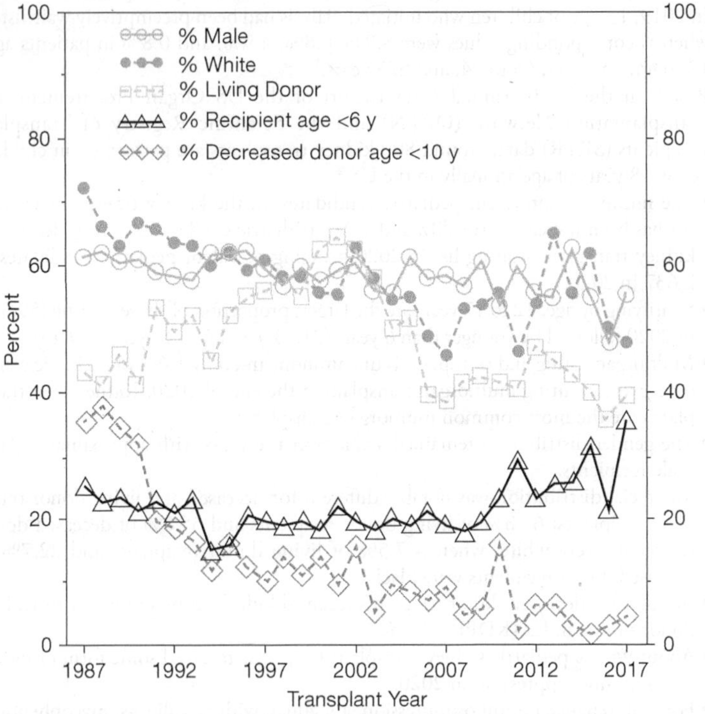

Figure 21-1. **Demographic characteristics of pediatric transplant recipients and donors between 1987 and 2017.** (Reproduced with permission from Chua A, Cramer C, Moudgil A, et al. Kidney transplant practice patterns and outcome benchmarks over 30 years: The 2018 report of the North American Pediatric Renal Trials and Collaborative Studies. *Pediatr Transplant.* 2019;23:e13597.)

- Proportions of children with congenital anomalies of the kidney and urinary tract (CAKUT) as the primary cause of disease increased from 29.0% in 2010 to 38.3% in 2020, and proportions with glomerulonephritis and FSGS decreased.[2]
- CAKUT is the primary cause of ESKD in 40% of children less than 6 years of age, whereas it is the etiology in only 20% of those between 11 and 17 years of age.[2]
- The most common primary renal diseases that lead to ESKD in adults are diabetic nephropathy, hypertension, and autosomal dominant polycystic kidney disease, which rarely cause ESKD in children.

PREEMPTIVE KIDNEY TRANSPLANT

- In preemptive renal transplantation, transplantation is the first mode of treatment for ESKD in children.
- Preemptive transplantation avoids the morbidity associated with dialysis as well as dialysis access and its complications but needs a predictable and steady decline of function rate and a good social support situation.
- The rate of preemptive transplants are higher in children. Twenty-two percent of incident ESKD patients <17 years received preemptive transplant compared with 6% in 18 to 44 age group, 4% in 46 to 64 year group, 2% in 65 to 74 year group.[1]
- Compared with children transplanted preemptively, children who received any dialysis prior to transplant experienced much higher rates of graft failure and death.[4]
- The Eurotransplant registry analysis demonstrated that children with a preemptive transplant had a higher acute rejection-free proportion at 3 years post transplant (52% vs. 37%). They also had improved 6-year allograft survival when compared with dialysis patients (82% vs. 69%).[5]

DONOR CONSIDERATIONS

- The transplanted kidney allograft has a finite survival, median being 12 to 14 years. Therefore, children transplanted early in life will probably have 2 or 3 kidney transplants in their lifetime.
- The median waiting time for a deceased donor kidney transplant in the US is 6.6 months as compared with median wait-time between 42.3 and 59.5 months in individuals >18 years of age.[1,2]
- Various organ-sharing organizations across the globe have allocation policies that prioritize pediatric patients. In Eurotransplant, for pediatric patients the points for HLA-antigen mismatches are doubled and they also receive bonus points for waiting time. Scandiatransplant prioritizes pediatric recipients when the donor is <40 years old.[6]
- In the US the Kidney Allocation System implemented on December 4, 2014, was based on KDPI scoring. It was designed to better match deceased donor kidneys with the longest expected graft survival to patients expected to live the longest post transplant.
- Pediatric patients receive the kidneys with lowest KDPI scores, preferentially allocated organs from donors with KDPI < 35%.
- Living donors have superior long-term survival compared with deceased donors.[2]
- Deceased donor transplantation rates are higher in developed countries, highest in Spain followed by the US.
- Parents are the majority of living donors to the pediatric recipient (77.3%).[3]

- Unrelated living donations increased from 1.3% of living donor transplants in 1987 to 31.4% in 2017.[3]
- Living donations are most common for recipients aged 0 to 5 years.[3] See **Figure 21-2** for donation by type and by age group.
- Developing countries rely more on living donor programs.
- Size-matched donors are at a higher risk of vascular complications such as thrombosis, primary graft nonfunction, and acute tubular necrosis in pediatric kidney transplant.[7]
- Use of adult-sized kidneys in pediatric patients is an established practice and is associated with superior graft outcome.[8]
- At our center, the minimum weight and height of children to receive an adult kidney is generally >75 cm and >10 kg.
- An important conundrum in pediatric kidney transplant is if there is only 1 possible living donor, should the first kidney transplant be from a living or a deceased donor?
  - The advantage for receiving a deceased organ first is that children get good-quality donors in a relatively short period of time.
  - An argument against this is that living donor survival rate is higher than deceased donors and the potential donor may be ineligible for donation when retransplantation is considered.

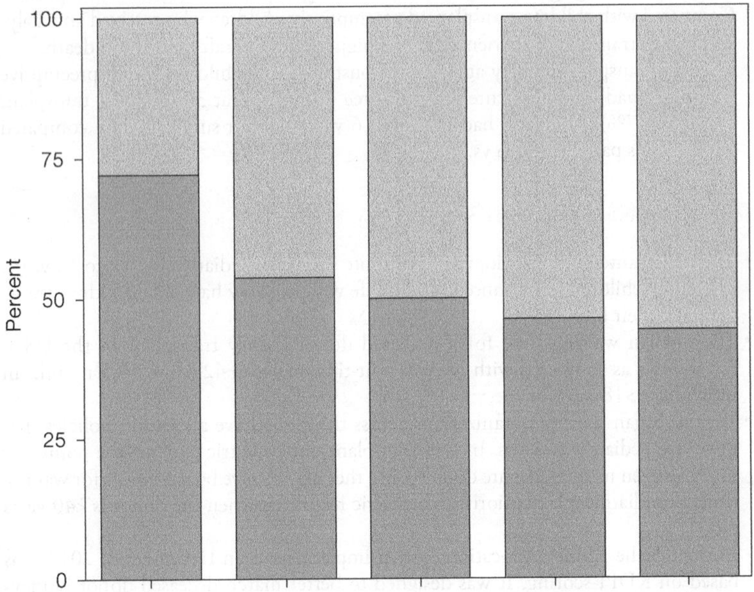

Figure 21-2. **Donor source by recipient age at transplant.** (Reproduced with permission from Chua A, Cramer C, Moudgil A, et al. Kidney transplant practice patterns and outcome benchmarks over 30 years: The 2018 report of the North American Pediatric Renal Trials and Collaborative Studies. *Pediatr Transplant.* 2019;23:e13597.)

- There are no differences in the cumulative graft life between children receiving deceased donor kidney transplant followed by living donor retransplantation and vice versa.[9]
- Very young pediatric deceased donor kidneys often get transplanted en bloc into adults, with good results.[10]

SURGICAL CONSIDERATIONS

Native Nephrectomy

- Indications for native nephrectomies include
  - Significant polyuria
  - Intractable proteinuria due to congenital nephrotic syndrome
  - Malignancy or conditions that may confer a high risk of future malignancy like Denys-Drash syndrome
- Loss of residual excretory capacity, erythropoietin production, and need for intermittent hemodialysis are potential complications of native nephrectomy prior to transplant.
- At our center, we consider unilateral nephrectomy for polyuria before the transplant and subsequent nephrectomy if needed 6 to 8 weeks post transplant. But other centers may perform bilateral nephrectomies 3 weeks before a scheduled living donor transplant and perform hemodialysis in the intervening 3 weeks in situations of polyuria or nephrotic range proteinuria with edema.

Transplant Surgical Considerations

- Size and age matching is generally not required in kidney transplantation as the allograft is placed in a different location from the failed native organ. The allograft only needs to be attached to the vascular tree and near enough for the donor ureter to be attached to the recipient's urinary bladder.
- At our center, infants weighing less than 10 kg usually undergo an intraperitoneal approach with midline laparotomy and vascular anastomosis of the adult-sized donor vessels to the recipient's inferior vena cava and the aorta.
- In teenagers and in children weighing more than 30 kg, the graft is placed extraperitoneally in the iliac fossa, like in adults. Anastomoses are performed between donor renal vein and recipient external iliac vein, and between donor renal artery and recipient internal or external iliac artery.
- In children between 10 and 30 kg, these surgical decisions are made on a case-by-case basis.
- At our center, we use prophylactic Aspirin for a month post transplant for the prevention of allograft thrombosis. In patients with a working arteriovenous fistula, we continue prophylactic anticoagulation for longer periods.
- Ureteral stents across the ureteral-vesicular anastomosis reduce the risk of urologic complications such as urinary leak or ureteral stenosis but may predispose to early urinary tract infections or BK virus DNAemia.
- Other complications of stent placement can include migration, stone formation, breakage, and hematuria.
- At our center, double-J ureteral stents are placed in all children and are removed via ureteroscope at 3 to 4 weeks post transplant.

Urologic Issues

- Children with congenital anomalies in the kidney and urinary tract require evaluation of their kidneys, ureters, and bladder by an ultrasound scan prior to transplant.

- We will obtain a micturating cystourethrogram if there is a history of recurrent urinary tract infections or urinary incontinence.
- Urodynamic studies are obtained prior to transplant if bladder dysfunction is suspected.
- Renal transplant patients should have a reliable urinary drainage system with low-pressure storage and adequate emptying.
- The most common bladder abnormality associated with ESKD is the low-capacity, hypertonic bladder with poor compliance. This is the typical picture with posterior urethral valves.
- The hypertonic bladder and low-volume bladder are managed by anticholinergics and clean intermittent catheterization as first-line therapy.
- An open vesicostomy may be required to decompress a dysfunctional bladder.
- Bladder augmentation with segments of ileum, stomach, or appendix to create a permanent cutaneous conduit that enables the child to be continent and to have clean, intermittent catheterization is the second-line therapy. An appendicovesical continent conduit is often known by its creator's name as a Mitrofanoff conduit.

CRITERIA FOR EVALUATION AND TRANSPLANT

Criteria for Evaluation

- Patients with chronic kidney disease (CKD) without known contraindications for transplantation should be referred to a transplant program when they approach CKD stage 4 or a glomerular filtration rate (GFR) less than 30 mL/min/1.73 m^2.
- Early referral will improve the chances of a patient receiving a preemptive transplant, especially those with a potential living donor.

Criteria for Transplantation

- End-stage kidney disease on dialysis
- Chronic renal failure with GFR < 20 mL/min/1.732 m^2

Contraindications

- Pediatric kidney transplantation is generally considered an elective procedure and contraindicated if transplant and lifelong immunosuppression result in more harm than benefit.
- There are few absolute contraindications to kidney transplantation in children, which include
  - Primary unresectable/untreatable malignancy
  - Metastatic malignancy
  - Progressive terminal nonrenal disease
  - Uncontrolled systemic infection
  - Mitochondrial disorders with progressive neurological involvement
- There are also a few relative contraindications to kidney transplantation in children, which include
  - Advanced or partially treated systemic infection
  - Body mass index >35 kg/m^2
  - HIV infection with high viral titers
  - Incomplete preventative vaccinations, without medical contraindication
  - ESKD from autoimmune disease with persistently high titers of autoantibody
  - Ongoing active infections

- Underlying kidney disease is still active
- Caregivers not ready
- Issues with adherence

IMMUNE SYSTEM IN THE PEDIATRIC AGE GROUP

- From birth to adulthood, the immune system undergoes significant change. The absolute counts and percentages of circulating T-cell and B-cell subtypes change, increasing the alloreactivity.
- Thymic activity decreases as we age, and this changes the composition of the T-cell pool to memory T cells from naive T cells.
- In contrast to adults, the alloimmune response in children has the following[11]:
  - Low expression of the CD40 ligand (CD40-L/CD154), a member of the TNF family. This is expressed more widely in activated $CD4^+$ T cells, and CD40-CD40-L interactions play a great role in immune regulation.
  - Fewer antigen-specific CD8(+) T cells.
  - Higher levels of Th2 and lower levels of the type 1 helper T cell.
  - Mitigated T-cell effector function.
  - Higher levels of the dendritic cells, which are specialized in antigen presentation and to drive T-cell priming and differentiation.
  - Lower titers of anti-HLA antibodies prior to transplantation.

Immunosuppression

- Our center's standard immunosuppression protocol is based on perceived risk of early acute rejection and will be determined for all patients at the time of transplant listing.
- We stratify patients based on risk factors to choose induction therapy and then titrate maintenance therapy to achieve optimal immunosuppression.
- Standard risk: Structural lesions or nonimmune complex glomerular diseases as primary renal disease, first transplant, negative or low panel reactive antibody (PRA).
- High risk: Glomerular or immune complex disease with risk of recurrence, retransplant (prior living or deceased transplant), PRA greater than 0%.

Induction Immunosuppression

- The aim of the induction therapy is to deplete or modify T cells before donor antigen presentation and reduce the risk of early rejection.
- Available induction agents in pediatric transplant include the following:
  - Antilymphocyte antibodies
    - Polyclonal antilymphocyte antibodies: Rabbit antithymocyte globulin (Thymoglobulin in the US, also Fresenius-ATG in Europe)
    - Monoclonal anti-CD52 lymphocyte antibodies: Alemtuzumab
  - IL-2 receptor antagonists: Monoclonal IL-2 receptor antibody: Basiliximab
  - Anti-CD20 antibodies: anti-CD20 monoclonal antibody: Rituximab
- According to 2018 OPTN and the SRTR database, 63% of pediatric kidney transplant recipients received T-cell depleting antibodies, 35% received anti-IL-2 receptor antibodies, and 2% received no induction therapy.[2]
- Our center's protocol
  - For all patients the initial dose of IV thymoglobulin (1.5 mg/kg) is given intraoperatively, in combination with IV methylprednisolone (7 mg/kg).

- Standard-risk patients receive 3 total doses of thymoglobulin with a cumulative dose of 4.5 mg/kg.
- High-risk patients receive 5 total doses of thymoglobulin with a cumulative dose of 7.5 mg/kg.
- For standard-risk patients we follow a rapid steroid taper maintenance regimen by tapering and stopping the steroids by day 5 post transplant.
- For high-risk patients we follow a steroid maintenance regimen by weaning the high-dose steroids (2 mg/kg/d) over a period of 3 months and maintaining the lower dose 5 to 10 mg once daily.

Maintenance Immunosuppression

- At our center, our initial maintenance immunosuppression calcineurin inhibitor is tacrolimus and our antimetabolite is either MMF, or enteric-coated mycophenolate sodium.
- MMF is started in the operating room at a daily dose of 600 mg/m^2. Mycophenolate sodium is used in cases of gastrointestinal intolerance to MMF. We do not routinely measure mycophenolic acid levels. We adjust doses based on leukopenia or gastrointestinal side effects.
- Tacrolimus is initiated at 0.05 mg/kg/dose twice daily (after serum creatinine improved below 1 mg/dL). The dose is adjusted based on the 12-hour trough blood level.
- Target tacrolimus levels
  - Posttransplant weeks 1 to 2: 8 to 10 ng/mL
  - Posttransplant weeks 3 to 26: 6 to 8 ng/mL
  - Posttransplant weeks 26 to 52: 5 to 7 ng/mL
  - Posttransplant week 52 onward: 4 to 6 ng/mL
- A stable maintenance immunosuppression regimen is established within the first year after transplantation.
- We only decrease the maintenance immunosuppression during the first year if opportunistic infections flare.
- After a year, we do not routinely reduce maintenance immunosuppression, even among stable patients.
- Our center's approach for adjusting maintenance immunosuppression
  - Biopsy-proven calcineurin inhibitor nephrotoxicity
    - Decrease the target calcineurin inhibitor level.
    - Switch to an mammalian target of rapamycin inhibitor (sirolimus or everolimus).
  - With significant gastrointestinal side effects, we change MMF to enteric-coated mycophenolate, and if the side effects persist we change to azathioprine.

OPPORTUNISTIC INFECTIONS AND VACCINATIONS

- Posttransplant infections now exceed acute rejection as the cause of hospitalization in the first 2 years following renal transplantation.[12]
- Our center's pretransplant screening includes the following:
  - Cytomegalovirus (CMV) IgG antibody
  - Epstein-Barr virus (EBV) antibody IgG
  - Herpes simplex virus IgG antibody
  - HIV antibody
  - Hepatitis B virus: Hepatitis B surface antigen (HBsAg), anti-hepatitis B surface Ag (anti-HBsAg), hepatitis B core antibody (HBcAb) IgM/IgG

  - Hepatitis C virus antibody test
  - Toxoplasma IgG and IgM
  - Measles, mumps, and rubella (MMR) antibody
  - Rapid plasma reagin test
  - Purified protein derivative skin test or interferon-γ release assays for latent tuberculosis.
- Hogan et al. reported an overall hospital admission rate of 38.7 per 100 person-years in a French cohort of 563 children with renal transplants.[13]
- A multicenter, prospective, observational cohort, Immune Development in Pediatric Transplantation (IMPACT) study, identified that 73% of patients developed viral DNAemia (EBV, 34%; CMV, 23%; BK virus, 23%; and JC virus, 21%).[14]
- During the first 30 days of transplant, bacterial, fungal, and donor-derived pathogens are the most common infections.
- After the first month and during the first year post transplant, opportunistic infections are prominent and latent pathogens previously present in the recipient or derived from the donor reactivate.
- Community-acquired viruses as well as infections associated with chronic graft dysfunction predominate the infectious scenario post first year of transplant.
- Recognized risk factors for opportunistic infections include younger age, EBV-negative serostatus, CMV donor (+)/recipient (−), biopsy-proven acute rejection, absolute neutrophil count less than 1,000, MMF dose greater than 500 mg/m^2, and any infection.[15]
- Urinary tract infections are the most common infection after kidney transplantation in children.
- At our center, standard-of-care posttransplant follow-up includes quantitative monthly nucleic acid testing by polymerase chain reaction assay for EBV, CMV, and BK virus.
- At our center, in the first year post transplant
  - Trimethoprim/sulfamethoxazole remains the prophylactic agent of choice to prevent both pneumocystis infection and toxoplasmosis posttransplant.
  - For patients allergic to sulfa drugs we use Pentamidine aerosol or IV every month for 12 months.
  - Valganciclovir is used for the prevention of CMV.
- BK polyoma virus
  - On detection of BK virus in urine we do not escalate the immunosuppression.
  - On detection of BK virus in blood we will decrease the immunosuppression.
  - For patients with biopsy-proven BK virus nephropathy or presumed BK virus nephropathy (>10,000 IU/mL with elevated creatinine) we administer intravenous immune globulin (IVIG) monthly (500 mg/kg) for 6 months.
  - Leflunomide is used as the second-line agent.
- Immunization
  - The Infectious Diseases Society of America and the American Society of Transplantation recommend vaccines prior to transplantation using age-appropriate guidelines.
  - The immune response mounted after vaccination is suboptimal in transplant candidates, compared with the general population, but they have better immune responses compared with patients after transplantation.
  - Nonlive vaccines can be administered safely.
  - Live vaccines are contraindicated post transplantation. Transplant should be delayed by a minimum of 4 weeks post live vaccine administration.

- For the live-attenuated vaccines MMR and varicella, waiting a minimum of 4 weeks between vaccine administration and transplantation is recommended, given the theoretical risk of developing disease from the vaccine strain.
- Rituximab usage can inhibit the immune response to vaccines for as long as 12 months, although the maximum effect occurs within the first 6 months.
- Inactivated influenza vaccine is recommended yearly to pediatric kidney transplant recipients, healthcare givers, and household contacts.
- At our center, we recommend the 9-valent human papillomavirus vaccine, a 3-dose series separated by 0, 1, and 6 months.

ALLOGRAFT REJECTION

- The proportion of all allograft failure due to acute rejection was 5% in children who received living donor kidneys and 8% in those with deceased donor kidneys as per the 2014 NARTCS report.[16]
- Acute rejection episodes are generally associated with a reduction in long-term allograft survival, although not all rejection episodes have the same impact on long-term graft function.
- Diagnosis of renal transplant rejection is based on interpretation of renal allograft biopsies by the Banff Classification of Allograft Pathology, similar to adults.[17]
- Recommended therapy for acute T-cell-mediated (cellular) rejection (TCMR) at our center
  - Banff grade IA—For patients with biopsy-proven Banff grade IA TCMR (with no evidence of antibody-mediated rejection [ABMR]), we treat with glucocorticoids pulse IV methylprednisolone at 3 to 5 mg/kg daily for 3 to 5 doses and retaper oral steroids.
  - Banff grade IB—For patients with Banff grade IB TCMR, we suggest treatment with antithymocyte globulin 1.5 mg/kg per dose for 3 days in addition to pulse glucocorticoids.
  - Banff grade II or III rejection: For patients with biopsy-proven Banff grade IIA, IIB, or III TCMR, we suggest treatment with Thymoglobulin 1.5 mg/kg per dose for 5 days, in addition to glucocorticoids.
- Recommended therapy for active (acute) ABMR at our center
  - Therapeutic plasma exchange—typically a 1½ volume exchange with albumin alternate days for 5 to 7 treatments.
  - We administer IVIG at a dose of 100 mg/kg after each session of plasmapheresis.
  - If there is severe allograft dysfunction, we administer a single dose of rituximab 375 mg/m^2 after completion of plasmapheresis and IVIG.
  - At our center, for mixed acute rejection, we administer thymoglobulin immediately after therapeutic plasma exchange.
- Subclinical rejection is defined as presence of histological features of acute rejection on surveillance renal biopsy in the absence of a decline in renal function. At our center, we perform 3-, 6-, and 12-month surveillance biopsies as standard of care. Other centers might differ in their frequency of surveillance biopsy, if at all done, due to lack of consensus.
  - In all patients with evidence of subclinical ABMR, we use the same therapeutic approach as that used to treat patients with clinical ABMR.
  - In all patients with evidence of subclinical T-cell-mediated rejection, we will optimize the maintenance immunosuppression.

POSTTRANSPLANT LYMPHOPROLIFERATIVE DISORDER

- Incidence rates of posttransplant lymphoproliferative disorder (PTLD) are higher in pediatric kidney transplant recipients than in adult kidney transplant recipients, ranging from 1.2% to 10%.[18,19]
- Majority of pediatric PTLDs are due to EBV-positive B-cell proliferation.
- Incidence of PTLD among EBV-negative recipients from 2008 to 2018 was 3.8% at 5 years post transplant, compared with 0.7% among EBV-positive recipients as per SRTR registry data.[2]
- Risk factors for EBV-associated PTLD include recipient EBV seronegativity, level of immunosuppression, acute rejection episodes, use of tacrolimus, recipient age and race, allograft type, and host genetic variations.
- Pediatric allograft recipients often experience primary EBV infection after transplantation compared with adults who have acquired immunity to EBV.
- Although EBV-infected transformed B cells are highly immunogenic and rapidly eliminated by EBV-specific T cells in healthy hosts, if immunosuppressed pediatric patients have primary EBV infection, then an inadequate immune response may result in massive infection of B cells.
- Primary EBV infection increases the chance of developing PTLD.[20]
- The occurrence of PTLD in kidney transplant recipients follows a bimodal distribution, with one peak in the first year and the second in the later posttransplantation period.
- Early PTLD, occurring within the first year of transplantation, is associated with EBV infection and tends to occur more commonly in children than in adults.
- The primary goal in the treatment of PTLD is cure, and a concomitant objective should be preservation of the allograft organ.
- The mainstay of treatment has been reduction in immunosuppression.
- Other treatment options include rituximab monoclonal antibody given combined or in sequence with combination chemotherapy, with cyclophosphamide, doxorubicin, vincristine, and prednisone (CHOP) being the most common.
- Novel therapeutic approaches continued to be explored, including adoptive immunotherapy, cytokine treatment, and anti-EBV-based therapy.

GROWTH AND NEUROCOGNITIVE DEVELOPMENT POST TRANSPLANT

- Poor linear growth and growth failure are frequent complications of CKD and have a profound impact on quality of life.
- Anthropometric analysis of children with ESKD revealed preferential shunting of leg growth and preserved trunk growth resulting in disproportionate stunting.[21]
- Catch-up growth post transplant is generally not enough to compensate for the deficit that happened before transplantation, and growth impairment persists even after transplant.
- Around 30% of pediatric renal transplant recipients do not achieve a normal adult height.[22]
- The mean height deficit was −1.75 standard deviations below the age- and sex-adjusted height level at the time of kidney transplant and remained relatively constant at follow-up post transplant.[16]
- Growth analysis in the North American Pediatric Renal Transplant Cooperative Study (NAPRTCS) 2018 annual report suggested that magnitude of pretransplantation

growth deficit, primary kidney disease, presence of comorbidities, age at the time of transplant, allograft function, and steroid exposure affect growth post transplant.[3,16]
- Prolonged steroid exposure hinders catch-up growth and restoration of body proportions and was associated with shorter leg length.
- Early/intermediate steroid withdrawal and complete steroid avoidance are associated with improved growth outcome after transplant in younger children.[23,24]
- Poor allograft function (GFR <50 mL/min per 1.73 m^2 in the first year post transplant) hampers catch-up growth post transplant.
- Posttransplant catch-up growth patterns are different among age groups.
- Children younger than 6 years have the greatest height deficits at the time of transplant but experienced a greater posttransplant height increase and attained normal height. Children who were 6 to 12 years of age showed very limited catch-up growth, and those older than 12 years at the time of transplant experienced no increase or even a slight decrease in height standard deviation.[3]
- Congenital primary renal diseases (CAKUT and hereditary nephropathies) were associated with greater growth impairment when compared with glomerular and vascular diseases, probably related to longer duration of the CKD and the tubular losses of the urinary electrolytes.
- Recombinant human growth hormone increases the linear growth in children with no increase in incidence of acute rejection.[22,25,26]
- Neurocognitive functions of pediatric kidney transplant recipients: Children with CKD have lower intellectual functioning, deficits in executive functions, and problematic academic progress.[27]
- Dialysis vintage and earlier onset of ESKD were associated with lower IQ scores.
- Kidney transplantation results in improved neurocognitive function, without negatively affecting neurocognitive function in kidney donors.
- Kidney transplant improves in addition to cognitive function, fatigue and depression scores, all of which are important contributors of quality of life of CKD.
- Earlier transplant and shorter dialysis improve neurocognitive outcome.

TRANSITION TO ADULT CARE

- Irrespective of the age at transplant, graft failure rates begin to increase around 12 years of age, peak at 17 to 24 years, and decline thereafter.[28,29]
- Transition is the step-by-step, phased preparation and movement of adolescents and young adults with chronic medical problems from a child-centered to an adult-centered healthcare system.
- At our center, the transition process begins around 14 years of age and is completed by age 18 to 24 years.
- Failure of proper transition increases the risk of medical nonadherence and subsequent loss of graft.
- At our center, phase 1 of the transition process involves recognition of their disease process, reason for transplant, and the short- and long-term impacts of the disease.
- Phase 2 of transition involves learning the names and doses of the immunosuppression, learning how to communicate with their healthcare team, self-advocating, and drug refilling. This is the phase when the adolescent starts developing competence in self-management. This is the phase of self-autonomy with supervision.
- Phase 3 of transition involves achieving educational and vocational goals, establishing healthy lifestyle choices, and transferring to adult transplant center. This is the phase of autonomy combined with providing support when need arises.

- Throughout all stages, the parent or primary care giver is there to offer additional support in times of physical and psychological stress, illness, or other life complications.
- An interdisciplinary pediatric nephrology team (nephrologists, nurses, nutritionist, social worker, psychologist, child-life workers) works with the patient and family throughout the transition process.

PREVENTIVE CARE

Hypertension

- Persistent posttransplant hypertension is a common complication and risk factor for adverse cardiovascular outcomes as an adult.
- In children we use left ventricular hypertrophy as the marker for cardiovascular risk stratification.
- To avoid detrimental effects of hypotension causing vascular thrombosis and graft loss we accept permissive hypertension in the immediate and early posttransplant period.
- Later in the transplant course, our treatment goals are <95th percentile by sex, age, and height.
- Yearly echocardiograms and ambulatory blood pressure monitoring are performed in hypertensive patients.

Malignancies

- Due to cumulative effect of immunosuppression, children have the highest risk for cancer post transplant.
- PTLD, squamous and basal cell carcinoma, and anogenital/gynecologic cancers associated with human papillomavirus (HPV) are the most common neoplasms reported in pediatric kidney transplant recipients.[30]
- At our center, we employ routine EBV DNA blood load screening, optimizing the immunosuppression regimens, and vaccination for HPV as preventive strategies.
- Adolescent female transplant recipients will have regular gynecological checkups with Pap and HPV screenings.

OUTCOMES

- Over the last few decades there is significant improvement in the outcomes of kidney transplant in children in terms of both allograft survival and patient survival. See **Figure 21-3**.
- For the cohort of pediatric recipients who underwent transplant in 2013 to 2015, 1-year graft survival of deceased donor recipients was comparable with that of living donor recipients (96.7% vs. 97%).[2]
- For the cohort of pediatric recipients who underwent transplant in 2013 to 2015, 5-year graft survival for living donor recipients (92.4%) is higher than that for deceased donor recipients (83.1%).[2]
- Estimated glomerular filtration rate (eGFR) at 12 months, an early surrogate allograft outcome, also improved over the decades. In pediatric transplant cohorts, younger recipients begin with a higher eGFR and are subject to greater absolute declines over time compared with older recipients.[3]
- In the year 2019, 70% of deceased donor recipients and 67% of living donor recipients had eGFR of 60 mL/min/1.73 m^2 or higher at a year post transplant.[2]

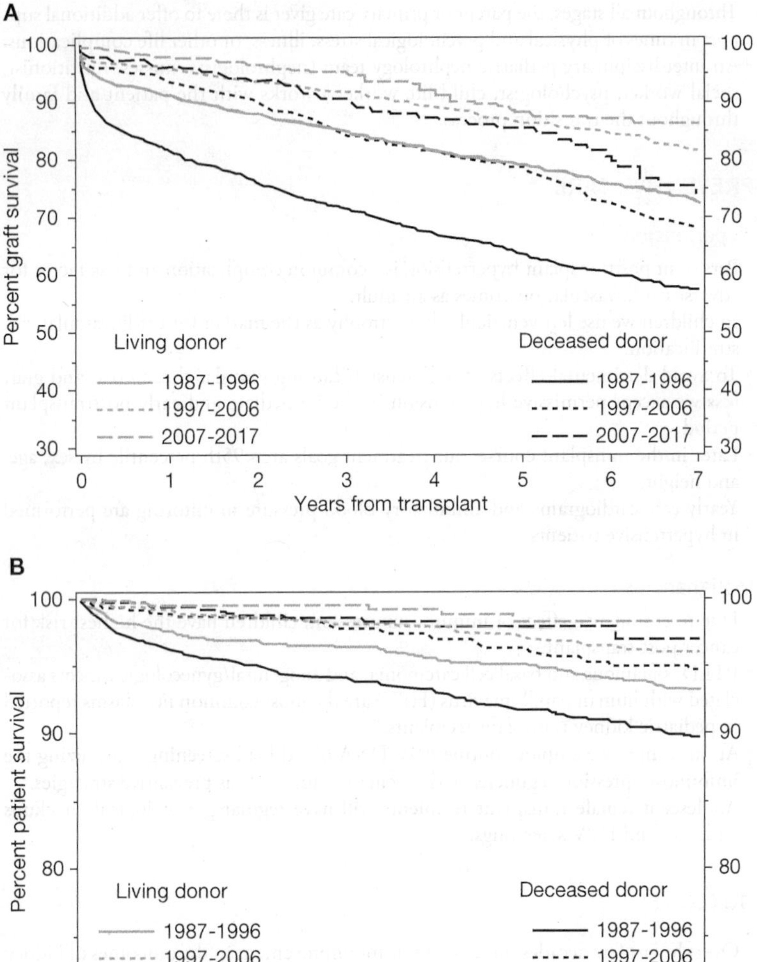

Figure 21-3. **A, Graft by transplant era, stratified by donor source. B, Patient survival by transplant era, stratified by donor source.** (Reproduced with permission from Chua A, Cramer C, Moudgil A, et al. Kidney transplant practice patterns and outcome benchmarks over 30 years: The 2018 report of the North American Pediatric Renal Trials and Collaborative Studies. *Pediatr Transplant.* 2019;23:e13597.)

REFERENCES

1. End stage renal disease among children and adolescents from the Annual Data Report of the U.S. Renal Data System (USRDS). Accessed April 17, 2023. https://usrds-adr.niddk.nih.gov/2022/end-stage-renal-disease/8-esrd-among-children-and-adolescents
2. OPTN/SRTR 2020 annual data report: preface. *Am J Transplant* 2022;22:1-10.
3. Chua A, Cramer C, Moudgil A, et al. Kidney transplant practice patterns and outcome benchmarks over 30 years: the 2018 report of the NAPRTCS. *Pediatr Transplant.* 2019;23(8):e13597.
4. Amaral S, Sayed BA, Kutner N, Patzer RE. Preemptive kidney transplantation is associated with survival benefits among pediatric patients with end-stage renal disease. *Kidney Int.* 2016;90(5):1100-8.
5. Cransberg K, Smits JM, Offner G, Nauta J, Persijn GG. Kidney transplantation without prior dialysis in children: the Eurotransplant experience. *Am J Transplant.* 2006;6(8):1858-64.
6. Capitaine L, Van Assche K, Pennings G, Sterckx S. Pediatric priority in kidney allocation: challenging its acceptability. *Transpl Int.* 2014;27(6):533-40.
7. Yaffe HC, Friedmann P, Kayler LK. Very small pediatric donor kidney transplantation in pediatric recipients. *Pediatr Transplant.* 2017;21:e12924.
8. Salvatierra O Jr, Singh T, Shifrin R, et al. Successful transplantation of adult-sized kidneys into infants requires maintenance of high aortic blood flow. *Transplantation.* 1998;66(7):819-23.
9. Van Arendonk KJ, James NT, Orandi BJ, et al. Order of donor type in pediatric kidney transplant recipients requiring retransplantation. *Transplantation.* 2013;96(5):487-93.
10. Dharnidharka VR, Stevens G, Howard RJ. En-bloc kidney transplantation in the United States: an analysis of united network of organ sharing (UNOS) data from 1987 to 2003. *Am J Transplant.* 2005;5(6):1513-7.
11. Dharnidharka VR, Fiorina P, Harmon WE. Kidney transplantation in children. *N Engl J Med.* 2014;371(6):549-58.
12. Dharnidharka VR, Stablein DM, Harmon WE. Post-transplant infections now exceed acute rejection as cause for hospitalization: a report of the NAPRTCS. *Am J Transplant.* 2004;4(3):384-9.
13. Hogan J, Pietrement C, Sellier-Leclerc A-L, et al. Infection-related hospitalizations after kidney transplantation in children: incidence, risk factors, and cost. *Pediatr Nephrol.* 2017;32(12):2331-41.
14. Ettenger R, Chin H, Kesler K, et al. Relationship among viremia/viral infection, alloimmunity, and nutritional parameters in the first year after pediatric kidney transplantation. *Am J Transplant.* 2017;17(6):1549-62.
15. Jordan CL, Taber DJ, Kyle MO, et al. Incidence, risk factors, and outcomes of opportunistic infections in pediatric renal transplant recipients. *Pediatr Transplant.* 2016;20(1):44-8.
16. Smith JM, Martz K, Blydt-Hansen TD. Pediatric kidney transplant practice patterns and outcome benchmarks, 1987-2010: a report of the North American Pediatric Renal Trials and Collaborative Studies. *Pediatr Transplant.* 2013;17(2):149-57.
17. Loupy A, Haas M, Roufosse C, et al. The Banff 2019 Kidney Meeting Report (I): updates on and clarification of criteria for T cell- and antibody-mediated rejection. *Am J Transplant.* 2020;20(9):2318-31.
18. Jeong HJ, Ahn YH, Park E, et al. Posttransplantation lymphoproliferative disorder after pediatric solid organ transplantation: experiences of 20 years in a single center. *Korean J Pediatr.* 2017;60(3):86-93.
19. McDonald RA, Smith JM, Ho M, et al. Incidence of PTLD in pediatric renal transplant recipients receiving basiliximab, calcineurin inhibitor, sirolimus and steroids. *Am J Transplant.* 2008;8(5):984-9.
20. Green M, Michaels MG. Epstein-Barr virus infection and posttransplant lymphoproliferative disorder. *Am J Transplant.* 2013;13(suppl 3):41-54; quiz 54.
21. Zivicnjak M, Franke D, Filler G, et al. Growth impairment shows an age-dependent pattern in boys with chronic kidney disease. *Pediatr Nephrol.* 2007;22(3):420-9.

22. Fine RN, Ho M, Tejani A; North American Pediatric Renal Transplant Cooperative Study NAPRTCS. The contribution of renal transplantation to final adult height: a report of the North American Pediatric Renal Transplant Cooperative Study (NAPRTCS). *Pediatr Nephrol.* 2001;16(12):951-6.
23. Grenda R, Watson A, Trompeter R, et al. A randomized trial to assess the impact of early steroid withdrawal on growth in pediatric renal transplantation: the TWIST study. *Am J Transplant.* 2010;10(4):828-36.
24. Sarwal MM, Ettenger RB, Dharnidharka V, et al. Complete steroid avoidance is effective and safe in children with renal transplants: a multicenter randomized trial with three-year follow-up. *Am J Transplant.* 2012;12(10):2719-29.
25. Maxwell H, Rees L. Randomised controlled trial of recombinant human growth hormone in prepubertal and pubertal renal transplant recipients. British Association for Pediatric Nephrology. *Arch Dis Child.* 1998;79(6):481-7.
26. Fine RN, Stablein D, Cohen AH, Tejani A, Kohaut E. Recombinant human growth hormone post-renal transplantation in children: a randomized controlled study of the NAPRTCS. *Kidney Int.* 2002;62(2):688-96.
27. Molnar-Varga M, Novak M, Szabo AJ, et al. Neurocognitive functions of pediatric kidney transplant recipients. *Pediatr Nephrol.* 2016;31(9):1531-8.
28. Foster BJ, Dahhou M, Zhang X, Platt RW, Samuel SM, Hanley JA. Association between age and graft failure rates in young kidney transplant recipients. *Transplantation.* 2011;92(11):1237-43.
29. Van Arendonk KJ, James NT, Boyarsky BJ, et al. Age at graft loss after pediatric kidney transplantation: exploring the high-risk age window. *Clin J Am Soc Nephrol.* 2013;8(6):1019-26.
30. Paramesh A, Cannon R, Buell JF. Malignancies in pediatric solid organ transplant recipients: epidemiology, risk factors, and prophylactic approaches. *Curr Opin Organ Transplant.* 2010;15(5):621-7.

22 Pancreas Transplantation

Massini Merzkani, Abdullah Jalal, and Tarek Alhamad

GENERAL PRINCIPLES

- Pancreas transplantation is among the most effective treatments for diabetes mellitus with the goal of achieving complete insulin independence.
- Pancreas transplantation has been shown to improve patient quality of life, reduce the progression of diabetic complications, and improve patient survival through the prevention of major life-threatening conditions including diabetic ketoacidosis and hypoglycemia unawareness.
- First performed on December 17, 1966 at the University of Minnesota by William Kelly and Richard Lillehei, pancreas transplantation has evolved from an experimental procedure to a potent cure for diabetes.[1]
- Pancreas transplants can be performed as simultaneous pancreas and kidney (SPKT), pancreas transplant alone (PTA), or pancreas after kidney transplant (PAK).
- Indication for PTA is hypoglycemia unawareness or brittle diabetes with a frequent incidence of diabetic ketoacidosis and hypoglycemia (**Figure 22-1**).
- Indication for SPKT is having a chronic kidney disease with a glomerular filtration rate of less than 20 mL/min or being on dialysis and a diagnosis of diabetes mellitus that meets the indication for PTA.
- Most of the SPKT is performed in type 1 diabetes mellitus (T1DM), but it could also be performed in selected patients with type 2 diabetes mellitus.[2]
- The International Pancreas Transplant Registry reports 63,871 pancreas transplants occurred between December 1966 and December 2020.[3]

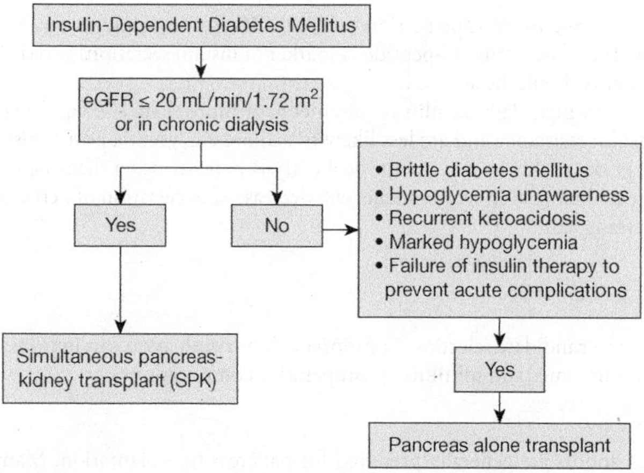

Figure 22-1. **Indications for a pancreas transplant.** eGFR, estimated glomerular filtration rate.

- Recent data trends show that the number of pancreas transplants has decreased from 1,177 in 2010 to 963 in 2021 (18.2%) with corresponding decreases in candidates on the pancreas transplant wait-lists. This can be partially attributed to significant improvements in the medical management of diabetes and its complications over the past decade.[2]

CANDIDATE ELIGIBILITY

- Candidate selection is an important determinant of allograft survival. A multidisciplinary team performs a pretransplant evaluation to determine the candidates' eligibility and ability to tolerate surgery and long-term immunosuppression.
- The primary determinants of candidate eligibility are generally similar to kidney transplantation. The major differences in eligibility are noted below.

Age

- Transplant centers have different cutoffs of age for pancreas transplantation. At Washington University, the age cutoff is 60 years.
- Younger patients have better patient and graft survival than patients >50 years.[4] This is likely related to fewer diabetic complications including cardiovascular complications and diabetic nephropathy.
- Patients between 50 and 65 years without significant comorbidities would still benefit from SPKT or PAK.[4]

Obesity

- Body mass index (BMI) requirements are variable between transplant centers. Generally, BMI thresholds for most centers are between 30 and 35 kg/m^2.
- BMI cutoff for pancreas transplantation at Washington University was increased recently to 32 kg/m^2.
- In a recent analysis of patients with T1DM, mildly obese patients with BMI 30 to 35 kg/m^2 have outcomes comparable with those of lean patients.[5]

Insulin Requirements

- The goal of pancreas transplantation in T1DM is restoring endogenous insulin production. Therefore, serum C-peptide (a marker of insulin secretion) and daily insulin requirements should be assessed.
- Patients with high daily insulin requirements of more than 1 U/kg/d may exhibit early insulin resistance and are less likely to achieve euglycemia post transplant.
- An exception to this involves peritoneal dialysis patients using dextrose-containing dialysate as their insulin requirements will decrease after cessation of peritoneal dialysis post transplant.

DONOR SELECTION

In addition to candidate selection, appropriate donor evaluation can improve pancreas transplant outcomes and minimize postoperative complications.

Age

- Younger donors are generally preferred for pancreas transplantation. Many studies have demonstrated an association between young donors and better graft survival.[6]

- Given the limited availability of donor organs, several studies have investigated broadening donor criteria. The EXPAND study investigated extended donor criteria (age 50-60 years, BMI 30-34 kg/m^2) and found no decrease in graft function at 3 and 12 months with similar rates of morbidity and rejection.[7]

Cold Ischemia Time

The pancreas is a highly vascular organ and is particularly susceptible to ischemia. Consequently, prolonged cold ischemic time and/or hemodynamic instability corresponding to donors on a high dose or multiple vasopressors at time of procurement have been associated with postoperative complications including graft thrombosis, pancreatitis, intra-abdominal infections, and anastomotic leaks.[8]

Cause of Death

Trauma and brain death donors without significant comorbidities are ideal candidates for pancreatic transplantation. Patients with cardiac arrest or stroke remain viable candidates but often have systemic vascular disease (coronary or intracranial artery atherosclerosis) requiring evaluation.[8,9]

Macroscopic Evaluation

- The transplant surgeon will perform a macroscopic examination of the pancreas to determine its viability. The pancreas is inspected for signs of trauma, inflammation, consistency (nodularity/masses, calcification, edema, fatty infiltration), vasculature, and coloration.
- Organs with trauma, masses (including pseudocysts or nodularity), or extensive fatty infiltration are excluded. Coloration can be an important indicator of ischemia (pale) versus fatty infiltration (yellow).[8]

BENEFITS OF PANCREAS TRANSPLANTATION

- SPKT is a well-established and effective treatment of patients with T1DM with chronic kidney disease. It allows for insulin independence and euglycemia. Consequently, it can stabilize or potentially reverse secondary diabetic complications improving patient morbidity and mortality and conferring improved quality of life.
- Pancreas transplantation improves the quality of life. It provides freedom from dietary restrictions, hypoglycemic episodes, frequent glucose monitoring, and insulin therapy.
- Pancreas transplantation is associated with decreased morbidity via stabilization or reversal of diabetic sequelae.
  - Diabetic nephropathy: Fioretto et al. demonstrated improvements in albuminuria in T1DM at 5 years after PTA with reversal of diabetic lesions at 10 years (although the use of calcineurin inhibitors is a confounding factor given its antiproteinuric effects).[10] Similarly, Lindahl et al. found that patients with DM1 who underwent kidney transplant alone (KTA) had wider glomerular basement membrane and mesangial volumes than those who underwent SPKT.[11]
  - Diabetic neuropathy and retinopathy: Data are less robust than in diabetic retinopathy. Some studies have shown stabilization in the progression of retinopathy lesions,[12,13] while others showed no benefit.[14,15] In some cases, there is a stabilization of diabetic neuropathy[16]; many others have demonstrated no benefit. These variable results are likely dependent on the length of diabetes.

- Improved metabolic profile—Improvements in lipid profile post transplantation may abate the progression of atherosclerosis, thereby reducing cardiovascular disease risk.[17,18]
- Cost-effectiveness: Douzdijan et al demonstrated that SPKT is among the most cost-effective strategies for the treatment of patients with T1DM and end-stage renal disease. In their analysis, the estimated costs per quality-adjusted year were $317,746 for dialysis, $156,042 for deceased donor KTA, $123,923 for living donor KTA, and $102,422 for SPKT.[19]

TECHNICAL COMPLICATIONS

- Pancreas transplants have higher technical failure rates than kidney transplants.
- It is estimated that approximately up to 10% of pancreas transplants in the US are lost due to technical failure during the first 12 months of transplantation, most commonly due to graft thrombosis.[20]
- While advancements in immunosuppression management have significantly reduced immunologic allograft loss, technical failure rates have remained stagnant.
- Currently, technical failure is the predominant cause of early graft failure (<1 year) and thus is a significant contributor to surgical morbidity and mortality in pancreas transplants.[20,21]
- Technical failure refers to intraoperative technical errors (i.e., anastomosis, vascular graft placement) and postoperative sequela of pancreas transplantation including vascular thrombosis, infections, exocrine leaks, pancreatitis, and bleeding (see **Table 22-1**).[20]
- Risk factors for technical failure include previously transplanted candidate and donor characteristics (as discussed above such as age, cold ischemia time).[20,21]
- Perioperative anticoagulation: The pancreas is a low-flow organ and highly susceptible to graft thrombosis (usually venous). Most centers will use perioperative anticoagulation with either antiplatelet agents or more commonly heparin.[22]
- Historically, allograft pancreas ductal secretions were managed with enteric drainage.
- In the early 1990s, most centers shifted toward bladder drainage due to more effective management of exocrine leaks (systemic vs. localized) and the ability to monitor for rejection (with urinary amylase).
- However, due to chronic bicarbonate loss (with corresponding dehydration, metabolic acidosis), pancreatitis, and enzymatic urothelial damage (cystitis, urethritis, hematuria), bladder drainage has fallen out of favor. Currently, the predominant surgical technique is enteric drainage (typically donor duodenum anastomosed to recipient small bowel).

TABLE 22-1 Etiology of Technical Failure in Pancreas Transplant

Causes of Technical Failure	Percentage From All Technical Failure (n = 123)
Thrombosis	52 (n = 64)
Pancreatitis	20.3 (n = 25)
Intra-abdominal infection	18.7 (n = 23)
Exocrine leak	6.5 (n = 8)
Bleed	2.4 (n = 3)

Data from Humar A, Ramcharan T, Kandaswamy R, Gruessner RW, Gruessner AC, Sutherland DE. Technical failures after pancreas transplants: Why grafts fail and the risk factors—a multivariate analysis. *Transplantation*. 2004;78:1188-1192. Table 3.

- Various composite risk models have been proposed to optimize allograft success through early identification of pancreas transplants at high risk of technical failure. These models can help guide candidate/donor selection criteria, modify posttransplant management, and potentially expand the pool of available organs.[21,23]
- One such model is the pancreas donor risk index (PDRI). This model is calculated using the donor risk factors sex, age, race, BMI, height, cause of death, preservation time, donation after cardiac death (DCD), and creatinine. Higher PDRI was associated with lower pancreas survival.[23]

DEATH-CENSORED GRAFT FAILURE

- A primary nonfunctional pancreas transplant is usually identified by the removal of the pancreas transplant within 14 days after the pancreas transplant (in these cases, the recipient will gain the waiting time for a pancreas transplant).[24]
- Pancreas graft failure is the removal of the allograft pancreas after 14 days, the use of insulin ≥0.5 U/kg/d for more than 90 consecutive days, or recipient death.[24]
- During the first 3 months post transplantation, technical complications are the most common complication.
- After 3 months, pancreas allograft rejection is the most common cause of pancreas allograft failure.
- In 2021, the incidence of 1-year pancreas transplant graft failure had increased: 10.5% for SPK, 15.6% for PTA, and 14.6% for PAK.[2]
- In 2018, the International Pancreas and Islet Transplant Association and the European Pancreas and Islet Transplant Association gave the classification of functional and clinical outcomes of β-cell therapy, as seen in **Table 22-2**.[25]

TABLE 22-2 Definition of Functional and Clinical Outcomes for β-cell Replacement Therapy

Graft Status	Hemoglobin A1C %	Severe Hypoglycemic Events per Year	Insulin Unit Requirements	C-Peptide	Treatment Success
Optimal graft function	≤6.5%	None	None	>Baseline	Yes
Good graft function	<7.0%	None	<50% Baseline	>Baseline	Yes
Marginal graft function	Baseline	<Baseline	≥50% Baseline	>Baseline	No
Failed graft	Baseline	Baseline	Baseline	Baseline	No

Adapted with permission from Rickels MR, Stock PG, de Koning EJP, et al. Defining outcomes for β-cell replacement therapy in the treatment of diabetes: a consensus report on the Igls criteria from the IPITA/EPITA opinion leaders workshop. *Transplantation.* 2018;102:1479-86.

- Various composite risk models have been proposed to optimize allograft success through early identification of pancreas transplants at high risk of technical failure. These models can help guide candidate/donor selection criteria, modify posttransplant management, and potentially expand the pool of available organs.[21,23]
- One risk model is the PDRI. This model is calculated using the donor risk factors sex, age, race, BMI, height, cause of death, preservation time, DCD, and creatinine. Higher PDRI was associated with lower pancreas survival.[23]

PANCREAS REJECTION

- Three months post transplant, pancreatic allograft rejection remains the first cause of death-censored pancreas allograft loss.
- The incidences of acute rejection in patients receiving a pancreas transplant are 12.5% for PAK, 21.8% for PTA, and 10.6% for SPKT.[26]
- Clinical manifestations can be from asymptomatic to pancreatitis of the allograft with abdominal pain, nausea, vomiting, fever, and tenderness of the allograft. Depending on the severity patient can present with clinical findings of hyperglycemia and even diabetic ketoacidosis.
- Laboratory findings show an elevation of pancreatic enzymes of the exocrine function such as serum amylase and lipase. One study showed the sensitivity of serum lipase for rejection is 71% and that of serum amylase is 50%. In SPKT, serum lipase and serum creatinine increased up to 86%.[27]
- In **Table 22-3**, we review the cause of elevated pancreatic enzymes in pancreas transplant according to the time period of transplant and etiology.[28]
- De novo donor-specific antibodies (DSAs) are strongly associated with pancreas rejection and death-censored allograft failure. A meta-analysis of 8 studies found higher odds of graft failure (odds ratio [OR] = 4.42) and rejection (OR = 3.35) compared with the ones without DSAs.
- One of the novel markers is plasma donor-derived cell-free DNA (dd-cfDNA).[29]
- There are not much data about the use of dd-cfDNA in pancreas transplantation surveillance protocol.
- In SPKT having dd-cfDNA >1% is associated with rejection.[30]
- dd-cfDNA has a sensitivity of 85.7% and a specificity of 93.7% of detecting pancreas rejection.[30]
- One important factor to assess chronicity is monitoring hemoglobin A1C, C-peptide, and history of hyperglycemia or requiring insulin.
- The gold-standard diagnosis of a pancreas transplant rejection is a pancreas biopsy. In cases of SPKT with acute kidney injury, it is preferable to do a kidney biopsy as it has less complications and has a 60% concurrence in diagnosis. Pancreas transplant biopsy has a higher risk for complications, up to 2.8%.
- The histological classification of pancreas transplant rejection is based on Banff classification and summarized in **Table 22-4**.[31]
- Treatment of indeterminate/borderline cellular rejection is preferred by the use of steroids.
- Treatment of acute cellular rejection grades I, II, and III is preferably thymoglobulin and steroids.
- For maintenance immunosuppression, there is a need to augment the level of tacrolimus, such as considering a target trough level of 8 to 10 ng/mL. Antimetabolite dose could be increased to a full dose (such as mycophenolate mofetil 1,000 mg bid); it was reduced earlier in the course of transplant.

TABLE 22-3 Common Diagnosis Contributed to Increase Pancreatic Enzymes After Pancreas Transplant

Diagnosis	Overall Frequency (%)	Frequency the Entity Presents With Elevated Enzymes
Perioperative < 45 d		
Enzyme leak (enteric or parenchymal)	~5	High
Infected fluid or abscess	~5	Moderate
Thrombosis	2-5	Low
Ileus	5-10, transient	Moderate
Acute rejection	1-2	High
Mild Postoperative (>45 d-1 y)		
Acute rejection	15-20	High
SBO	5	Low-moderate
Pseudocyst	2-5	High
Constipation	2-5	Low-moderate
Abscess	2-5	Low-moderate
CMV pancreatitis	~1	High
Late Postoperative (>1 y)		
Acute rejection	5-10	High
Chronic rejection	~5	Moderate-high
SBO/ventral hernia	~10	Low-moderate
Intrinsic pancreatic abnormality	~5	Moderate-high
Native pancreatitis	1	High
CMV pancreatitis	<1	High

CMV, cytomegalovirus; SBO, small bowel obstruction.
Adapted with permission from Redfield RR, Kaufman DB, Odorico JS. Diagnosis and treatment of pancreas rejection. *Curr Transplant Rep.* 2015;2:169-75.

- For antibody-mediated rejection (AMR), the treatment is similar to kidney transplant AMR.
- In general, AMR could be treated with a combination of plasmapheresis, intravenous immune globulin (IVIG), and rituximab for patients within the first year. For recipients with AMR after the first year of transplant, treatment with IVIG and rituximab can be considered.

POSTTRANSPLANT DIABETES AFTER PANCREAS TRANSPLANT

- Some patients may develop hyperglycemia post pancreas transplant without necessarily having pancreas rejection. This could be related to pancreas dysfunction or the development of type 2 diabetes.

TABLE 22-4 Histological Classification of Pancreas Rejection

Classification of Rejection	
Acute cellular rejection	
Borderline/indeterminate	Active septal inflammation (activated lymphocytes with or without eosinophils)
Grade I/mild acute T-cell-mediated rejection	Active septal inflammation (activated, blastic lymphocytes and with or without eosinophils) involving septal structures; venulitis (subendothelial accumulation of inflammatory cells and endothelial damage in septal veins) or ductitis (epithelial inflammation and damage of ducts) and/or Focal acinar inflammation. No more than 2 inflammatory foci per lobule with absent or minimal acinar cell injury
Grade II/moderate acute T-cell-mediated rejection	Multifocal (but not confluent or diffuse) acinar inflammation (≥3 foci per lobule) with spotty (individual) acinar cell injury and dropout and/or Mild intimal arteritis (with minimal, <25% luminal compromise)
Grade III/severe acute T-cell-mediated rejection (requires differentiation from AMR)	Diffuse (widespread, extensive) acinar inflammation with focal or diffuse multicellular/confluent acinar cell necrosis and/or Moderate or severe intimal arteritis, >25% luminal compromise and/or Transmural inflammation—Necrotizing arteritis
Antibody-mediated rejection (3 criteria to meet the diagnosis)	1. Confirmed circulating donor-specific antibody 2. Morphological evidence of tissue injury (interacinar inflammation/capillaritis, acinar cell damage swelling/necrosis/apoptosis/dropout, vasculitis, thrombosis) 3. C4d positivity in interacinar capillaries (≥5% of acinar lobular surface)
Grade I/mild acute AMR	Well-preserved architecture, mild monocytic-macrophagic or mixed (monocytic-macrophagic/neutrophilic) infiltrates with rare acinar cell damage

TABLE 22-4 Histological Classification of Pancreas Rejection (Continued)

Classification of Rejection	
Grade II/moderate acute AMR	Overall preservation of the architecture with interacinar monocytic-macrophagic or mixed (monocytic-macrophagic/neutrophilic) infiltrates, capillary dilatation, capillaritis, congestion, multicellular acinar cell dropout, and extravasation of red blood cells
Grade III/severe acute AMR	Architectural disarray, scattered inflammatory infiltrates in a background of interstitial hemorrhage, multifocal and confluent parenchymal necrosis, arterial and venous wall necrosis and thrombosis

AMR, antibody-mediated rejection.
Data from Drachenberg CB, Torrealba JR, Nankivell BJ, et al. Guidelines for the diagnosis of antibody-mediated rejection in pancreas allografts—updated Banff grading schema. *Am J Transplant.* 2011;11:1792-802. Tables 2 and 4.

- Risk factors for posttransplant hyperglycemia include high pretransplant insulin dose, pretransplant obesity, and acute rejection episodes.[32]
- The insulin requirement for pancreas transplant candidate should be less than 1 U/kg/d as higher insulin requirement means higher incidence of insulin resistance.
- Early treatment of hyperglycemia after a pancreas transplant with a DPP-4 inhibitor, such as sitagliptin, prolongs the survival of a pancreas transplant (time to insulin therapy) compared with a standard observation approach.[33]
- Causes of pancreas graft failure should be assessed to determine reversible causes of posttransplant diabetes.

DEATH WITH FUNCTIONAL GRAFT

- The most common causes of death include cardio/cerebrovascular disease, infection, and malignancies.
- Cardiovascular mortality has improved over time but remained one of the leading causes of death.[11]
- The survival of those who received SPKT with a functional pancreas at 3 months is better than those who received a living or deceased kidney transplant alone.[34]
- Pancreas transplants are susceptible to infectious agents including bacteria, viruses, and fungi.
- Cytomegalovirus (CMV) infection is a commonly seen infection. Patients with CMV seronegativity have a higher risk of infection.
- The incidence of posttransplant malignancy increases over time. The incidence increases from 2% at 5 years to 9% at 10 years and reaches 20% at 25 years.[35] Among malignancies, skin cancers are the most common, accounting for more than 50% of cases.[35]

REFERENCES

1. Laftavi MR, Gruessner A, Gruessner R. Surgery of pancreas transplantation. *Curr Opin Organ Transplant.* 2017;22(4):389-97.
2. Kandaswamy R, Stock PG, Miller JM, et al. OPTN/SRTR 2021 annual data report: pancreas. *Am J Transplant.* 2023;23(2 suppl 1):S121-77.
3. Gruessner AC, Gruessner RWG. The 2022 international pancreas transplant registry report-A review. *Transplant Proc.* 2022;54(7):1918-43.
4. Siskind E, Maloney C, Akerman M, et al. An analysis of pancreas transplantation outcomes based on age groupings—an update of the UNOS database. *Clin Transplant.* 2014;28(9):990-4.
5. Merzkani M, Murad H, Wang M, et al. Outcomes in obese patients with diabetes mellitus type 2 that received simultaneous pancreas and kidney transplant. *Am J Transplant.* 2022;22(suppl 3).
6. Andreoni KA, Brayman KL, Guidinger MK, Sommers CM, Sung RS. Kidney and pancreas transplantation in the United States, 1996-2005. *Am J Transplant.* 2007;7(5 pt 2):1359-75.
7. Proneth A, Schnitzbauer AA, Schenker P, et al. Extended pancreas donor program-the EXPAND study: a prospective multicenter trial testing the use of pancreas donors older than 50 years. *Transplantation.* 2018;102(8):1330-7.
8. Muñoz-Bellvís L, López-Sánchez J. Donor risk factors in pancreas transplantation. *World J Transplant.* 2020;10(12):372-80.
9. Blundell J, Shahrestani S, Lendzion R, Pleass HJ, Hawthorne WJ. Risk factors for early pancreatic allograft thrombosis following simultaneous pancreas-kidney transplantation: a systematic review. *Clin Appl Thromb Hemost.* 2020;26:1076029620942589.
10. Fioretto P, Steffes MW, Sutherland DE, Goetz FC, Mauer M. Reversal of lesions of diabetic nephropathy after pancreas transplantation. *N Engl J Med.* 1998;339(2):69-75.
11. Lindahl JP, Hartmann A, Aakhus S, et al. Long-term cardiovascular outcomes in type 1 diabetic patients after simultaneous pancreas and kidney transplantation compared with living donor kidney transplantation. *Diabetologia.* 2016;59(4):844-52.
12. Königsrainer A, Miller K, Steurer W, et al. Does pancreas transplantation influence the course of diabetic retinopathy? *Diabetologia.* 1991;34(suppl 1):S86-8.
13. Pearce IA, Ilango B, Sells RA, Wong D. Stabilisation of diabetic retinopathy following simultaneous pancreas and kidney transplant. *Br J Ophthalmol.* 2000;84(7):736-40.
14. Ramsay RC, Goetz FC, Sutherland DE, et al. Progression of diabetic retinopathy after pancreas transplantation for insulin-dependent diabetes mellitus. *N Engl J Med.* 1988;318(4):208-14.
15. Wang Q, Klein R, Moss SE, et al. The influence of combined kidney-pancreas transplantation on the progression of diabetic retinopathy. A case series. *Ophthalmology.* 1994;101:1071-6.
16. Navarro X, Sutherland DE, Kennedy WR. Long-term effects of pancreatic transplantation on diabetic neuropathy. *Ann Neurol.* 1997;42(5):727-36.
17. Larsen JL, Stratta RJ, Ozaki CF, Taylor RJ, Miller SA, Duckworth WC. Lipid status after pancreas-kidney transplantation. *Diabetes Care.* 1992;15(1):35-42.
18. Katz HH, Nguyen TT, Velosa JA, Robertson RP, Rizza RA. Effects of systemic delivery of insulin on plasma lipids and lipoprotein concentrations in pancreas transplant recipients. *Mayo Clin Proc.* 1994;69(3):231-6.
19. Douzdjian V, Ferrara D, Silvestri G. Treatment strategies for insulin-dependent diabetics with ESRD: a cost-effectiveness decision analysis model. *Am J Kidney Dis.* 1998;31(5):794-802.
20. Humar A, Ramcharan T, Kandaswamy R, Gruessner RWG, Gruessner AC, Sutherland DER. Technical failures after pancreas transplants: why grafts fail and the risk factors—a multivariate analysis. *Transplantation.* 2004;78(8):1188-92.
21. Finger EB, Radosevich DM, Dunn TB, et al. A composite risk model for predicting technical failure in pancreas transplantation. *Am J Transplant.* 2013;13(7):1840-9.
22. Sharma S, Barrera K, Gruessner RWG. Chapter 13: surgical techniques for deceased donor pancreas transplantation. In: Orlando G, Piemonti L, Ricordi C, Stratta RJ, Gruessner RWG, eds. *Transplantation, Bioengineering, and Regeneration of the Endocrine Pancreas.* Academic Press; 2020:149-67.

23. Axelrod DA, Sung RS, Meyer KH, Wolfe RA, Kaufman DB. Systematic evaluation of pancreas allograft quality, outcomes and geographic variation in utilization. *Am J Transplant.* 2010;10(4):837-45.
24. *Definition of Pancreas Graft Failure by the Organ Procurement Transplant Tetwork (OPTN).* 2014. Accessed April 15, 2023. https://optn.transplant.hrsa.gov/media/1572/policynotice_20150701_pancreas.pdf
25. Rickels MR, Stock PG, de Koning EJP, et al. Defining outcomes for β-cell replacement therapy in the treatment of diabetes: a Consensus report on the Igls criteria from the IPITA/EPITA opinion Leaders Workshop. *Transplantation.* 2018;102(9):1479-86.
26. Kandaswamy R, Stock PG, Miller J, et al. OPTN/SRTR 2020 annual data report: pancreas. *Am J Transplant.* 2022;22(suppl 2):137-203.
27. Sugitani A, Egidi MF, Gritsch HA, Corry RJ. Serum lipase as a marker for pancreatic allograft rejection. *Clin Transplant.* 1998;12(3):224-7.
28. Redfield RR, Kaufman DB, Odorico JS. Diagnosis and treatment of pancreas rejection. *Curr Transplant Rep.* 2015;2:169-75.
29. Khan SM, Sumbal R, Schenk AD. Impact of anti-HLA de novo donor specific antibody on graft outcomes in pancreas transplantation: a meta-analysis. *Transplant Proc.* 2021;53(10):3022-9.
30. Ventura-Aguiar P, Ramirez-Bajo MJ, Rovira J, et al. Donor-derived cell-free DNA shows high sensitivity for the diagnosis of pancreas graft rejection in simultaneous pancreas-kidney transplantation. *Transplantation.* 2022;106(8):1690-7.
31. Drachenberg CB, Torrealba JR, Nankivell BJ, et al. Guidelines for the diagnosis of antibody-mediated rejection in pancreas allografts—updated Banff grading schema. *Am J Transplant.* 2011;11(9):1792-802.
32. Dean PG, Kudva YC, Larson TS, Kremers WK, Stegall MD. Posttransplant diabetes mellitus after pancreas transplantation. *Am J Transplant.* 2008;8(1):175-82.
33. Jang HW, Jung CH, Ko Y, et al. Beneficial effects of posttransplant dipeptidyl peptidase-4 inhibitor administration after pancreas transplantation to improve β cell function. *Ann Surg Treat Res.* 2021;101(3):187-96.
34. Ji M, Wang M, Hu W, et al. Survival after simultaneous pancreas-kidney transplantation in type 1 diabetes: the critical role of early pancreas allograft function. *Transpl Int.* 2022;35:10618.
35. Krendl FJ, Messner F, Bösmüller C, et al. Post-transplant malignancies following pancreas transplantation: incidence and implications on long-term outcome from a single-center perspective. *J Clin Med.* 2021;10(21):4810.

23 Multiorgan Transplantation

Sri Mahathi Kalipatnapu, Ojaswi Tomar, and
Rowena Delos Santos

GENERAL PRINCIPLES

- There has been an increase in the number of patients being considered for heart and liver transplants, many of whom have multiple comorbidities including kidney dysfunction.[1]
- The number of combined liver-kidney transplants has increased in the last 2 decades from fewer than 200 transplants in 2000 to 400 transplants in 2010, and more than 800 transplants in 2020.[2]
- The number of combined heart-kidney transplants has also increased in the last 2 decades, from fewer than 50 transplants in 2000 to almost 300 transplants in 2020.
- There are defined criteria for liver-kidney transplant as detailed later this chapter, but criteria are still evolving for heart-kidney transplant.[2]
- Multiple organ transplant is beneficial to an individual patient with multiorgan failure. However, it remains to be seen whether this outweighs the risk of limiting access to the general pool for a kidney transplant alone (KTA).[2]
- **Ethical considerations**
  - Because there is no standardization of criteria for multiorgan transplants (with the exception of liver-kidney), there is potential for disparities between patients awaiting single organ transplant and those awaiting multiorgan transplant.
  - The disparity can happen in terms of frequency of transplantation itself and time to transplant.
  - Patients awaiting multiorgan transplants tend to have shorter wait times due to being more ill, compared with those awaiting a single organ transplant.
  - Organ Procurement and Transplantation Network's (OPTN) strategic plan is to minimize disparities and improve equity in organ allocation.

Liver-Kidney Transplantation

GENERAL PRINCIPLES

- Renal failure in cirrhosis is mainly hemodynamically mediated, resulting from marked reduction in systemic vascular resistance due to arterial vasodilation in the splanchnic circulation triggered by portal hypertension.[3]
- In patients with orthotopic liver transplantation, the percentage of primary graft nonfunction, 30-day mortality, long-term graft function, and patient survival was significantly lower in patients with mean creatinine clearance (CrCl) < 35 mL/min compared with CrCl > 48 mL/min[4-6]

Epidemiology

- Simultaneous liver-kidney transplantation (SLK) comprises 10% of all the liver transplants and is the most common multiorgan transplant performed in the US.

- There has been a steady increase in the number of SLK procedures since 1988, with a distinct deviation developing between SLK and kidney after liver transplant (KAL) after the adoption of the model for end-stage liver disease (MELD) score in 2002. See **Figure 23-1**.
- There was a 233% increase in the number of SLK procedures, coinciding with a 74% decrease in the number of KAL procedures from 2001 to 2007.[3]

Eligibility Criteria for Simultaneous Liver-Kidney Transplant

- In 2017, the United Network for Organ Sharing (UNOS) enacted a policy for the allocation of SLK based on medical eligibility (**Table 23-1**) and introduced the "safety net" for patients with marginal renal function who received a liver transplant alone (LTA), so that they have priority access to kidney transplantation (KT) (**Table 23-2**) should the renal function worsen after the LTA.
- To qualify for the "safety net" provision, these LTA patients have glomerular filtration rate (GFR) <20 mL/min or remain dialysis dependent 2 to 12 months after the LTA.

Timing of Surgery

- Hemodynamic instability and coagulopathy in liver transplant patients construe an unfavorable milieu for the newly implanted kidney allograft at the time of liver transplant.
- In a study of 1998 SLK patients, 5-year kidney graft was 64% for SLK recipients versus 75% for KTA ($P < .001$).[7]
- Patient survival was 66% for SLK recipients versus 81% KTA ($P < .001$).[7]

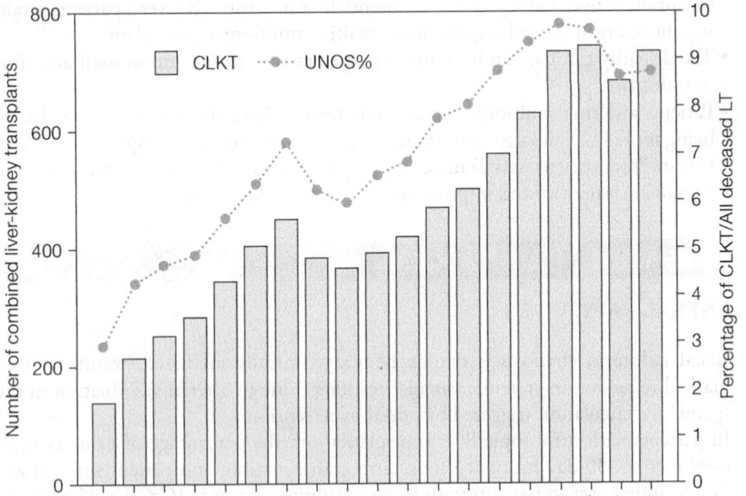

Figure 23-1. **Number of combined liver kidney transplants (CLKT) from 2001 to 2019.** LT, liver transplant. (Reproduced with permission from Ekser B, Contreras AG, Andraus W, et al. Current status of combined liver-kidney transplantation. *Int J Surg* 2020;82:149-54. Figure 1.)

TABLE 23-1 Medical Eligibility Criteria for Combined Liver-Kidney Transplantation

Categories	Transplant Program Must Document at Least One of the following
Chronic kidney disease with a measured or calculated glomerular filtration rate (GFR) ≤60 mL/min for >3 mo	• Candidate is on regular hemodialysis • Candidate's most recent GFR is ≤30 mL/min at the time of registration for kidney transplant
Sustained acute kidney injury	• Candidate is on dialysis at least 6 wk • Candidate's GFR is ≤25 mL/min for at least 6 wk (as documented in weekly measurements) • Candidate has any combination of above 2 criteria for 6 wk
Metabolic disease	• Hyperoxaluria • Atypical hemolytic syndrome from mutations in factor H or I • Familial nonneuropathic systemic amyloidosis • Methylmalonic aciduria

Reproduced with permission from Ekser B, Contreras AG, Andraus W, et al. Current status of combined liver-kidney transplantation. *Int J Surg*. 2020;82:149-54. Table 1.

- Survival was significantly lower in SLK versus kidney-alone recipients of the contralateral kidney.[7]
- This gives rise to the consideration of delaying kidney transplant surgery in SLK recipients.
- The "Indiana approach," whereby KT was placed on a hypothermic perfusion machine and delayed by 48 to 72 hours after liver transplant, showed lower rates of delayed graft function (DGF) (0% vs. 7.3%, $P < .01$) and higher patient survival (91%, $P = .0019$) in the delayed group, despite the increased cold ischemia time (10 ± 3 and 50 ± 15 hours). This was attributed to increased time to wean off vasopressor support and improve hemodynamic stability.[8]

OUTCOMES

- A study comparing LTA with SLK and KAL reported that patient survival for KAL recipients was worse than for SLK recipients at <3 months of transplantation and >12 months of transplantation. There was no difference observed between 6 and 12 months.[9] See **Figure 23-2** and **Table 23-3**.
- There was no difference in recipient mortality between LTA and SLK ($P = .024$).
- There was a 15% decreased risk of graft loss in SLK compared with LTA (hazard ratio [HR] = 0.85, $P < .0001$).
- SLK recipients had higher patient survival (81.8% vs. 71%) and graft survival (HR 0.85 vs. 1.34) compared with liver after kidney transplantation.[9]

TABLE 23-2 "Safety-Net" Kidney Transplantation Allocation Sequences for Liver Transplant Recipients With Nonrecovery of Renal Function

Sequence A (KDPI ≤ 20%)	Sequence B (KDPI > 20% < 35%)	Sequence C (KDPI > 35% < 85%)	Sequence D (KDPI > 85%)
Highly sensitized	Highly sensitized	Highly sensitized	Highly sensitized
0-ABDR mismatch	0-ABDR mismatch	0-ABDR mismatch	0-ABDR mismatch
Prior living donor KT	Prior living donor KT	Prior living donor KT	Local CLKT safety net
Local pediatrics	Local pediatrics	Local CLKT safety net	Local + regional
Local top 20% EPTS	Local CLKT safety net	Local candidates	National candidates
0-ABDR mismatch (all)	Local adults	Regional candidates	
Local (all)	Regional pediatrics	National candidates	
Regional pediatrics	Regional adults		
Regional (to 20%)		National pediatrics	
Regional (all)		National adults	
National pediatrics			
National (top 20%)			
National (all)			

EPTS, Estimated post-transplant survival; CLKT; combined liver kidney transplants, KDPI; kidney donor profile index; KT, kidney transplant.
Reproduced with permission from Ekser B, Contreras AG, Andraus W, et al. Current status of combined liver-kidney transplantation. *Int J Surg.* 2020;82:149-54. Table 2.

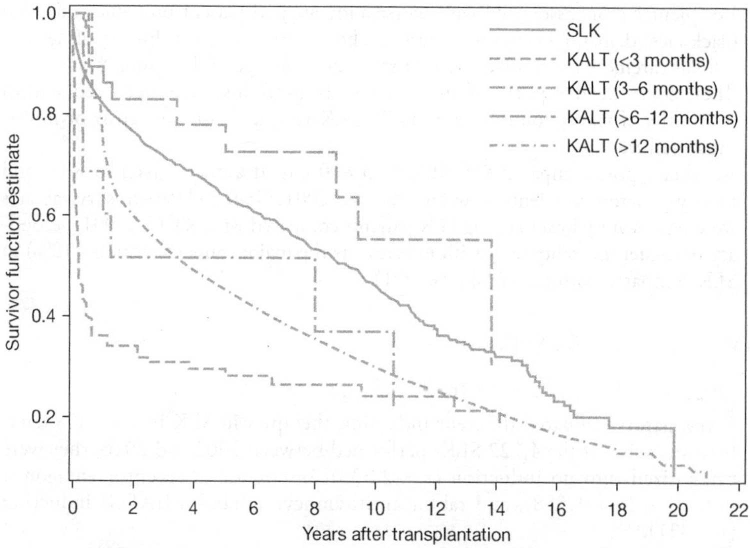

Figure 23-2. **Overall recipient survival in SLK compared with KALT.** KALT, kidney after liver transplant; SLK, simultaneous liver-kidney transplants. (Reproduced with permission from Martin EF, Huang J, Xiang Q, et al. Recipient survival and graft survival are not diminished by simultaneous liver-kidney transplantation: an analysis of the United Network for Organ Sharing database. *Liver Transpl.* 2012;18:914-29. Figure 3.)

- A retrospective analysis was done between 2002 and 2011, comparing 3026 subjects who received SLK from donation after brain death (DBD) and 98 from donation after cardiac death (DCD). The study showed that kidney, liver, and patient survival of recipients of DCD organs were inferior to DBD recipients at 1, 3, and 5 years ($P < .02$).[10]

TABLE 23-3 Predictors of Recipient Mortality and Graft Loss

Recipient age ≥ 65 y
Male
Black
Hepatitis C/diabetes mellitus status
Donor age ≥ 60 y
Serum creatinine ≥ 2 mg/dL
Cold ischemia time > 12 h
Warm ischemia time > 60 min

Data from Martin EF, Huang J, Xiang Q, et al. Recipient survival and graft survival are not diminished by simultaneous liver-kidney transplantation: an analysis of the United Network for Organ Sharing database. *Liver Transpl.* 2012;18:914-29.

- Recipient factors associated with worse allograft and patient outcomes included black race, diabetes, being on a ventilator, hospitalization, DGF, history of hepatocellular carcinoma, intensive care unit stay, and older age of the donor.[10]
- There have been reports of increased early graft loss that occurred within 6 months of transplantation among 99 SLK recipients due to sepsis or multiorgan failure.[11]
- Another report compared 800 SLK with 800 paired kidneys given to KTA and kidney-pancreas recipients between 1987 and 2001. Graft and patient survival rates were significantly lower among SLK patients compared with KT ($P < .001$) secondary to higher mortality rates with infection as the major cause of mortality (8%) in SLK compared with KT (2%) ($P < .001$).[12]

IMMUNOLOGIC CONSIDERATIONS

Induction and Maintenance Immunosuppression

- Investigators evaluated different induction therapies in SLK in a UNOS database analysis. Of the 4,722 SLKs performed between 2002 and 2016, they were categorized into no induction (n = 2,333), interleukin 2-receptor antagonist induction (n = 1,558), and rabbit antithymocyte globulin (rATG) induction (n = 831).[13]
- The rATG group had more kidney-machine perfusion (34% vs. 20% in other groups; $P < .001$), longer kidney cold ischemia time (15.7 vs. 11.5 hours in other groups; $P < .001$), and less DGF (18% vs. 19% and 25% in other groups; $P < .001$) but higher mortality (29% vs. 27% and 23% in other groups).[13]
- In a study with 45 SLK recipients, between January 1997 and October 2011, 13 patients received induction with alemtuzumab compared with no induction therapy followed by maintenance with tacrolimus and steroids, mycophenolate mofetil (MMF), or sirolimus.[14]
- Overall survival for the alemtuzumab versus no induction therapy groups were 100% versus 76% at 1 year, 85.7% versus 76% at 3 years, and 85.7%, versus 70% at 5 years of follow-up ($P = .04$).[14]
- Recipient age > 60 years, MELD score > 20, donor age > 60 years, indications for SLKs, and use of MMF or sirolimus for maintenance immunosuppression did not show a difference in overall survival.[14]

Rejections and Long-Term Allograft Survival

- In a study, 68 consecutive SLK recipients (14 with donor-specific alloantibodies at transplantation [DSA+], 54 with low or no DSA [DSA−]) were compared with biopsies of a matched cohort of KTA recipients (28 DSA+, 108 DSA−).
- The cumulative incidence of antibody-mediated rejection was lower in DSA+ SLK versus DSA+ KTA (7% vs. 46%, $P = .01$), and cumulative incidence of T-cell-mediated rejection was lower in DSA- SLK versus DSA- KTA (7% vs. 31%, $P < .0007$).[15]
- Molecular markers of inflammation and T-cell activation are significantly less common in kidney biopsies of SLK recipients compared with KTA recipients as evidenced by decreased expression of transcripts of the endothelial cell activation and inflammation/rejection gene sets and DSA-selective transcripts on biopsies.[16]

- It has also been shown that a simultaneous or partial auxiliary liver transplant with a kidney transplant can turn a positive crossmatch before transplant into a negative one,[17] which has been proposed to be secondary to the liver absorbing or neutralizing the donor-specific antibodies.[18]

Heart-Kidney Transplantation

GENERAL PRINCIPLES

- Patients with end-stage heart failure commonly have kidney dysfunction.
- In severe heart failure, both arterial underfilling from impaired cardiac output and increased venous pressures from venous congestion result in decreased glomerular filtration and elevation in serum creatinine.
- Conversely, progressive renal dysfunction causes atherosclerotic changes and metabolic disturbances that further exacerbate heart failure. This complex cardiorenal pathophysiology is the basis of cardiorenal syndrome.[19]
- For selected patients with end-stage heart disease, heart transplant is the treatment of choice.
- In patients with end-stage heart disease, renal dysfunction with a serum creatinine of >1.5 mg/dL is an independent predictor and risk factor for death within 2 months of listing for a heart transplant in UNOS.[20]
- One of the initial studies that compared outcomes of heart transplants alone with simultaneous heart-kidney transplants (SHK) on a national level showed that patients with lower GFR (<37 mL/min/m^2) undergoing heart transplant alone (HTA) have a significantly increased risk of requiring dialysis in the early posttransplant period (odds ratio 2.093; 95% confidence interval [CI], 1.835-2.386; $P < .001$).[21]
- A conclusion of this study was that, in potential heart transplant recipients with an estimated GFR (eGFR) of <37 mL/min/m^2, SHK should be recommended instead of HTA because SHK has been shown to improve posttransplant survival in this group of low-eGFR patients.[21]

EPIDEMIOLOGY

- The first SHK using the same donor was described in 1978 by Norman and colleagues.[22]
- Between 2000 and 2019, the annual number of heart transplants performed increased by 61%, but a dramatic increase of 650% was seen in the number of SHK performed during this time.[23] See **Figure 23-3**.
- From 2010 to 2018 alone, at least more than 5% of all heart transplants were SHK.[19] See **Figure 23-4**.
- Among multiorgan transplants, SHK has shown the largest increase in frequency between 2015 and 2020.[24]

CRITERIA

- There are no universally agreed upon guidelines to establish appropriate eligibility criteria for SHK. This has led to SHK being performed on nondialysis patients with a wide range of eGFR.[24]

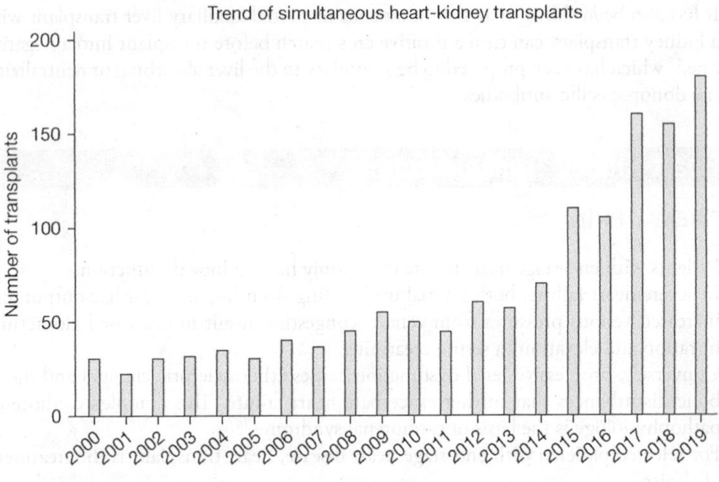

Figure 23-3. Trends of simultaneous heart-kidney transplants. (Reproduced with permission from Agarwal KA, Patel H, Agrawal N, et al. Cardiac outcomes in isolated heart and simultaneous kidney and heart transplants in the United States. *Kidney Int Rep*. 2021;6:2348-57. Figure 2A.)

- It is challenging to determine which patients may have reversible kidney dysfunction and hence could benefit from heart transplantation alone rather than SHK. Similarly, it is also challenging to determine the true benefit of the kidney in patients receiving SHK.[25]

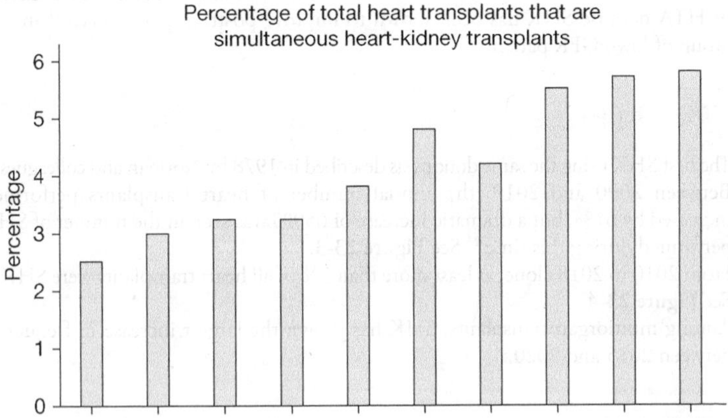

Figure 23-4. Trends of simultaneous heart-kidney transplants. (Reproduced with permission from Kobashigawa J, Dadhania DM, Farr M, et al. Consensus conference on heart-kidney transplantation. *Am J Transplant*. 2021;21:2459-67. Figure 1B.)

- A consensus conference on SHK was held in June 2019 in Boston. The objective of the heart/kidney workgroup at the consensus conference was to make uniform suggestions to help patients who will benefit from SHK and to prevent unnecessary kidney transplants by developing a safety net.[19]
- It is important to understand that these should be considered only as suggestions by the heart/kidney workgroup. These should not be used as set criteria as there are no definite guidelines in UNOS.

Heart and Kidney Workgroup

- According to the heart/kidney workgroup, the following factors need to be considered when evaluating a pre–heart transplant patient for SHK.[19]
- Presence of chronic kidney disease (CKD): By definition, this means an eGFR of <60 mL/min/1.73 m^2 for at least 90 days. However, these data are not always available to us at the time of evaluation. The presence of long-standing risk factors for CKD, renal ultrasound findings consistent with CKD, and proteinuria >0.5 g/d could be used as surrogate markers to suggest the presence of CKD.[19]
- Duration of acute kidney injury and potential for recovery of renal function: Acute kidney injury requiring dialysis or one that does not recover despite correcting the contributing factors could be considered irreversible kidney dysfunction and may be considered for SHK. In situations when there is insufficient time to wait for renal recovery, a multidisciplinary approach should be taken, involving a transplant nephrologist and cardiologist to determine whether it is reasonable to proceed with SHK.[19]
- Accurate measurement of renal function: 2 separate measurements of eGFR at least 2 weeks apart are suggested. The first one could be an modification of diet in renal disease or chronic kidney disease epidemiology collaboration (CKD-EPI) equation. The second or confirmatory measurement should be either measured eGFR or calculated eGFR using serum creatinine and cystatin C levels in the CKD-EPI equation.[19]

Current Consensus

The following considerations are, again, not solidified as criteria for SHK selection and still undergoing discussions.

- eGFR 45 to 59 mL/min/1.73 m^2: should not be considered for SHK. The safety net policy could be applied to these patients (see below).
- eGFR < 45 mL/min/1.73 m^2: should begin evaluation by nephrologist for potential SHK candidacy.
- eGFR 30 to 44 mL/min/1.73 m^2: consider SHK evaluation in presence of other findings suggestive of CKD (proteinuria > 0.5 g/d, small kidneys on ultrasound) on a case-by-case basis.
- eGFR < 30 mL/min/1.73 m^2: reasonable to be listed for SHK.[19]

Safety Net Policy

- This is adapted from the safety net policy for liver-kidney transplants. The objective is to decrease the number of unnecessary kidney transplants by providing time for renal recovery after HTA.[19]
- The safety net policy suggests that patients on chronic dialysis or those with eGFR < 20 mL/min/1.73 m^2 for 6 weeks between postoperative day 30 and day 365 after a heart transplant should be given priority for kidney transplant (donors with a kidney donor profile index >20%).[19]

IMMUNOLOGIC CONSIDERATIONS

- There are no established guidelines on appropriate immunosuppression management for patients after SHK transplant.
- The heart/kidney workgroup suggests carefully choosing the appropriate induction immunosuppression based on various patient factors including immunologic status and risk of infections.[19]
- Note that center protocols will differ from one another, and one may encounter different protocols depending on the center.
- Consider basiliximab for patients with low immunologic or infection risk.
- Consider rATG induction for patients who have a high probability of developing DGF and are sensitized.
- Calcineurin inhibitor (CNI) initiation can be safely delayed by 1 to 2 days if renal function remains impaired after transplantation and if anti-thymocyte globulin (ATG) was used for induction immunosuppression.
- If basiliximab was used for induction immunosuppression though, there should be no delay in starting a CNI. It is recommended to be given within 24 hours of SHK.
- There is no consensus on the goal CNI level.
- In select patients with low immunologic risk, steroids can be carefully weaned off.
- Novel immunosuppressant agents, such as belatacept and extended-release tacrolimus, as well as mTOR inhibitors, have not been studied in this patient population.

OUTCOMES

- One of the initial and largest studies analyzed data from 26,183 heart transplant recipients, among which 593 were heart-kidney transplant recipients, and compared outcomes among the 2 groups.[21]
- Among isolated heart transplant recipients, the mean eGFR for grouped quintiles in ascending order was 36.6 ± 8.9 mL/min, 54.8 ± 4.1 mL/min, 68.9 ± 4.2 mL/min, 87.1 ± 6.6 mL/min, and 140.3 ± 56.4 mL/min, respectively.
- Among isolated heart transplant recipients, the risk of requiring early dialysis was highest among the lowest quintile group (22%) versus 16% and 11% in the next 2 quintiles. This study showed that the likelihood of requiring posttransplant dialysis was reduced among patients who had a higher eGFR before transplant (odds ratio 0.647; 95% CI 0.574-0.72; $P < .001$).[21]
- Among patients with eGFR < 37 mL/min/m^2, those with isolated heart transplants had worse median survival when compared with patients with SHK (7.1 years vs. 7.7 years).[21]
- This further emphasizes that pretransplant estimated GFR is an important factor in determining posttransplant survival among patients with isolated heart transplants and serves as a predictor of early renal failure requiring dialysis.
- Risk-unadjusted survival in patients with isolated heart transplants and SHK was found to be similar (8.4 years for heart transplant recipients and 7.7 years for SHK recipients; $P = .76$).[21]
- There is increased cardiac graft survival in patients with SHK (12.5 years) when compared with ones with heart transplants alone (11.2 years); $P = .008$.[23]

- SHK should be recommended in potential heart transplant recipients with kidney dysfunction. SHK has been shown to improve posttransplant survival in this category of patients.[21]

Lung-Kidney Transplantation

- There have been 110 lung-kidney transplants in the US since 1995.
- Indications include kidney and lung failure due to a number of underlying causes, including cystic fibrosis, restrictive or obstructive lung disease for lung failure and diabetes, tubular or interstitial diseases, glomerulonephritis, hypertensive nephrosclerosis, and calcineurin-induced kidney disease for kidney failure.
- There are limited data on immunosuppression regimens. Most regimens consist of induction with either basiliximab or ATG followed by maintenance triple immunosuppression therapy with a calcineurin inhibitor, antimetabolite, and corticosteroid.
- One study looked at 31 lung-kidney transplants performed between 1995 and 2013. Mean recipient age was 45.4 ± 13.5 years; 48.3% were male.[26]
- Retransplantation for graft failure was the leading indication for lung-kidney transplant (n = 13), and the most common renal indication was CNI nephrotoxicity (n = 11).[26]
- Patient survival after lung-kidney transplant was 93%, 71.0%, and 71.0% at 1 month, 6 months, and 1 year, with a median survival of 95.2 months.[26]
- Patient survival after lung-kidney transplant was similar to isolated lung transplant, and these results suggest that lung-kidney transplant is a feasible therapeutic option for lung transplant candidates with significant renal dysfunction.[26]

Heart-Liver-Kidney Transplant

GENERAL PRINCIPLES

- There have been 39 heart-liver-kidney transplants in the US since 1989 to 2022 as per the UNOS OPTN database.[2]
- Cardiac cirrhosis caused by congestive hepatopathy due to congenital heart disease, amyloidosis, familial hypercholesterolemia, hypertrophic cardiomyopathy, and dilated cardiomyopathy are the most common indications. See **Figure 23-5** and **Table 23-4**.

OUTCOMES

- A study of 7 heart-liver-kidney transplant patients at University of Chicago from 2008 to 2020 had 100% survival rate at 1 year with mean hospital stay of 32 days.[27]
- In the same cohort, basiliximab and methylprednisolone 1000 mg IV was used for induction and MMF and tacrolimus were used for maintenance therapy.[27]

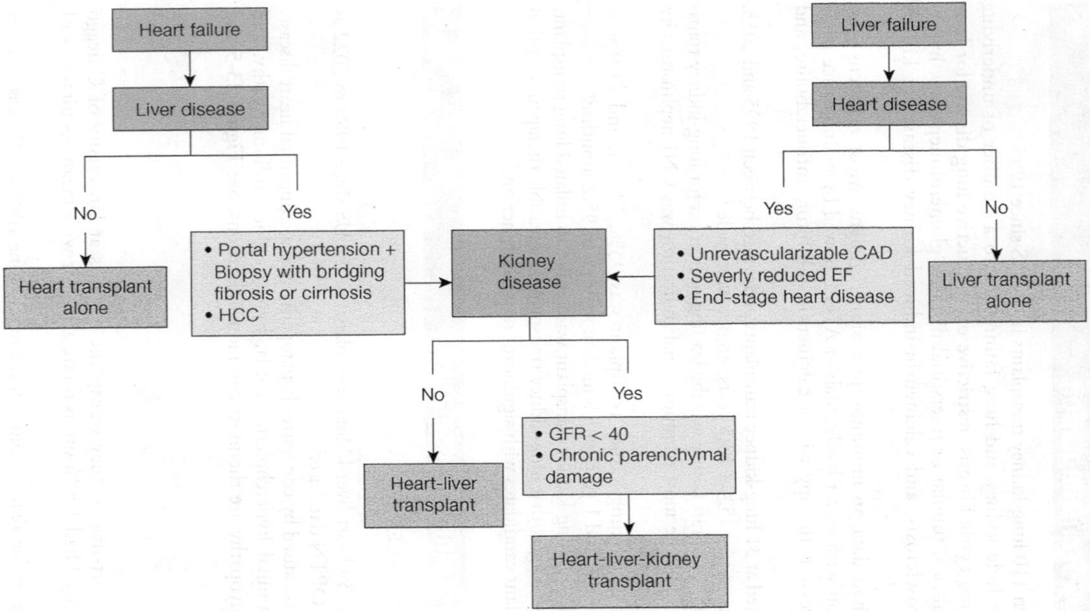

Figure 23-5. **Criteria for heart-liver-kidney transplant.** CAD, coronary artery disease; EF, ejection fraction; GFR, glomerular filtration rate; HCC, hepatocellular carcinoma. (Reproduced with permission from Perez-Gutierrez A, Siddiqi U, Kim G, et al. Combined heart-liver-kidney transplant: the University of Chicago medicine experience. *Clin Transplant.* 2022;36:e14586. Figure 1.)

TABLE 23-4 Workup for Combined Heart, Liver, and Kidney Transplant Candidates

Heart	Liver	Kidney
Echocardiography	Cross-sectional imaging: triple-phasic CT or MRI	Abdomen and pelvis noncontrast CT
Right-sided heart catheterization	Doppler US imaging of the liver	
Electrocardiogram	HCC panel: α-fetoprotein, descarboxy prothrombin and AFP-L3	
CXR		

HCC, hepatocellular carcinoma; US, ultrasound.
Reproduced with permission from Perez-Gutierrez A, Siddiqi U, Kim G, et al. Combined heart-liver-kidney transplant: The University of Chicago medicine experience. *Clin Transplant*. 2022;36:e14586. Table 1

REFERENCES

1. Stites E, Wiseman AC. Multiorgan transplantation. *Transplant Rev*. 2016;30(4):253-60.
2. Organ Procurement and Transplantation Network. Based on data obtained as of February 2, 2023. https://optn.transplant.hrsa.gov/data/view-data-reports/build-advanced/.
3. Ekser B, Contreras AG, Andraus W, Taner T. Current status of combined liver-kidney transplantation. *Int J Surg*. 2020;82S:149-54.
4. Gines P, Schrier RW. Renal failure in cirrhosis. *N Engl J Med*. 2009;361(13):1279-90.
5. Stepanova M, Wai H, Saab S, Mishra A, Venkatesan C, Younossi ZM. The outcomes of adult liver transplants in the United States from 1987 to 2013. *Liver Int*. 2015;35(8):2036-41.
6. Zarrinpar A, Busuttil RW. Liver transplantation: past, present and future. *Nat Rev Gastroenterol Hepatol*. 2013;10(7):434-40.
7. Choudhury RA, Reese PP, Goldberg DS, Bloom RD, Sawinski DL, Abt PL. A paired kidney analysis of multiorgan transplantation: implications for allograft survival. *Transplantation*. 2017;101(2):368-76.
8. Ekser B, Mangus RS, Fridell W, et al. A novel approach in combined liver and kidney transplantation with long-term outcomes. *Ann Surg*. 2017;265(5):1000-8.
9. Martin EF, Huang J, Xiang Q, Klein JP, Bajaj J, Saeian K. Recipient survival and graft survival are not diminished by simultaneous liver-kidney transplantation: an analysis of the united network for organ sharing database. *Liver Transplant*. 2012;18(8):914-29.
10. Alhamad T, Spatz C, Uemura T, Lehman E, Farooq U. The outcomes of simultaneous liver and kidney transplantation using donation after cardiac death organs. *Transplantation*. 2014;98(11):1190-8.
11. Ruiz R, Kunitake H, Wilkinson AH, et al. Longterm analysis of combined liver–kidney transplantation at a single center. *Arch Surg*. 2006;141:1-8.
12. Fong TL, Bunnapradist S, Jordan SC, Selby RR, Cho YW. Analysis of the United Network for Organ Sharing database comparing renal allografts and patient survival in combined liver–kidney transplantation with the contralateral allografts in kidney alone or kidney–pancreas transplantation. *Transplantation*. 2003;76(2):348-53.
13. AbdulRahim N, Anderson L, Kotla S, et al. Lack of benefit and potential harm of induction therapy in simultaneous liver-kidney transplants. *Liver Transplant*. 2019;25(3):411-24.
14. Del Gaudio M, Ravaioli M, Ercolani G, et al. Induction therapy with alemtuzumab (campath) in combined liver-kidney transplantation: University of Bologna experience. *Transplant Proc*. 2013;45(5):1969-70.

15. Taner T, Heimbach JK, Rosen CB, Nyberg SL, Park WD, Stegall MD. Decreased chronic cellular and antibody-mediated injury in the kidney following simultaneous liver-kidney transplantation. *Kidney Int.* 2016;89(4):909-17.
16. Taner T, Park WD, Stegall MD, et al. Unique molecular changes in kidney allografts after simultaneous liver-kidney compared with solitary kidney transplantation. *Kidney Int.* 2017;91(5):1193-202.
17. Olausson M, Mjörnstedt L, Nordén G, et al. Successful combined partial auxiliary liver and kidney transplantation in highly sensitized cross-match positive recipients. *Am J Tranplant.* 2007;7(1):130-6.
18. Manez R, Kelly RH, Kobayashi M, et al. Immunoglobulin G lymphocytotoxic antibodies in clinical liver transplantation: studies toward further defining their significance. *Hepatology.* 1995;21(5):1345-52.
19. Kobashigawa J, Dadhania DM, Farr M, et al. Consensus conference on heart-kidney transplantation. *Am J Transplant.* 2021;21(7):2459-67.
20. Lietz K, Miller LW. Improved survival of patients with end-stage heart failure listed for heart transplantation: analysis of organ procurement and transplantation network/U.S. United Network of Organ Sharing data, 1990 to 2005. *J Am Coll Cardiol.* 2007;50(13):1282-90.
21. Karamlou T, Welke KF, McMullan DM, et al. Combined heart-kidney transplant improves post-transplant survival compared with isolated heart transplant in recipients with reduced glomerular filtration rate: analysis of 593 combined heart-kidney transplants from the United Network Organ Sharing Database. *J Thorac Cardiovasc Surg.* 2014;147(1):456-61.e1.
22. Norman JC, Brook MI, Cooley DA, et al. Total support of the circulation of a patient with post-cardiotomy stone–heart syndrome by a artificial heart (ALVAD) for 5 days followed by heart and kidney transplantation. *Lancet.* 1978;311(8074):1125-27.
23. Agarwal KA, Patel H, Agrawal N, Cardarelli F, Goyal N. Cardiac outcomes in isolated heart and simultaneous kidney and heart transplants in the United States. *Kidney Int Rep.* 2021;6(9):2348-57.
24. Shaw BI, Sudan DL, Boulware LE, McElroy LM. Striking a balance in simultaneous heart kidney transplant: optimizing outcomes for all wait-listed patients. *JASN (J Am Soc Nephrol).* 2020;31(8):1661-4.
25. Kumar V, Tallaj JA. To transplant a kidney with the heart or not—that is the real question. *Am J Transplant.* 2014;14(2):253-4.
26. Reich HJ, Chan JL, Czer LSC, et al. Combined lung-kidney transplantation: an analysis of the UNOS/OPTN database. *Am Surg.* 2015;81(10):1047-52.
27. Perez-Gutierrez A, Siddiqi U, Kim G, et al. Combined heart-liver-kidney transplant: the University of Chicago medicine experience. *Clin Transplant.* 2022;36(4):e14586.

24 Outcomes of Kidney Transplantation

Gaurav Rajashekar, Su-Hsin Chang, and
Massini Merzkani

GENERAL PRINCIPLES

- On December 31, 2020, there were 127,003 patients waiting for a kidney transplant, and in the same year, there were a total of 23,643 transplants.[1]
- For patients wait-listed from 2015 to 2017, by 2020, 34.6% were still waiting 3 years after listing; 25.0% had undergone deceased donor kidney transplant (DDKT), 14.0% had undergone living donor kidney transplant (LDKT), 6.4% died on the waiting list, and 20.0% were removed from the waiting list.
- One of the unmet needs in kidney transplantation (KT) is to improve long-term graft and patient survival.
- Graft and patient survival have improved over the last 10 years. The 10-year graft survival rate was 42.3% for DDKT between 1996 and 1999 and increased to 53.6% for DDKT between 2008 and 2011. Similarly, the 10-year patient survival rate was 60.5% for LDKT between 1996 and 1999 and increased to 66.9% for LDKT between 2008 and 2011.[2] See **Figure 24-1** for improvement in graft survival over the years.[3]
- The rate of graft loss and death at different time points (<1 year, 1-<5 years, 5-<10 years, and 10-<20 years after KT) improved over time during the last decades.[2]
- This improvement has occurred despite increases in the recipients' age, body mass index, prevalence of diabetes, length of time undergoing dialysis, and proportion of recipients with a previous kidney transplant as well as increases in the donors' age, percentage of donations after circulatory death, and the degree of HLA presensitization (expressed as calculated panel-reactive antibody levels).[2]
- There was a higher percentage of improvement at 1- and 5-year graft survival comparing 1995 to 1999 with 2014 to 2017. Similar improvement in survival was seen in the subgroups of deceased donors, liver donors, different races, different ages, and different etiologies of end-stage kidney disease (ESKD).[3]
- **Figure 24-2** shows the improvement in death-censored graft survival in DDKT over the different follow-up time up to 2020.[3]
- In 2019, among DDKT recipients, 63.8% had a 12-month estimated glomerular filtration rate (eGFR), an early surrogate allograft outcome, of 45 mL/min/1.73 m^2 or higher, slightly lower than the 65.6% in 2018; furthermore, among LDKT recipients, 76.9% had 12-month eGFR of 45 mL/min/1.73 m^2 or higher, slightly lower than the 77.7% in 2018.[2]
- There has been an increase in the survival of DDKT recipients. The median graft survival increased from 8.2 years in the era of 1995 to 1999 to 9.7 years in the era of 2005 to 2009, an 18.3% improvement over a 10-year period. The predicted half-life for those transplanted in the era of 2014 to 2017 was 11.7 years, representing a 43% increase in half-life over a 20-year period.[3]
- Similarly, in LDKT recipients, the median graft survival increased from 12.1 years during 1995 to 1999 to 12.9 years during 2000 to 2004, a 6.6% increase over a

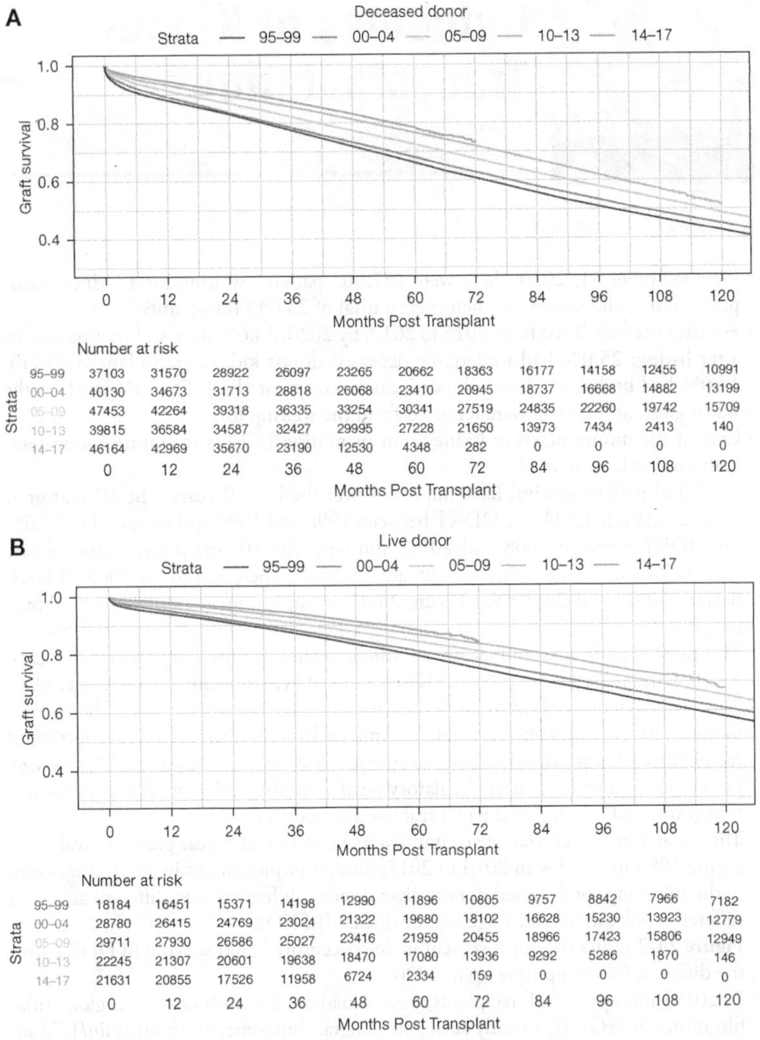

Figure 24-1. **Graft survival after kidney transplantation in the US stratified by year of transplant.** A, Deceased donor. B, Live donor. (Reproduced with permission from Poggio ED, Augustine JJ, Arrigain S, Brennan DC, Schold JD. Long-term kidney transplant graft survival—Making progress when most needed. *Am J Transplant.* 2021;21:2824-32. Figure 1.)

5-year period. For those transplanted after 2009, the median graft survival has not been reached, but the projected half-life for those transplanted in the era of 2014 to 2017 is 19.2 years, representing a 59% improvement over a 20-year period.[3]

- In recent United Network Organ Sharing data, 74.3% of DDKT recipients and 83.9% of LDKT recipients aged ≥65 years were alive after 5 years, compared with 95.8% and 97.8% of those aged 18 to 34 years.[1]

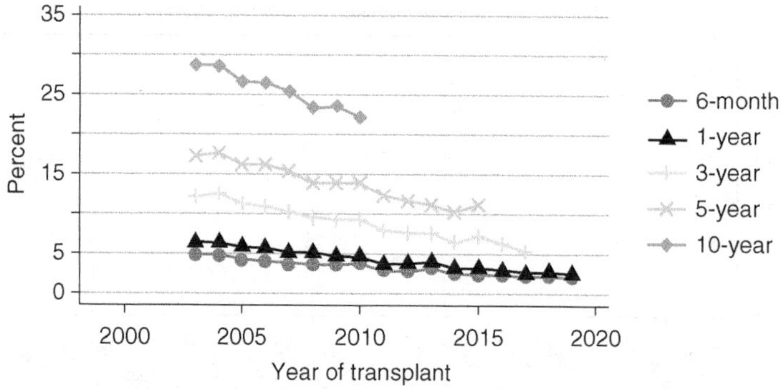

Figure 24-2. **Death-censored graft failure among adult deceased donor kidney transplant recipients.** (Reproduced with permission from Lentine KL, Smith JM, Hart A, et al. OPTN/SRTR 2020 annual data report: kidney. *Am J Transplant.* 2022;22(suppl 2):21-136. doi:10.1111/ajt.16982. Figure KI 87.)

- Five-year patient survival was lowest among recipients with diabetes as the cause of kidney disease, at 81.1% for DDKT recipients and 88.3% of LDKT recipients, and with kidney donor profile index ≥85 among DDKT recipients, at 75.9%.[1]

GRAFT FAILURE

- Death-censored graft failure is defined as a return to dialysis or subsequent transplantation. The incidence of death-censored graft failure has decreased over the years (across different follow-ups in the last 20 years) in **Figure 24-3.**[3]
- The causes of graft failure are different across follow-up times. The most common causes of graft loss in the first year post transplant were primary dysfunction and surgical complications accounting for 60.3%[4] (**Table 24-1**).
- Rejection is the most common cause of death-censored graft failure. It contributes to 40% to 65% of all graft failure. About 57% to 79% of graft rejection is attributed to antibody-mediated injury.[4-6]
- Glomerular diseases are the second most common cause of death-censored graft failure, accounting for 11.9% to 18.6%.[4,7]
- Mayrdorfer et al demonstrated that the most common cause leading to graft failure as primary or secondary cause (overall) in a single center was intercurrent medical events (medical events that lead to acute renal failure as infections or cardiorenal syndrome) 36.3% (n = 110/303), followed by T cell–mediated rejection (TCMR) 34% (n = 103/303) and antibody-mediated rejection (ABMR) 30.7% (n = 93/303). Combining TCMR and ABMR, these 2 causes of rejection as a group were the number 1 cause with 64.68% (n = 196/303).[8]
- Renal tubular injury could cause graft failure. Renal tubular injury could be associated with severe acute kidney injury and related to infection or cardiorenal syndrome. Renal tubular injury accounts for 14% of all the death-censored graft losses.[4]
- In the past, there was a terminology of chronic allograft nephropathy that was defined as interstitial fibrosis and tubular atrophy (IFTA) without evidence of specific etiology. However, in recent studies it is known that the IFTA lesion is a final common pathway for many different types of injuries (rejection, viral nephropathies,

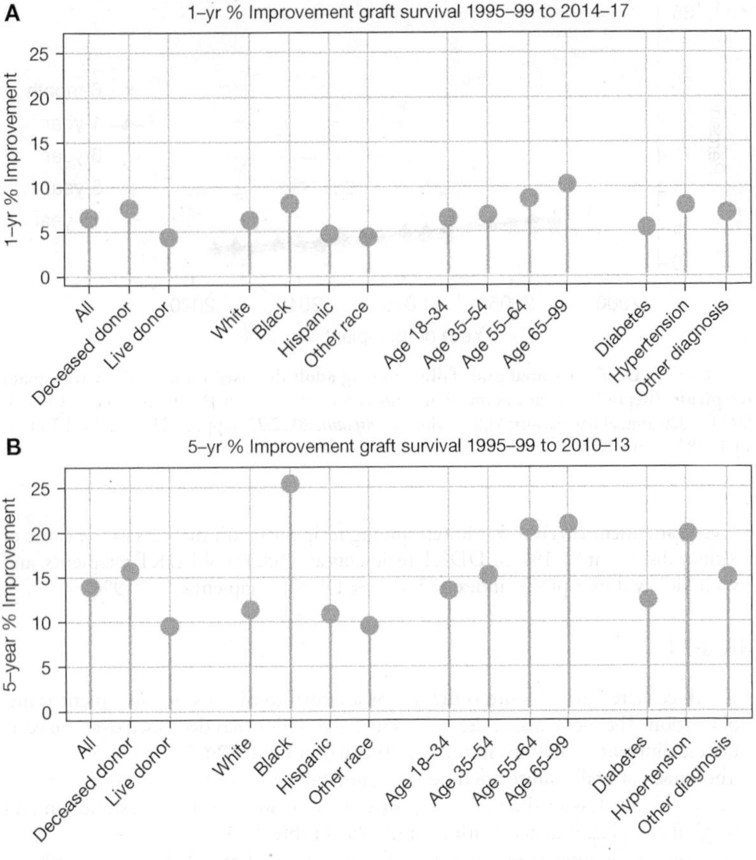

Figure 24-3. **Percentage of improvement of graft survival from 1995 to 1999 to 2014 to 2017.** A, Within 1 y; B, within 5 y of transplant. (Reproduced with permission from Poggio ED, Augustine JJ, Arrigain S, Brennan DC, Schold JD. Long-term kidney transplant graft survival—Making progress when most needed. *Am J Transplant.* 2021;21:2824-32. Figure 2.)

calcineurin inhibitor toxicity, chronic obstruction, recurrent bacterial infections, recurrent acute tubular necrosis, and others).[9]

- Risk factors for death-censored graft loss were younger age, history of pretransplant dialysis, time on dialysis, history of previous transplant, having delayed graft function, African American recipients, history of cardiovascular disease, and history of diabetes mellitus as a cause of ESKD.[4,7]

ALLOIMMUNE CAUSES (REJECTION)

- Rejection is the most common cause of graft loss accounting for 38.7% to 64.7%.[4,7,8]
- In 2018 to 2019, there were 6.8% of adult KT recipients who experienced acute rejection during the first year post transplantation. During the same time, the

TABLE 24-1 Causes of Death-Censored Graft Failure in Patients Transplanted From 2006 to 2018

	Time after Kidney Transplantation			
Cause	Total	Less Than 1 y	1-5 y	Greater Than 5 y
Total	553	131	235	188
Alloimmune	38.7%	12.2%	49.8%	43.3%
Glomerular diseases	18.6%	13.7%	17.4%	23.5%
Renal tubular injuries	13.9%	9.2%	17.4%	12.8%
Primary dysfunction/ surgical	14.3%	60.3%	0%	0%
BK nephropathy	4.3%	3.1%	4.3%	5.3%
Unknown/other	10.1%	1.5%	11.1%	15.0%

Reproduced with permission from Merzkani MA, Bentall AJ, Smith BH, et al. Death with function and graft failure after kidney transplantation: risk factors at baseline suggest new approaches to management. *Transplant Direct.* 2022;8:e1273. Table 3.

incidence was higher in younger recipients aged 18 to 34 years and lower in older recipients aged ≥65 years.

- Acute rejection at 1 year post transplant occurred in 8.4% of KT recipients who received induction with interleukin-2 receptor antibody and 6.6% in T-cell-depleting induction.[1]
- One of the highest risk factors for rejection is nonadherence to immunosuppression medication. This accounts for 40% to 47% of KT failure related to alloimmune causes.[4,10]
- Among all causes of graft loss due to rejection, 79.4% were associated with ABMR injury.[4]
- Acute rejection episodes decrease long-term allograft survival.[11]
- Risk factors for allograft loss due to alloimmune causes are younger age, DDKT, pre-transplant dialysis, African American recipients, HLA DR mismatch, and calculated panel reactive antibody >80%.[4]
- The costs for antibody-treated (year 1, $22,407; year 2, $18,803; year 3, $13,909) and non-antibody-treated (year 1, $14,122; year 2, $7,852 year 3, $8,234) acute rejection events were associated with significant increases in the cost of care.
- Further discussion of diagnosis and management could be found in Chapters 12 and 13.

GLOMERULAR DISEASES

- Recurrent or de novo glomerular disease is the second most common cause of death-censored graft loss.
- Approximately 18% to 22% of the causes of graft loss are due to recurrent or de novo glomerular disease.[4,10,12]
- The distinction between recurrent and de novo allograft glomerulonephritis is important but likely not very precise because pretransplantation native kidney biopsies are

often not performed.[13] Therefore, many cases of glomerulonephritis remained undiagnosed at the time of transplantation.

- The relative risk for allograft failure was 1.9 for those with glomerular disease compared with those without. At 5 years after KT, patients with glomerular disease had a much higher rate of allograft failure (60% vs. 32% in those without glomerular disease).[14]
- Recurrent glomerulonephritis in recipients with glomerulonephritis in the native kidney was associated with an increased risk of graft failure (which was highest in patients with recurrent membranoproliferative glomerulonephritis type 1 and focal segmental glomerulonephritis).[13]
- Recurrent IgA nephropathy was also associated with a higher risk of graft failure.[13,15]
- The most common cause of recurrent glomerular disease leading to graft loss was focal segmental glomerulosclerosis, membranoproliferative glomerulonephritis, and IgA nephropathy.
- More discussion regarding glomerular disease can be found in Chapter 14.

DEATH WITH FUNCTIONAL GRAFT

- It is defined as death with a functioning kidney graft. A study using a cohort from the Mayo Clinic showed that there are more deaths with functioning graft compared with graft failure.[4]
- Trends in adult patient survival are generally paralleled to those of graft survival. At 5 years, 74.3% of DDKT recipients and 83.9% of LDKT recipients aged ≥65 years were alive, compared with 95.8% of DDKT recipients and 97.8% of LDKT recipients aged 18 to 34 years.
- The cause of ESKD plays a role in patient survival following KT. Patients with cystic kidney disease, glomerulonephritis, hypertension, and other/unknown have the best survival, while patients with diabetes mellitus as a cause of ESKD have the worst survival.
- In 2020, the 5-year patient survival was lowest among recipients with diabetes as the cause of kidney disease, at 81.1% for DDKT recipients and 88.3% of LDKT recipients.
- Even though cardiac causes have been the most common cause of graft failure in the last 40 years, the incidence of cardiovascular death for those 1 to 5 years post transplant fell from 2.87 per 100 patient-years in 1980 to 1984 to 0.28 in 2015 to 2018.[16]
- Death related to cancer declined from 0.51 per 100 patient-years in 1980 to 1984 to 0.36 in 2015 to 2018.[17]
- The most common causes of death with functional graft are malignancy 20.0% (*n* = 138), infection 19.7% (*n* = 136), cardiac disease 12.6% (*n* = 87), and unknown 37.0% (*n* = 256); see **Table 24-2.**[4]
- For further details about infection or malignancies outcomes, see Chapter 17.

Cardiovascular Disease

- Cardiovascular disease is one of the most common causes of death with functional graft overall, even though the incidence of cardiovascular death for those 1 to 5 years post transplant fell from 2.87 per 100 patient-years in 1980 to 1984 to 0.28 in 2015 to 2018.[17]
- The ALERT trial demonstrated in renal transplant recipient there was no difference in its primary end point (combined cardiovascular end point) but a favorable

TABLE 24-2 Death With Functioning Graft After Solitary Kidney Transplantation (2006-2018)

	Time After Kidney Transplantation			
Cause	Total (%)	Less than 1 y (%)	1-5 y (%)	Greater Than 5 y (%)
All DWFG	12.0	12.3	45.4	42.3
Malignancy	20.0	11.8	21.0	21.2
Infection	19.7	34.1	20.1	15.1
Cardiac	12.6	12.9	10.2	15.1
Other	10.7	23.5	9.9	7.9
Unknown	37.0	17.6	38.9	40.8

DWFG, death with functioning graft.
Reproduced with permission from Merzkani MA, Bentall AJ, Smith BH, et al. Death with function and graft failure after kidney transplantation: risk factors at baseline suggest new approaches to management. *Transplant Direct.* 2022;8:e1273. Table 2.

reduction in the separate outcomes of cardiac death and nonfatal myocardial infarction with fluvastatin therapy.[16]

- Other studies have shown that cardiovascular cause of death has decreased to the third cause of death with functioning graft after infection and malignancy.[4]
- The incidence of death from cardiovascular disease is less frequent in younger kidney transplant recipients compared with older recipients.[18]
- Nimmo et al conducted a national prospective study of 2,572 kidney transplant recipients to assess whether pretransplant screening for coronary artery disease (CAD) in asymptomatic patients had any difference in major adverse cardiac events (MACE).[19]
  - The incidence of MACE was low with 0.9% at 90 days, 2.1% at 1 year, 9.4% at 5 years.
  - There was no association between screening and nonscreening strategies in major cardiovascular events at 5 years.
  - It is still unclear if screening asymptomatic patient with high-risk transplant candidates for CAD will decrease the incidence of MACE.
- A recent meta-analysis by Siddiqui et al that included 8 studies with 945 patients found no difference in MACE, cardiovascular mortality, or all-cause mortality in kidney transplant recipients with established CAD who underwent revascularization versus patients who were on optimal medical therapy alone before transplant. On the basis of these findings, revascularization should be limited to those high-risk CAD subsets that would yield substantial survival advantage with bypass, independent of a planned noncardiac surgery.[20]
- Of note, Kidney Disease Improving Global Outcomes guidelines recommend against routine coronary revascularization to reduce perioperative cardiac events in those asymptomatic kidney transplant candidates with known CAD.[21]
- Risk factors associated with posttransplant myocardial infarction include older age, history of angina, peripheral vascular disease, dyslipidemia, pretransplant myocardial infarction, and arrhythmia.[22]

- The treatment of CAD has not been extensively studied exclusively in kidney transplant recipients.
  - Subsequent meta-analyses including ALERT suggested a likely benefit for statin use in reducing the outcome of major vascular event, coronary revascularization or stroke, and mortality.[23]
  - Overall, given the likely benefit and little harm, initiation and continuation of statin therapy in patients with functioning kidney transplants are recommended.[24]
- The benefit of aspirin for primary prevention of CAD has not been studied in a randomized controlled trial of kidney transplant recipients.
- A retrospective study using propensity score matching analysis of aspirin use in the FAVORIT trial showed no benefit from baseline aspirin use on cardiovascular disease or mortality outcomes.[23]
- Given limited data in general kidney transplant recipients, guidelines generally recommend aspirin use to be considered in patients with diabetes or known atherosclerotic cardiovascular disease, unless contraindicated.
- The survival of the kidney transplant recipients who required either bypass surgery or angioplasty was 89%, 77%, and 65% at 1, 3, and 5 years post procedure, respectively.[25]

ESTIMATED POSTTRANSPLANT SURVIVAL

- The core concept was that the best 20% of kidneys would be preferentially allocated to the 20% of wait-listed patients with the highest estimated posttransplant survival (EPTS).
- The EPTS contains 4 elements: patient age, prior organ transplant, diabetic status, and dialysis time. The score even was validated using an outside dataset. The EPTS score was moderately good at discriminating posttransplant survival of adult kidney-only transplant recipients.[26]

MALIGNANCIES

- The risk of certain malignancies due to immunosuppression use is higher in kidney transplant recipients, compared with the general population.
- Cancer is the second leading cause of death (following cardiovascular disease) among recipients of transplants in most Western countries.[27]
- In other countries such as Australia, New Zealand, South Korea, Belgium, and Spain, a multicenter study showed that the death rate due to posttransplant malignancy after the first year of KT has surpassed the cardiovascular death rate as a result of a relatively greater reduction in cardiovascular death and increased use of KT in older and high-risk population.
- The most common malignancy is skin cancer, which includes squamous cell carcinoma, basal cell carcinoma, Kaposi sarcoma, and malignant melanoma, accounting for 90% to 95% of these skin cancers.
- Observational data showed that the standard mortality ratios for all cancer types are at least 1.8 to 1.9 times higher compared with the age- and sex-matched general population. The standardized mortality ratio is 2.6 for kidney transplant recipients.[28]
- Risk factors for malignancy included older age, recipient male sex, previous cancer history, T-cell-depleting antibodies, and dialysis at the time of transplant.
- There is a lack of clinical trials in kidney transplant recipients to suggest the frequency of routine population-based cancer screening for breast, colorectal, and

cervical cancers. The current recommendation is aligned with the guidelines as per the general population.[29]

- The cumulative incidence of cancer at 3 years post transplant was 5.7% for nonmelanoma skin cancers, 1.9% for viral-linked cancer, and 6.3% for almost all other cancers.
- Cancer also significantly increases the costs of posttransplant care. Newly diagnosed viral-linked cancer was associated with increased costs, i.e., \$22,000-\$27,000/y higher inpatient costs and \$9,000 to 11,000/y higher outpatient costs per case.
- There will be more discussion about transplant malignancies after Chapter 16, Posttransplant Malignancies.

INFECTIONS

- Infection is 1 of the 3 most common causes of death with functional graft in KT.
- Infection can occur in 10% to 30% of recipients in the first year after a kidney transplant. Among Medicare-insured kidney transplant recipients in 2000 to 2011, an increased mortality was found in the first year after transplant, ranging from 41% for urinary tract infection alone, 6-fold for pneumonia, 12-fold risk for sepsis, and 34-fold for those with all 3 infections in the first year.
- Infectious complications are categorized as occurring in 3 time periods post transplant: early posttransplant infections (0-30 days), infections during peak immunosuppression (30-365 days), and late-onset infections (above 1 year).
- Risk factor for increased risk of death for infection included older age, dialysis at the time of transplant, female sex, diabetes mellitus as a cause of ESKD, use of T-cell-depleting therapy, and prednisone as maintenance therapy.
- Infections increase the first-year cost of kidney transplant care by \$17,691 for urinary tract infection alone, \$40,000 to \$50,000 for pneumonia or sepsis alone, and \$134,773 for those with urinary tract infection, pneumonia, and sepsis. Clinical and economic impacts persist in years 2 to 3 post transplant.
- More discussion on infections can be found in Chapter 16.

REFERENCES

1. Lentine KL, Smith JM, Hart A, et al. OPTN/SRTR 2020 annual data report: kidney. *Am J Transplant.* 2022;22(suppl 2):21-136.
2. Hariharan S, Israni AK, Danovitch G. Long-term survival after kidney transplantation. *N Engl J Med.* 2021;385(8):729-43.
3. Poggio ED, Augustine JJ, Arrigain S, Brennan DC, Schold JD. Long-term kidney transplant graft survival—making progress when most needed. *Am J Transplant.* 2021;21(8):2824-32.
4. Merzkani MA, Bentall AJ, Smith BH, et al. Death with function and graft failure after kidney transplantation: risk factors at baseline suggest new approaches to management. *Transplant Direct.* 2022;8(2):e1273.
5. Chand S, Atkinson D, Collins C, et al. The spectrum of renal allograft failure. *PLoS One.* 2016;11(9):e0162278.
6. Gaston R, Cecka J, Kasiske B, et al. Evidence for antibody-mediated injury as a major determinant of late kidney allograft failure. *Transplantation.* 2010;90(1):68-74.
7. Gaston RS, Fieberg A, Helgeson ES, et al. Late graft loss after kidney transplantation: is "death with function" really death with a functioning allograft? *Transplantation.* 2020;104(7):1483-90.
8. Mayrdorfer M, Liefeldt L, Wu K, et al. Exploring the complexity of death-censored kidney allograft failure. *J Am Soc Nephrol.* 2021;32(6):1513-26.
9. Langewisch E, Mannon RB. Chronic allograft injury. *J Am Soc Nephrol.* 2021;16(11):1723-9.

10. Sellares J, de Freitas DG, Mengel M, et al. Understanding the causes of kidney transplant failure: the dominant role of antibody-mediated rejection and nonadherence. *Am J Transplant.* 2012;12(2):388-99.
11. Opelz G, Döhler B; Collaborative Transplant Study Report. Influence of time of rejection on long-term graft survival in renal transplantation. *Transplantation.* 2008;85(5):661-6.
12. El-Zoghby ZM, Stegall MD, Lager DJ, et al. Identifying specific causes of kidney allograft loss. *Am J Transplant.* 2009;9(3):527-35.
13. Cosio FG, Cattran DC. Recent advances in our understanding of recurrent primary glomerulonephritis after kidney transplantation. *Kidney Int.* 2017;91(2):304-14.
14. Hariharan S, Adams MB, Brennan DC, et al. Recurrent and de novo glomerular disease after renal transplantation: a report from Renal Allograft Disease Registry (RADR). *Transplantation.* 1999;68(5):635-41.
15. Moroni G, Longhi S, Quaglini S, et al. The long-term outcome of renal transplantation of IgA nephropathy and the impact of recurrence on graft survival. *Nephrol Dial Transplant.* 2013;28(5):1305-14.
16. Holdaas H, Fellström B, Jardine AG, et al. Effect of fluvastatin on cardiac outcomes in renal transplant recipients: a multicentre, randomised, placebo-controlled trial. *Lancet.* 2003;361(9374):2024-31.
17. Ying T, Shi B, Kelly PJ, Pilmore H, Clayton PA, Chadban SJ. Death after kidney transplantation: an analysis by era and time post-transplant. *J Am Soc Nephrol.* 2020;31(12):2887-99.
18. Briggs JD. Causes of death after renal transplantation. *Nephrol Dial Transplant.* 2001;16(8):1545-9.
19. Nimmo A, Forsyth JL, Oniscu GC, et al. A propensity score–matched analysis indicates screening for asymptomatic coronary artery disease does not predict cardiac events in kidney transplant recipients. *Kidney Int.* 2021;99(2):431-42.
20. Siddiqui MU, Junarta J, Marhefka GD. Coronary revascularization versus optimal medical therapy in renal transplant candidates with coronary artery disease: a systematic review and meta-analysis. *J Am Heart Assoc.* 2022;11(4):e023548.
21. Chadban SJ, Ahn C, Axelrod DA, et al. KDIGO clinical practice guideline on the evaluation and management of candidates for kidney transplantation. *Transplantation.* 2020;104(4S1 suppl 1):S11-03.
22. Lentine KL, Brennan DC, Schnitzler MA. Incidence and predictors of myocardial infarction after kidney transplantation. *J Am Soc Nephrol.* 2005;16(2):496-506.
23. Dad T, Tighiouart H, Joseph A, et al. Aspirin use and incident cardiovascular disease, kidney failure, and death in stable kidney transplant recipients: a post hoc analysis of the folic acid for vascular outcome reduction in transplantation (FAVORIT) trial. *Am J Kidney Dis.* 2016;68(2):277-86.
24. Cholesterol Treatment Trialists' CTT Collaboration; Herrington W, Emberson J, Mihaylova B. Impact of renal function on the effects of LDL cholesterol lowering with statin-based regimens: a meta-analysis of individual participant data from 28 randomised trials. *Lancet Diabetes Endocrinol.* 2016;4(10):829-39.
25. Black D, Levine DA, Nicoll L, et al. Low risk of complications associated with the fenestrated peritoneal catheter used for intraperitoneal chemotherapy in ovarian cancer. *Gynecol Oncol.* 2008;109(1):39-42.
26. Clayton PA, McDonald SP, Snyder JJ, Salkowski N, Chadban SJ. External validation of the estimated posttransplant survival score for allocation of deceased donor kidneys in the United States. *Am J Transplant.* 2014;14(8):1922-6.
27. Krynitz B, Edgren G, Lindelöf B, et al. Risk of skin cancer and other malignancies in kidney, liver, heart and lung transplant recipients 1970 to 2008: a Swedish population-based study. *Int J Cancer.* 2013;132(6):1429-38.
28. Au EH, Chapman JR, Craig JC, et al. Overall and site-specific cancer mortality in patients on dialysis and after kidney transplant. *J Am Soc Nephrol.* 2019;30(3):471-80.
29. Wong G, Chapman JR, Craig JC. Cancer screening in renal transplant recipients: what is the evidence? *J Am Soc Nephrol.* 2008;3(suppl 2):S87-100.

25

Management of Failing Kidney Transplant

Charbel C. Khoury

GENERAL PRINCIPLES

- Despite marked improvement in immunosuppression management, 20% of recipients will require renal replacement therapies within 5 years of transplantation and more than 50% will experience allograft loss by 10 years.[1]
- Patients with failing allografts are at risk for worsening quality of life and functional status. Their course may be complicated by increased hospitalizations, primarily due to infections.[2,3]
- Patients who return to dialysis may have an increased mortality when compared with patients with functioning allografts or nontransplant patients on the waiting list.[4]
- While there is no consensus definition in the literature, a failing allograft can be defined as[5]:
  - An allograft with a reduced yet stable function estimated glomerular filtration rate (eGFR) <30 mL/min/1.73 m^2 (chronic kidney disease [CKD] stage 4-5).
  - An allograft with an irreversible decline in function with anticipated allograft survival of <1 year.
  - A return to renal replacement therapy (either dialysis or retransplantation).

MANAGEMENT OF IMMUNOSUPPRESSION

- *Management of immunosuppression in patients with failing allografts should be individualized by weighing the benefits of continuing immunosuppression against the risks.*
- While there are no guidelines for the management of immunosuppression, a suggested plan is listed in **Figure 25-1**.[5] The goal is to withdraw the immunosuppression without precipitating rejection, causing any adverse effects related to drug withdrawal, or exacerbating allosensitization.
- Factors to consider in establishing a plan for immunosuppression include[5]:
  - Risk of complications from an immunosuppressed state
  - Candidacy for and timing of subsequent kidney transplantation
  - Residual renal allograft function and modality of dialysis

RISK OF COMPLICATIONS FROM AN IMMUNOSUPPRESSED STATE

- Potential complications are the main reason to withdraw immunosuppressive medications in dialysis patients. Many of these drugs promote diabetes, dyslipidemia, hypertension, and accelerated atherosclerotic vascular disease.
- Long-term immunosuppression is associated with increased risk of infection. Patients returning to dialysis after graft loss have higher rates of sepsis compared with patients without prior transplant or ones needing dialysis within 3 to 6 months after transplantation.

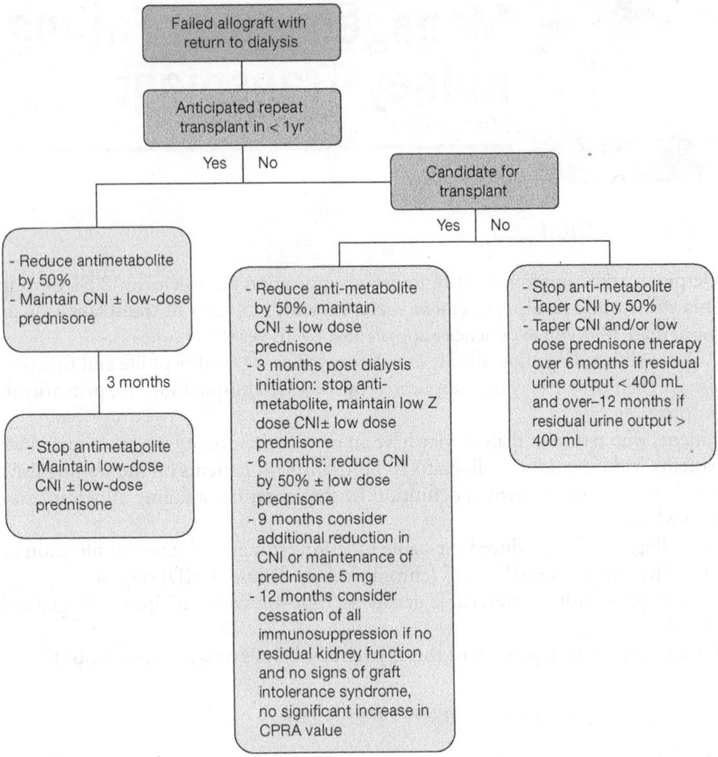

Figure 25-1. **Proposed immunosuppression management in failing kidney allograft.** CNI, calcineurin inhibitor; CPRA, calculated panel reactive antibody. (Data from Lubetzky M, Tantisattamo E, Molnar MZ, Lentine KL, Basu A, Parsons RF, et al. The failing kidney allograft: a review and recommendations for the care and management of a complex group of patients. *Am J Transplant.* 2021;21:2937-49. Figure 2.)

- Infection is a leading cause of death in the setting of failing allogrant.[6] This is especially concerning in the failed transplant patient utilizing a venous catheter for hemodialysis.
- Immunosuppression is associated with an increase in malignancy. However, this may be nuanced in patients with failing allografts on dialysis who have higher rates of leukemia and lung, kidney, urinary tract, and thyroid cancers. Kaposi sarcoma, non-Hodgkin lymphoma, lip cancer, and melanoma were all higher during transplantation.[7]
- Failing allografts compound the risk of immunosuppression drugs. Kidney failure decreases protein binding and increases free mycophenolic acid concentrations.[8]
- While calcineurin inhibitors are not metabolized or excreted by the kidney, their neurotoxicity may mimic uremic encephalopathy.[9]
- Tacrolimus is associated with an increased accumulation of certain uremic toxins compared with cyclosporine. Steroids, on the other hand, complicate bone health, muscle wasting, and hyperglycemia in patients reinitiating dialysis.

CANDIDACY FOR SUBSEQUENT KIDNEY TRANSPLANTATION

- Withdrawal of immunosuppression is associated with a higher risk of sensitization with the formation of HLA antibodies.[10] This is especially true for shorter withdrawal intervals (<3 months).[11]
- Sensitization generally decreases the chances of future transplantation. Thus, patients who are anticipated to have short time (generally less than a year) before a subsequent transplant may not need a complete withdrawal from immunosuppression.
- However, patients with graft loss due to polyomavirus BK may require more aggressive decrease in immunosuppression to reduce BK levels before a subsequent transplant.[12]

RESIDUAL RENAL FUNCTION AND MODALITY OF DIALYSIS

- Preserving residual kidney function can improve the quality of life of patients on dialysis. It helps maintain fluid balance, provides some solute clearance (mainly middle molecules), and limits the need for phosphorous and anemia management. It may be associated with a survival benefit especially in patients on peritoneal dialysis.[13]
- Maintaining immunosuppression can help preserve residual kidney function. However, this also depends on whether the underlying etiology of graft failure was immunologic in nature.[5]

REJECTION AND GRAFT INTOLERANCE SYNDROME

- Withdrawal of immunosuppression may result in graft intolerance syndrome in up to 30% to 50% of patients within 1 year of transplant failure and dialysis initiation.[14]
- This chronic inflammatory state can occur regardless of the immunosuppression withdrawal protocol used.
- Common symptoms of graft intolerance include fever, malaise, gross hematuria, and weight loss.
- Less common clinical findings include allograft enlargement, localized edema and tenderness, thrombocytopenia, erythrocyte stimulating agent resistance, elevated inflammatory markers such as ferritin and C-reactive protein, and elevated erythrocyte sedimentation rate. Other rare systemic inflammatory conditions such as bullous pemphigoid have been reported.

MANAGEMENT OF GRAFT INTOLERANCE

- A course of high-dose steroids (eg, prednisone 0.3-1.0 mg/kg/d) should be tried for treatment of symptomatic rejection.
- In many cases, transplant nephrectomy or graft embolization should be considered. Steroids may still be necessary especially in an edematous kidney at risk of rupture.
- The most significant indications for transplant nephrectomy include the following:
  - Hemorrhage (ongoing hematuria or, more urgently, intra-abdominal bleeding)
  - Uncontrolled pain
  - Persistent infection and sepsis
- Nephrectomy has been associated with improved mortality and may limit sensitization.[15] Complications include postoperative bleeding and hematoma, infection, lymphocele, abscess formation, and deep vein thrombosis.

- Radiologic embolization is an alternative to surgical nephrectomy and is achieved by the injection of ethanol followed by stainless steel coils into the branches of the renal artery. While generally associated with less morbidity and complications, it may be followed by a postembolization syndrome. This is characterized by fever 24 to 48 h after the procedure. The use of pulse steroids preprocedure may limit the risk of this syndrome.[16]
- Embolization followed by nephrectomy is sometimes considered to limit the risk of hemorrhage.

MANAGEMENT OF TRANSPLANT CHRONIC KIDNEY DISEASE

- Management of transplant CKD should involve a strong communication between the transplant team and general nephrologist. Alternatively, a multidisciplinary clinic dedicated to patients with low-functioning kidney allograft can help coordinate care.
- Management of transplant CKD and the associated anemia and bone mineral disease should follow the current Kidney Disease: Improving Global Outcomes guidelines.
- Caveats to evaluating transplant CKD include the following:
  - Compared with nontransplant patients, the performance of the chronic kidney disease epidemiology collaborative eGFR equations based upon creatinine and/or cystatin C have not been fully validated in kidney transplant patients.[17] However, they continue to be favored over the Modification in Diet in Renal Disease study equation to determine the stage of CKD.
  - Earlier attention should be paid to markers of graft failure, such as proteinuria, recurrent disease, or transplant glomerulopathy, to estimate the risk and speed of progression.

RENAL REPLACEMENT THERAPY PLANNING

- Referral for retransplantation should be sent when eGFR <20 mL/min/1.73 m^2. Preemptive second transplantation has been shown to have better graft and patient survival compared with patients who receive a second transplant after a period of dialysis.
- Transplant patients should be referred for dialysis education and receive appropriate dialysis modality counseling, regardless of their prior experience with dialysis.
- While there may be no significant differences in mortality among dialysis modalities, the quality of life in patients on home hemodialysis or peritoneal dialysis is overall better than that of patients on in-center dialysis.[18]
- Peritoneal dialysis catheters can be inserted percutaneously with the assistance of ultrasound and fluoroscopy in most kidney transplant patients.[19] Surgical placement should be favored in patients with hernias or who have undergone abdominal surgeries putting them at risk for adhesions.
- Patients planning for hemodialysis should be referred for vascular access planning when eGFR is 15 to 20 and/or declining, if there is no living donor, or if they are not being considered for retransplantation.
- The timing of initiation of dialysis should be based on clinical factors once volume overload, hyperkalemia, and/or acidosis can no longer be medically managed. There is no benefit and potential harm from starting dialysis at higher eGFR levels.[20]
- Overall dialysis modality and timing need to be individualized to each patient.

REFERENCES

1. Saran R, Robinson B, Abbott KC, et al. US Renal Data System 2016 Annual Data Report: epidemiology of kidney disease in the United States. *Am J Kidney Dis.* 2017;69(3 suppl 1):A7-8.
2. Perl J, Zhang J, Gillespie B, et al. Reduced survival and quality of life following return to dialysis after transplant failure: the Dialysis Outcomes and Practice Patterns Study. *Nephrol Dial Transplant.* 2012;27(12):4464-72.
3. Huml AM, Sehgal AR. Hemodialysis quality metrics in the first year following a failed kidney transplant. *Am J Nephrol.* 2019;50(3):161-7.
4. Kabani R, Quinn RR, Palmer S, et al. Risk of death following kidney allograft failure: a systematic review and meta-analysis of cohort studies. *Nephrol Dial Transplant.* 2014;29(9):1778-86.
5. Lubetzky M, Tantisattamo E, Molnar MZ, et al. The failing kidney allograft: a review and recommendations for the care and management of a complex group of patients. *Am J Transplant.* 2021;21(9):2937-49.
6. Gill JS, Abichandani R, Kausz AT, Pereira BJ. Mortality after kidney transplant failure: the impact of non-immunologic factors. *Kidney Int.* 2002;62(5):1875-83.
7. van Leeuwen MT, Webster AC, McCredie MR, et al. Effect of reduced immunosuppression after kidney transplant failure on risk of cancer: population based retrospective cohort study. *BMJ.* 2010;340:c570.
8. Meier-Kriesche HU, Shaw LM, Korecka M, Kaplan B. Pharmacokinetics of mycophenolic acid in renal insufficiency. *Ther Drug Monit.* 2000;22(1):27-30.
9. Burn DJ, Bates D. Neurology and the kidney. *J Neurol Neurosurg Psychiatry.* 1998;65(6):810-21.
10. Nimmo A, McIntyre S, Turner DM, Henderson LK, Battle RK. The impact of withdrawal of maintenance immunosuppression and graft nephrectomy on HLA sensitization and calculated chance of future transplant. *Transplant Direct.* 2018;4(12):e409.
11. Casey MJ, Wen X, Kayler LK, Aiyer R, Scornik JC, Meier-Kriesche HU. Prolonged immunosuppression preserves nonsensitization status after kidney transplant failure. *Transplantation.* 2014;98(3):306-11.
12. Geetha D, Sozio SM, Ghanta M, et al. Results of repeat renal transplantation after graft loss from BK virus nephropathy. *Transplantation.* 2011;92(7):781-6.
13. Davies SJ. Peritoneal dialysis in the patient with a failing renal allograft. *Perit Dial Int.* 2001;21(suppl 3):S280-4.
14. Pham PT, Everly M, Faravardeh A, Pham PC. Management of patients with a failed kidney transplant: dialysis reinitiation, immunosuppression weaning, and transplantectomy. *World J Nephrol.* 2015;4(2):148-59.
15. Ayus JC, Achinger SG, Lee S, Sayegh MH, Go AS. Transplant nephrectomy improves survival following a failed renal allograft. *J Am Soc Nephrol.* 2010;21(2):374-80.
16. Cofan F, Real MI, Vilardell J, et al. Percutaneous renal artery embolisation of non-functioning renal allografts with clinical intolerance. *Transpl Int.* 2002;15(4):149-55.
17. Delanaye P, Mariat C. The applicability of eGFR equations to different populations. *Nat Rev Nephrol.* 2013;9:513-22.
18. Perl J, Hasan O, Bargman JM, et al. Impact of dialysis modality on survival after kidney transplant failure. *Clin J Am Soc Nephrol.* 2011;6(3):582-90.
19. Quach T, Tregaskis P, Menahem S, Koukounaras J, Mott N, Walker RG. Radiological insertion of Tenckhoff catheters for peritoneal dialysis: a 1-year single-centre experience. *Clin Kidney J.* 2014;7(1):23-6.
20. Molnar MZ, Streja E, Kovesdy CP, et al. Estimated glomerular filtration rate at reinitiation of dialysis and mortality in failed kidney transplant recipients. *Nephrol Dial Transplant.* 2012;27(7):2913-21.

Index

Note: Page numbers followed by '*f*' indicate figures and '*t*' indicate tables.

D

R

U

V

W

X